INTRODUCTION TO DRUG METABOLISM

INTRODUCTION TO
DRUG METABOLISM

G. Gordon Gibson, PhD
Lecturer in Pharmacological Biochemistry
University of Surrey

AND

Paul Skett, Fil. dr.
Lecturer in Pharmacology
University of Glasgow

LONDON   NEW YORK

CHAPMAN AND HALL

First published in 1986 by
Chapman and Hall Ltd
11 New Fetter Lane, London EC4P 4EE
Published in the USA by
Chapman and Hall
29 West 35th Street, New York, NY 10001
© *1986 G. G. Gibson and P. Skett*
Printed in Great Britain at the
University Press, Cambridge

ISBN 0 412 26390 4 (Hb)
ISBN 0 412 26400 5 (Pb)

British Library Cataloguing in Publication Data

Gibson, G. G.
   Introduction to drug metabolism.
   1. Drugs—Metabolism
   I. Title   II. Skett, P.
       615'.7   RM301.55

   IBSN 0-412-26390-4
     0-412-26400-5 Pbk

Library of Congress Cataloging in Publication Data

Gibson, G. Gordon.
   Introduction to drug metabolism.

   Includes bibliographies and index.
   1.. Drugs—Metabolism. I. Skett, Paul. II. Title.
   [DNLM: 1. Drugs—metabolism. QV 38 G448i]
   RM301.55.G53 1986   615.7   85-15181
   ISBN 0-412-26390-4
   ISBN 0-412-26400-5 (pbk.)

Contents

Preface

v

Preface

Although the scientific literature on drug metabolism is extensive, it suffers from the disadvantage that the material is diffuse and consists largely of specialist monographs dealing with particular aspects of the subject. In addition, although there are a few excellent texts on drug metabolism in print, these tend to be earlier publications and hence do not take into account the many recent advances in this area. Our motivations for writing this book therefore arose from the clear need for a recent and cohesive introductory text on this subject, specifically designed to cater for the needs of undergraduate and postgraduate students. Much of the subject matter in this text is derived from various courses on drug metabolism given at the University of Surrey and the University of Glasgow to basic science students in pharmacology, biochemistry, nutrition and nursing studies, to pre-clinical medical students and to undergraduate and post-graduate students in toxicology. Therefore, it is our intention that this text will serve as a primer in drug metabolism to a variety of students in the life sciences taking courses in this subject.

The term 'drug metabolism' in its broadest sense may be considered as the absorption, distribution, biotransformation and excretion of drugs. To cover all these facets of drug metabolism in a single text is a voluminous task and therefore we have focused primarily on the biotransformation aspects of the subject. Having said this, the text is not solely a list of drug metabolism pathways, but rather it uses biotransformation reactions to rationalize many pharmacological and toxicological manifestations of drug action, clearly an important consideration in the clinical use of drugs.

The subject of drug metabolism or drug biotransformation is introduced in Chapter 1 by considering the relevant pathways, i.e. the enzyme-catalysed changes in drug structure. Wherever possible, currently used drugs are given as examples. Consideration is also given to the classification and functional role of the enzymes involved in these pathways. This is of importance as many of the drug-metabolizing enzymes are also involved in the metabolism of endogenous compounds and the chapter concludes by drawing attention to the competition between endogenous and exogenous substrates of these enzymes. Chapter 2 continues on the enzyme theme and considers, in detail, the enzymology of drug metabolism reactions including the molecular mechanisms involved. This chapter concludes by considering drug metabolism pathways not as separate events, but rather from the viewpoint of the interaction of the various pathways both with each other and with the pathways of endogenous, intermediary metabolism. Detailed consideration is also given to the overall control and regulation of drug metabolism pathways from various levels of integration.

Having established the basic chemistry and enzymology of drug metabolism, the three following chapters (3, 4 and 5) discuss factors that modulate drug metabolism, including induction and inhibition and external and internal factors. These are important aspects of any consideration of drug metabolism as the enzymes catalysing the various reactions are susceptible to changes in their activity or concentration, and are particularly influenced by other drugs or chemicals. Accordingly, these chapters are designed to rationalize, on an enzymatic or molecular level, why certain drugs, when given in combination, result in a response that could not be easily predicted by considering each drug in isolation. In view of the widespread use of polypharmacy where several drugs are given simultaneously, it is clear that the student should not only be aware of potential drug–drug interactions but should also be able to rationalize and explain why combination drug therapy interactions occur. These chapters conclude with a consideration of some of the internal or physiological factors that influence or regulate drug metabolism. A knowledge of these physiological factors is of utmost importance in clinical pharmacology in that, depending on the age, sex, hormonal status or genetic background of the patient, drug biotransformation pathways may either be switched on or turned off, thus influencing the clinical usage of drugs. In addition, patients on drug therapy for a particular ailment may have additional disorders of the heart, liver or kidney systems, defects which may subsequently influence drug disposition in the original disease, and attention is therefore drawn to the role of disease states in drug metabolism.

No matter how extensive or informative a test in drug metabolism is at the basic or theoretical level, a major consideration of this subject must include the the *raison d'etre* of drug biotransformation pathways. For example, the earlier chapters in this text highlight that one of the roles of drug metabolism is to make lipid-soluble drugs more polar, hence more readily excreted from the body. Thus if an efficient 'removal mechanism' did not exist for drugs, these highly lipid-soluble drugs would remain in the body for long time periods. Providing that the retained drug was maintained at sufficiently high concentrations at its site of action, then a prolonged pharmacological response would result. The majority of drugs have a half-life of only several hours in man and do not, in general, persist in the body; this underlines the important role of drug metabolism in clearing drugs from the body and hence terminating the pharmacological response. However, it should be emphasized that drug metabolism has additional, equally important roles to play in the overall, biological response to drugs. For example, as considered in Chapter 6, drug biotransformation may result in changes in both pharmacological and toxicological responses to drugs, an important consideration in drug therapy. From the pharmacological viewpoint, many drugs are inactivated by drug metabolism, probably as a result of the chemically changed drug metabolite not being recognized by the appropriate receptor system. Conversely, many 'pro-drugs' are inactive *per se*, and absolutely require biotransformation to release the pharmacologically active drug. Drug metabolism also has an important role to play in the side effects or toxicity of drugs. There are many well-documented examples where drug metabolism results in the transformation of a totally innocuous drug to a metabolite that is highly biologically reactive, and by a variety of mechanisms, can result in an overt toxicological response. Therefore in Chapter 6, we have emphasized that drug metabolism not only facilitates drug excretion, but is also an important determinant of pharmacological and toxicological responses to drugs.

One of the goals in the study of drug metabolism is to understand biotransformation pathways and biological responses to drugs in man. Unfortunately, there are many obvious practical and ethical constraints limiting our study of drug metabolism in man. Chapter 7 deals primarily with *in vivo* drug metabolism in man, and draws attention to the problems and advantages of applying *in vitro* drug metabolism data to man. Emphasis is placed on pharmacokinetics and the clinical relevance of drug metabolism in the human situation, drawing on the knowledge and information built up from previous chapters. Pharmacokinetics is not exclusively considered from a mathematical viewpoint but rather from a physiological/clinical stance. In this way, it is our intention to highlight the importance of pharmacokinetics in drug action, without placing an undue demand on the student to struggle with unnecessary mathematical formulae.

The final chapter in this text is concerned with the more practical aspects of drug metabolism and outlines several experiments that may be undertaken by practical classes. This chapter should not be considered in isolation but rather is designed to demonstrate experimentally some of the concepts developed in the remainder of the text. Rigid experimental practicals are not extensively described and we have devised this chapter on a 'menu' basis. This was achieved by initially detailing the methodology associated with the study of the enzymes and metabolites of drug biotransformation pathways, and subsequently applying these methodologies to highlight some concepts in drug metabolism. In this manner, the organisers of class practicals can devise their own experiments, tailored to their own needs and constraints placed upon them by factors such as class size and availability of facilities (including instrumentation). This chapter should also be of use to postgraduate students who require a detailed laboratory manual of experimental techniques to assay both the content and functional expression of the drug-metabolizing enzymes. The detailed methodology, analytical techniques and class practicals described in this chapter are based on both our own research activities and experience of undergraduate and postgraduate practical classes; and it should be emphasized that these have successfully run in our laboratories for several years.

In compiling this text, we have made liberal use of both tables and figures. We feel this is an important aspect of an introductory text of this nature in that a concept is more readily appreciated and remembered if numerical data or a simple figure can exemplify the point being made. In addition, we have included an extensive further reading section at the end of each chapter. Where possible, we have included all the text books, monographs and symposium proceedings relevant to each chapter, in addition to recent review articles. Where necessary, we have also included references to original articles to highlight a particular point being made in the chapter. In this way, we hope we have provided reference to sufficient additional reading material such that the interested reader can further pursue any particular area of interest in drug metabolism and related subjects.

Acknowledgements

In producing this text, the authors would like to acknowledge the expert secretarial assistance of Mrs Valerie Saunders and Mrs Marjory Wright in typing the initial drafts. We would also like to thank our present and past students who made so many constructive suggestions as to the content and emphasis of this book. Their help was indispensable and hopefully has helped us to identify the focus of this text. We also wish to thank both our colleagues and associates in the publishing area for their advice and permission to use some of their published material. Finally, we express our thanks to the staff of Chapman and Hall for their excellent co-operation and for giving us the opportunity to bring this project to fruition.

1
Pathways of drug metabolism

1.1 Introduction

Drug metabolism is an immense area of study and this is reflected in the range of chemical reactions the substrates can undergo during metabolism, e.g. oxidation, reduction, hydrolysis, hydration, conjugation and condensation. Drug metabolism is normally divided into two phases: phase I (or functionalization reactions) and phase II (or conjugative reactions). The division between phase I and II is given in Table 1.1.

Recently the existence of a third phase of metabolism has been postulated involving metabolism of conjugate (excreted in the bile) by the intestinal microflora and subsequent re-absorption and metabolism (see section on phase III metabolism).

There is great interest in the inter-relationship of the various metabolic routes in terms of competing reactions of the substrate for phase II enzymes. There is much evidence to suggest that the phase I reactions create a reactive functional group on the molecule so that it can be attacked by the phase II enzymes. Thus, the phase II reactions are the true 'detoxification' pathways and give products that account for the bulk of the inactive, excreted products of a drug.

This chapter will examine the different types of reactions involved in drug metabolism using the phase I and II classification as a basis. Examples of each type of reaction will be given and, where possible, these will be actual reactions

Table 1.1 Reactions classed as phase I or phase II metabolism

Phase I	Phase II
Oxidation	Glucuronidation/glucosidation
Reduction	Sulfation
Hydrolysis	Methylation
Hydration	Acetylation
Dethioacetylation	Amino acid conjugation
Isomerization	Glutathione conjugation
	Fatty acid conjugation
	Condensation

of drug substrates rather than model substrates. This will show the pharmacological, toxicological and clinical relevance of the reactions. Attention will be drawn to competing reactions for the same substrate where appropriate. A brief discussion of the postulated phase III metabolism will be included.

Many of the enzymes involved in drug metabolism are, in fact, principally involved in the metabolism of, or are capable of metabolizing, endogenous compounds. Thus a separate section of the chapter will be devoted to the metabolism of endogenous compounds by 'drug-metabolizing' enzymes. The interaction of drugs and endogenous compound metabolism will be highlighted.

It will be appreciated at this stage that, in a limited space, not every reaction undergone by every drug can be covered and that inevitably there will be omissions. This chapter is designed to give a feel for the possible metabolism of drugs and information regarding specific drugs will be found in specialist publications. A list of further reading material will be found at the end of the chapter, from which further information on specific pathways can be obtained.

1.2 Phase I metabolism

Phase I metabolism includes oxidation, reduction, hydrolysis and hydration reactions as well as isomerization and other rarer miscellaneous reactions. The reactions will be discussed in terms of reaction type and, with respect to oxidation, site of enzyme – the classification of phase I reactions can be found in Table 1.2. Oxidation performed by the microsomal mixed-function oxidase system (cytochrome P-450-dependent) is considered separately because of the diversity of reactions performed by this enzyme system.

1.2.1 OXIDATIONS INVOLVING THE MICROSOMAL MIXED-FUNCTION OXIDASE

The mixed-function oxidase system found in microsomes (endoplasmic reticulum) of many cells (notably those of liver, kidney, lung and intestine)

Table 1.2 Sub-classification of phase I reactions

Oxidation involving cytochrome P-450
Oxidation – others
Reduction
Hydrolysis
Hydration
Isomerization
Miscellaneous

performs many different functionalization reactions (summarized in Table 1.3). An example of each reaction is given below.

(a) AROMATIC HYDROXYLATION

This is a very common reaction for drugs and xenobiotics containing a benzene ring. In this example (Figure 1.1) the local anaesthetic and antidysrhythmic drug lignocaine is converted to its 3-hydroxy derivative.

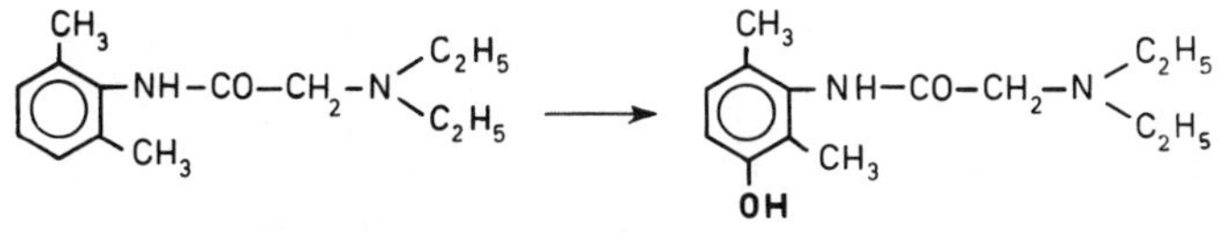

Figure 1.1 The 3-hydroxylation of lignocaine.

(b) ALIPHATIC HYDROXYLATION

Another very common reaction, e.g. pentobarbitone hydroxylated in the pentyl side chain (Figure 1.2).

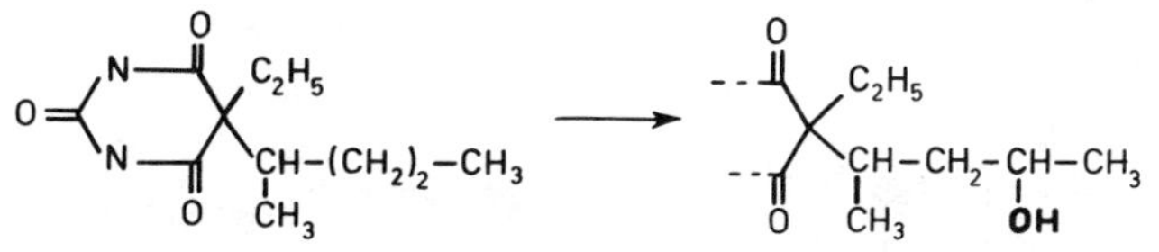

Figure 1.2 The side-chain hydroxylation of pentobarbital.

(c) EPOXIDATION

Epoxides are normally unstable intermediates but may be stable enough to be isolated from polycyclic compounds (e.g. the precarcinogenic polycyclic hydrocarbons). Epoxides are substrates of epoxide hydratase (discussed later) forming dihydrodiols; they may also spontaneously decompose to form hydroxylated products. It has been suggested that epoxide formation is the first step in aromatic hydroxylation but this remains an area of debate. Figure 1.3 shows the epoxidation of benzo[a]pyrene to its 4,5-epoxide.

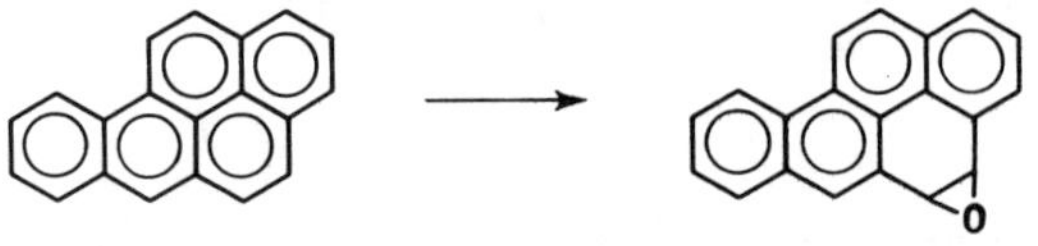

Figure 1.3 The formation of benzo[a]pyrene-4,5-epoxide.

(d) N-DEALKYLATION

This reaction occurs very readily with most drugs containing an alkyl group attached to an amine or ring nitrogen, leading to the formation of a primary or secondary amine. The alkyl group is lost as the corresponding aldehyde. In the example in Figure 1.4 diazepam is converted to N-desmethyldiazepam with the loss of formaldehyde.

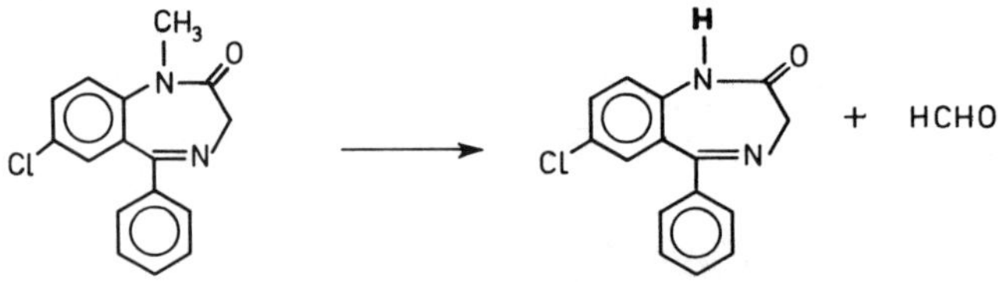

Figure 1.4 The N-demethylation of diazepam.

The reaction is considered to occur in two steps, the first being hydroxylation of the methyl group on the nitrogen, and the second a decomposition of this intermediate (see Figure 1.5).

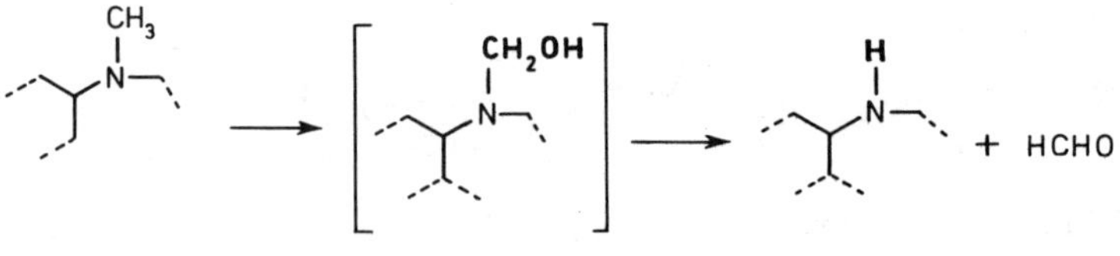

Unstable intermediate

Figure 1.5 The mechanism of N-demethylation of diazepam.

(e) O-DEALKYLATION

A very similar reaction to (d) above. Figure 1.6 shows the O-demethylation of codeine to yield morphine.

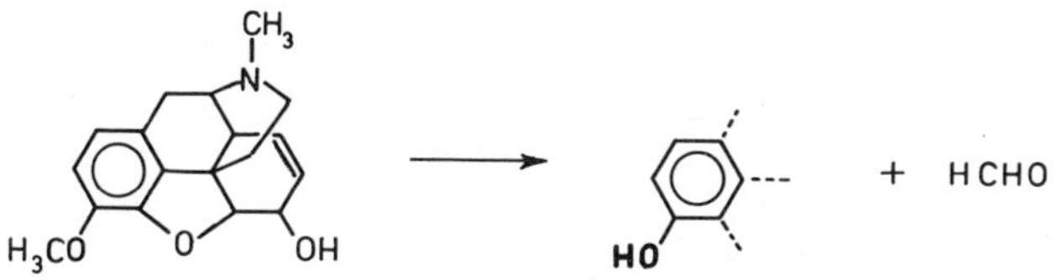

Figure 1.6 The O-demethylation of codeine.

The reaction proceeds via a hydroxy intermediate as N-dealkylation.

(f) S-DEALKYLATION

Various S-methyl compounds can be S-demethylated by hepatic microsomes but a soluble factor appears to be necessary as well. This reaction may not, therefore, be a true microsomal one. The S-demethylation of S-methyl-thiopurine is illustrated in Figure 1.7.

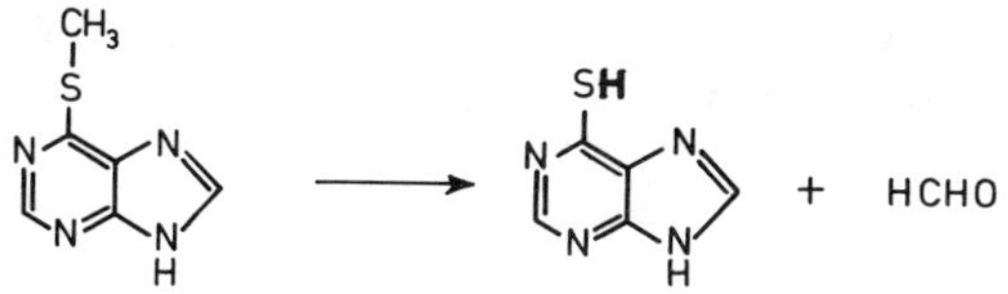

Figure 1.7 The S-demethylation of S-methylthiopurine.

(g) OXIDATIVE DEAMINATION

Amines containing the structure $-\underset{\underset{CH_3}{|}}{CH}-NH_2$ are metabolized by the micro-somal mixed-function oxidase system to release ammonia and leave the corresponding ketone. This is a different substrate specificity to the other amine metabolizing enzymes, namely monoamine oxidase (MAO – see later) and the two enzymes do not compete for the same substrates. Figure 1.8 shows the deamination of amphetamine.

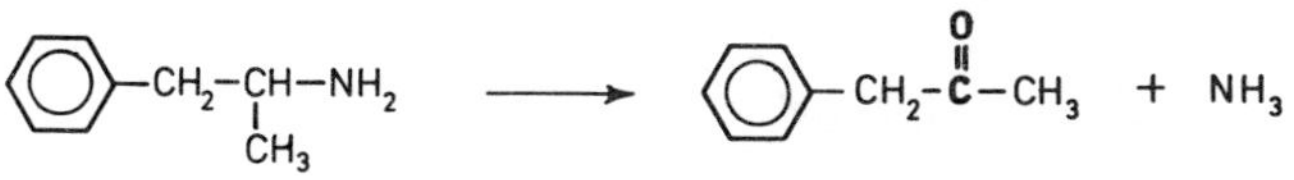

Figure 1.8 The oxidative deamination of amphetamine.

The ketone formed in this case is phenylacetone. As with dealkylation, oxidative deamination involves an intermediate hydroxylation step (Figure 1.9) with subsequent decomposition to yield the final products.

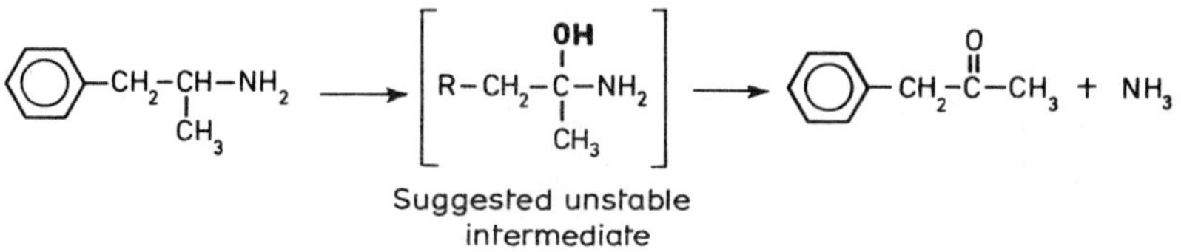

Suggested unstable
intermediate

Figure 1.9 The mechanism of oxidative deamination of amphetamine.

(h) N-OXIDATION

Hepatic microsomes in the presence of oxygen and NADPH can form N-oxides. These oxidation products may be formed by the mixed-function oxidase system or by separate flavoprotein N-oxidases (see later). The enzyme involved in N-oxidation depends on the substrate under study. Many different chemical groups can be N-oxidized including amines, amides, imines, hydrazines and heterocyclic compounds. In Figure 1.10 the N-oxidation of 3-methylpyridine (a cytochrome P-450-dependent reaction) is illustrated.

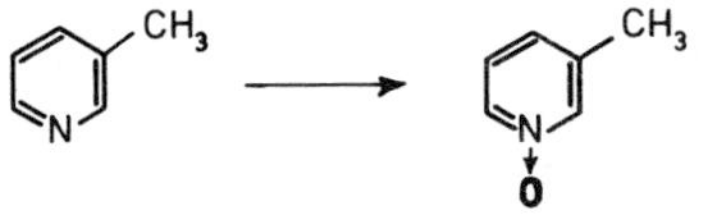

Figure 1.10 The N-oxidation of 3-methylpyridine.

N-Oxidation may manifest itself as the formation of a hydroxylamine as in the metabolism of 2-acetylaminofluorene (2-AAF) (Figure 1.11). This is of interest as the hydroxylamine of 2-AAF is thought to be a proximate carcinogen giving the toxicity of 2-AAF.

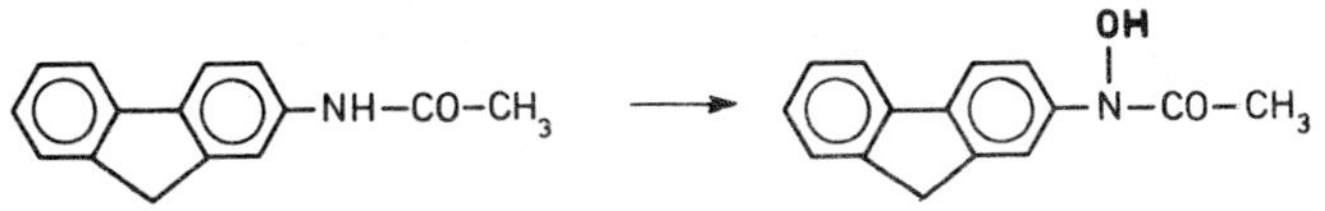

Figure 1.11 The N-hydroxylation of 2-acetylaminofluorene.

(i) S-OXIDATION

Phenothiazines can be converted to their S-oxides by the microsomal mixed-function oxidase system. As an example the S-oxidation of chlorpromazine is shown in Figure. 1.12.

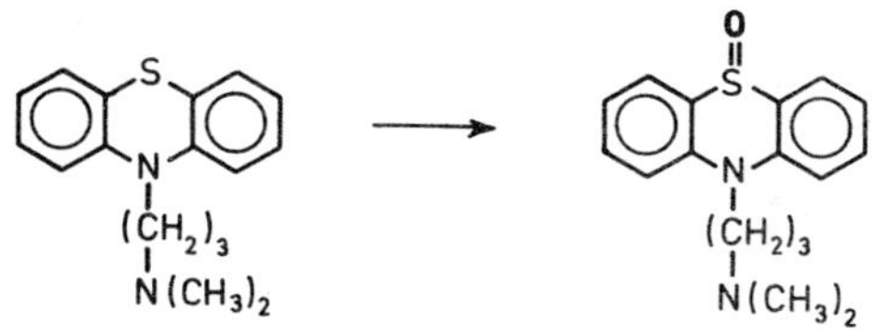

Figure 1.12 The S-oxidation of chlorpromazine.

(j) PHOSPHOTHIONATE OXIDATION

The replacement of a phosphothionate sulfur atom with oxygen is a reaction common to the phosphothionate insecticides, e.g. parathion (Figure 1.13). The product paraoxon is a potent anticholinesterase.

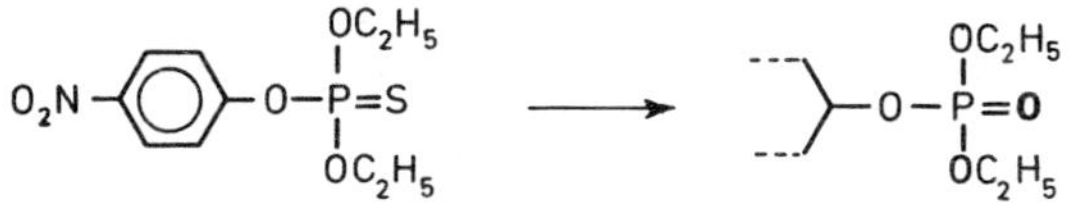

Figure 1.13 The oxidation of parathion.

(k) DEHALOGENATION

The halogenated general anaesthetics, e.g. halothane, undergo oxidative dechlorination and debromination to yield the corresponding alcohol or acid (Figure 1.14).

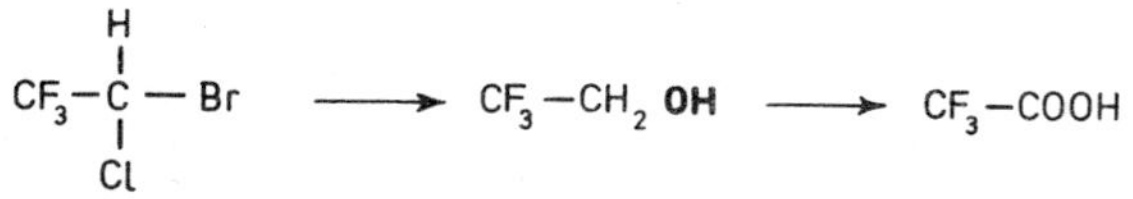

Figure 1.14 The oxidative dehalogenation of halothane.

All of the above reactions require the presence of molecular oxygen and NADPH as well as the complete mixed-function oxidase system. It is seen that all reactions involve the initial insertion of a single oxygen atom into the drug molecule. A subsequent rearrangement and/or decomposition of this product may occur leading to the final products seen. The mechanism of insertion of this single oxygen atom is discussed at length in Chapter 2.

One unusual oxidation reaction performed by the mixed-function oxidase system is the conversion of ethanol to acetaldehyde (Figure 1.15). In this case the microsomal ethanol-oxidizing system (MEOS) dehydrogenates ethanol. This may still be a hydroxylation reaction, however, as illustrated in Figure 1.15 but no proof exists to support this mechanism of reaction; indeed, other

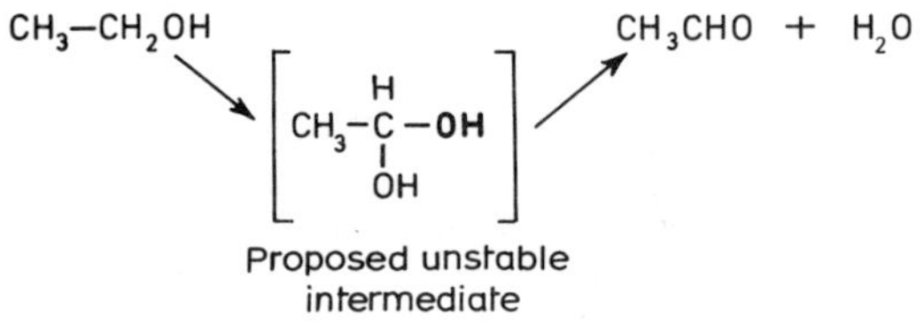

Figure 1.15 The oxidation of ethanol.

mechanisms have been proposed. In naive animals the cytochrome *P*-450-mediated oxidation of ethanol is thought to be of minor importance but following induction by ethanol, the microsomal oxidation of ethanol increases dramatically and may account for 80% of ethanol clearance in certain cases. In uninduced situations, alcohol dehydrogenase is the major metabolizer of ethanol (see next section).

Table 1.3 Reactions performed by the microsomal mixed-function oxidase system

Reaction	Substrate
Aromatic hydroxylation	Lignocaine
Aliphatic hydroxylation	Pentobarbitone
Epoxidation	Benzo[*a*]pyrene
N-Dealkylation	Diazepam
O-Dealkylation	Codeine
S-Dealkylation	6-Methylthiopurine
Oxidative deamination	Amphetamine
N-Oxidation	3-Methylpyridine
	2-Acetylaminofluorene
S-Oxidation	Chlorpromazine
Phosphothionate oxidation	Parathion
Dehalogenation	Halothane
Alcohol oxidation	Ethanol

The microsomal mixed-function oxidase system can, thus, catalyse a large range of oxidation reactions on a variety of substrates (Table 1.3). The mitochondrial mixed-function oxidase is more selective in its substrates and is mainly involved in endogenous steroid metabolism (see section on endogenous metabolism in this chapter).

1.2.2 OXIDATION OTHER THAN THE MICROSOMAL MIXED-FUNCTION OXIDASE

A number of enzymes in the body not related to mixed-function oxidases can oxidize drugs, and these are listed in Table 1.4.

Most of these enzymes are primarily involved in endogenous compound metabolism and will be dealt with in the section related to that topic. A number

Table 1.4 Oxidative enzymes other than
mixed-function oxidase

Alcohol dehydrogenase
Aldehyde dehydrogenase
Xanthine oxidase
Amine oxidases
Aromatases
Alkylhydrazine oxidase

---

however, are more intimately involved in drug metabolism and are discussed
below:

(a) ALCOHOL DEHYDROGENASE

This enzyme catalyses the oxidation of many alcohols to the corresponding
aldehyde and is localized in the soluble fraction of liver, kidney and lung cells.
Unlike the microsomal ethanol oxidizing system (MEOS) mentioned above, this
enzyme uses NAD^+ as co-factor (Figure 1.16) and is a true dehydrogenase (the
MEOS is an oxidase).

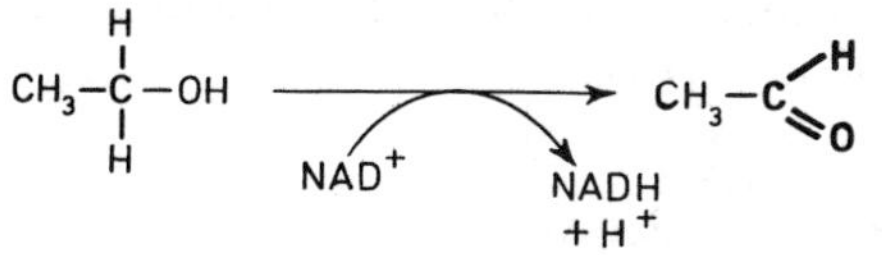

Figure 1.16 The oxidation of ethanol by alcohol dehydrogenase.

(b) ALDEHYDE OXIDATION

Aldehydes can be oxidized by a variety of enzymes involved in intermediary
metabolism, e.g. aldehyde dehydrogenase, aldehyde oxidase and xanthine
oxidase (the latter two being soluble metalloflavoproteins). The product of the
reaction is the corresponding carboxylic acid (Figure 1.17).

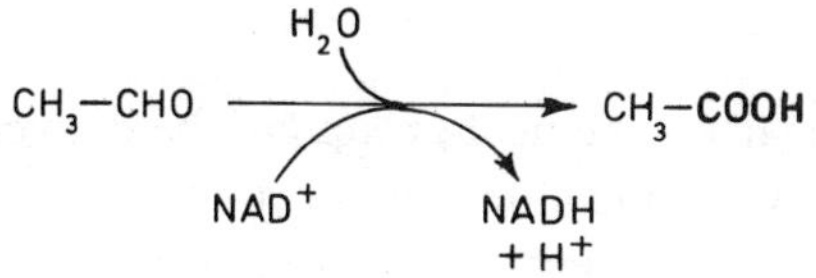

Figure 1.17 The oxidation of acetaldehyde.

(c) XANTHINE OXIDASE

This enzyme will metabolize the xanthine-containing drugs, e.g. caffeine,
theophylline and theobromine, and the purine analogues to the corresponding
uric acid derivative (Figure 1.18).

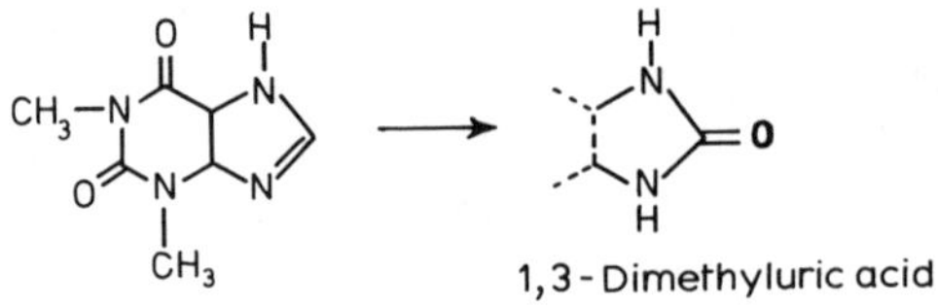

Figure 1.18 The oxidation of theophylline.

(d) AMINE OXIDASES

This group of enzymes can be subdivided into monoamine oxidases (responsible for the metabolism of endogenous catecholamines), diamine oxidases (deaminating endogenous diamines, e.g. histamine) and the flavoprotein N-oxidases and N-hydroxylases (which have been discussed above).

Monoamine oxidase metabolizes dietary exogenous amines, e.g. tyramine (found in cheese) to the corresponding aldehyde (cf. oxidative deamination by the mixed-function oxidase) and is found in mitochondria, at nerve endings and in the liver. The enzyme does not metabolize the amphetamine class of drugs that are metabolized by the mixed-function oxidase.

Diamine oxidase is primarily involved with endogenous metabolism and is of little relevance here, whereas the N-oxidases are of importance in the metabolism of drugs, e.g. imipramine (Figure 1.19).

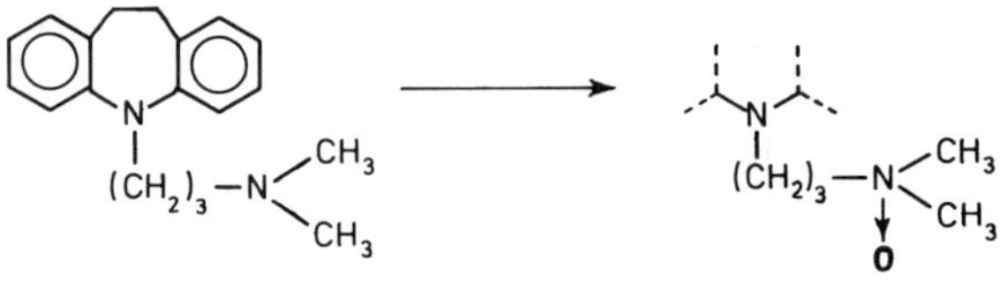

Figure 1.19 The N-oxidation of imipramine.

These enzymes are found in liver microsomes. They appear to require NADPH and molecular oxygen, but are not mixed-function oxidases.

(e) AROMATASES

Xenobiotics containing a cyclohexanecarboxylic acid group can be converted to the corresponding benzoic acid by a liver and kidney mitochrondrial enzyme. The enzyme requires the coenzyme A derivative of the acid as substrate, and oxygen and FAD as cofactors (Figure 1.20).

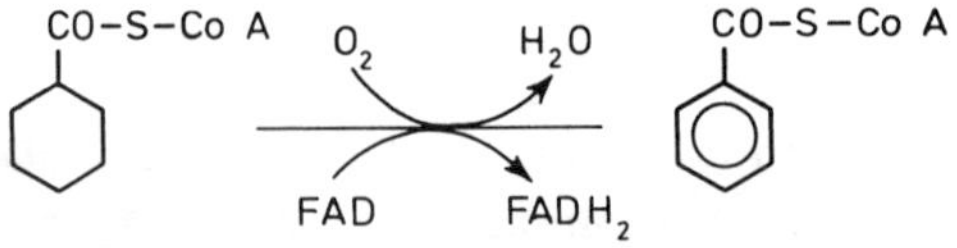

Figure 1.20 The aromatization of cyclohexanecarboxylic acid CoA.

(f) ALKYLHYDRAZINE OXIDASE

Carbidopa can be converted to 2-methyl-3′-4′-dihydroxyphenylpropionic acid (Figure 1.21) by oxidation of the nitrogen function and subsequent rearrangement and decomposition of the intermediate. The exact mechanism is not known.

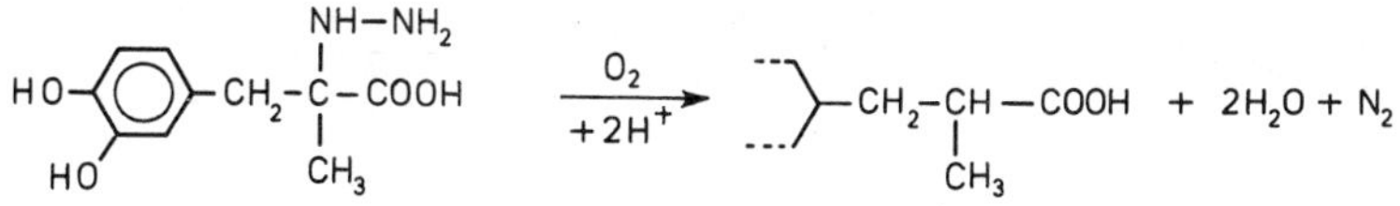

Figure 1.21 The oxidation of carbidopa.

1.2.3 REDUCTIVE METABOLISM

A number of reductive reactions can be catalysed by hepatic microsomes; these reactions require NADPH but are generally inhibited by oxygen. A list of the types of compounds undergoing reduction is given in Table 1.5. Other compounds such as disulfides, unsaturated ring compounds and sulfoxides and N-oxides can undergo reduction but the nature and location of the enzymes involved is unclear.

Table 1.5 Compounds undergoing reduction
by hepatic microsomes

Azo-compounds
Nitro-compounds
Epoxides
Heterocyclic ring compounds
Halogenated hydrocarbons

Azo- and nitro-reduction is catalysed by cytochrome *P*-450 (but can also be catalysed by NADPH-cytochrome c-reductase) and can involve substrates such as prontosil red (forming sulfanilamide) and chloramphenicol (Figure 1.22). The former reaction led to the discovery of the sulfonamides. The latter reaction is thought to occur in a stepwise fashion as in the reduction of nitrobenzene (Figure 1.23).

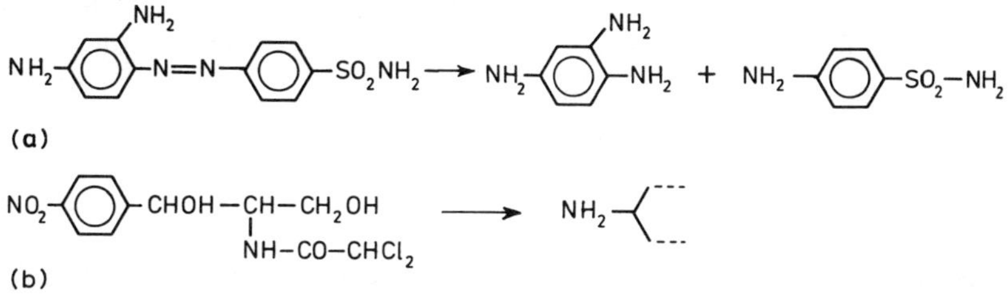

(a)

(b)

Figure 1.22 Reduction of (a) prontosil red and (b) chloramphenicol.

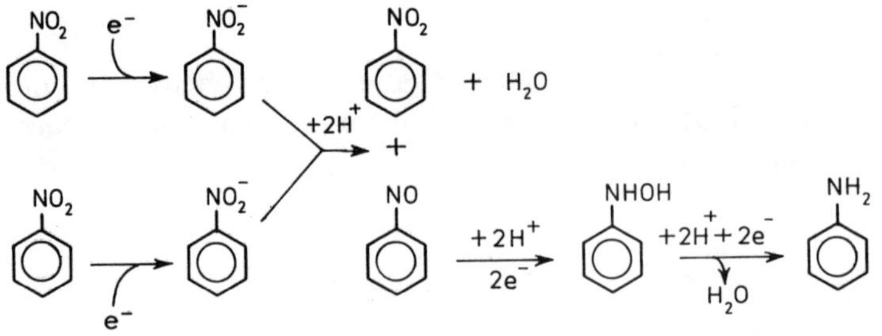

Figure 1.23 Stepwise reduction of aromatic nitro-group.

Epoxides can be converted back to the parent hydrocarbon, e.g. benzo[*a*]-anthracene-8,9-epoxide, whereas some heterocyclic compounds can be ring cleaved by reduction (Figure 1.24). The products of the latter reaction are unstable and break down further to yield rearrangement and hydrolysis products.

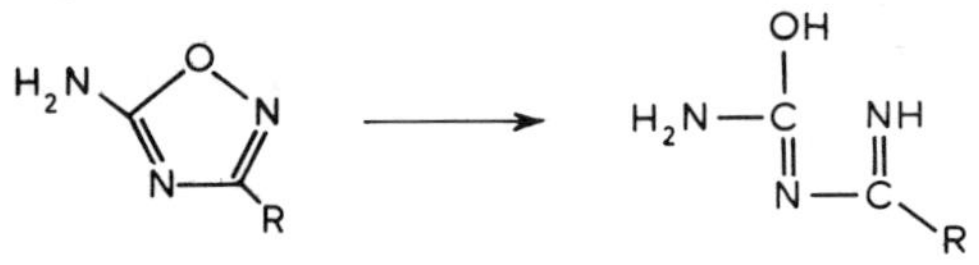

Figure 1.24 Ring cleavage of oxadiazoles.

Fluorocarbons of the halothane type can be defluorinated by liver microsomes in anaerobic conditions (cf. oxidative dehalogenation of halothane) as shown in Figure 1.25.

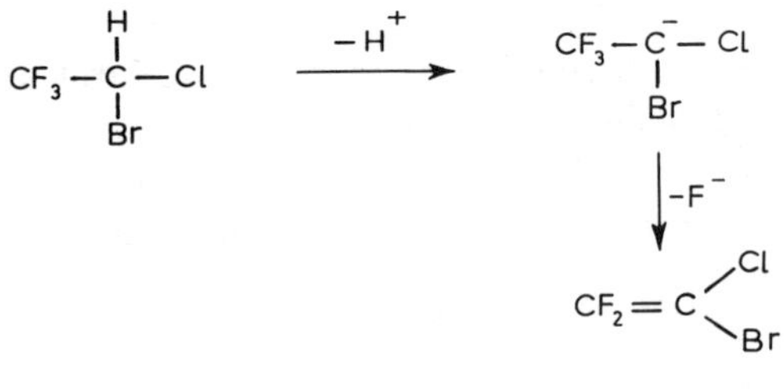

Figure 1.25 Reductive defluorination of halothane.

1.2.4 HYDROLYSIS

Esters, amides, hydrazides and carbamates can readily be hydrolysed by various enzymes.

(a) ESTER HYDROLYSIS

The hydrolysis of esters can take place in the plasma (non-specific acetyl-cholinesterases, pseudocholinesterases and other esterases) or in liver (specific esterases for particular groups of compounds). Procaine is metabolized by the plasma esterase (Figure 1.26) whereas pethidine (meperidine) is only metabolized by the liver esterase.

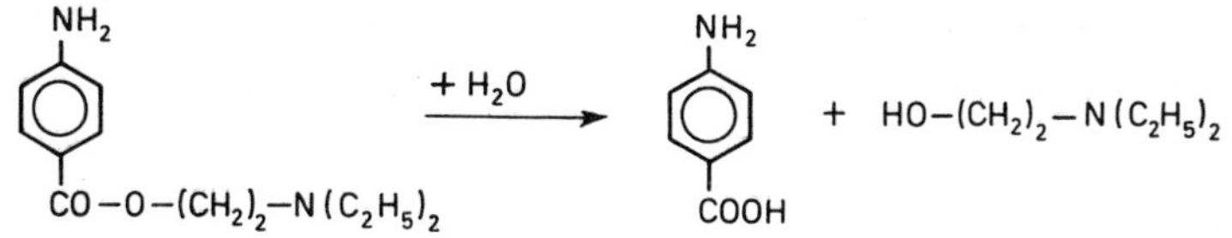

Figure 1.26 Hydrolysis of procaine.

(b) AMIDE HYDROLYSIS

Amides may be hydrolysed by the plasma esterases although more slowly than the corresponding esters but are more likely to be hydrolysed by the liver amidases. Ethylglycylxylidide, the N-de-ethylated phase I product of ligno-caine, is hydrolysed by the liver microsomal fraction to yield xylidine and ethylglycine (Figure 1.27).

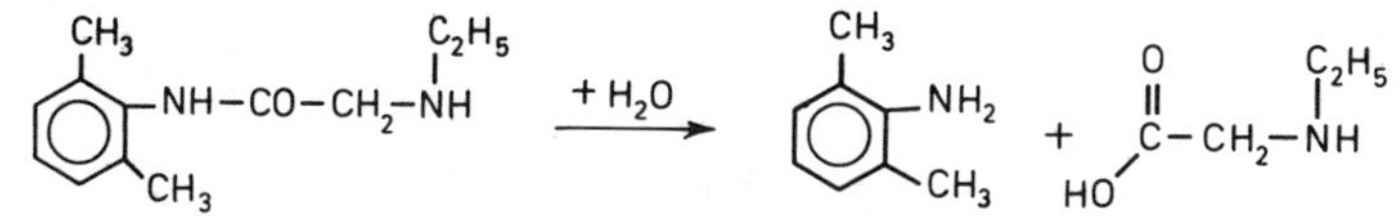

Figure 1.27 Hydrolysis of monoethylglycylxylidide.

(c) HYDRAZIDE AND CARBAMATE HYDROLYSIS

Less common functional groups in drugs can also be hydrolysed such as the hydrazide group in isoniazid (Figure 1.28) or the carbamate group in the previously used hypnotic, hedonal.

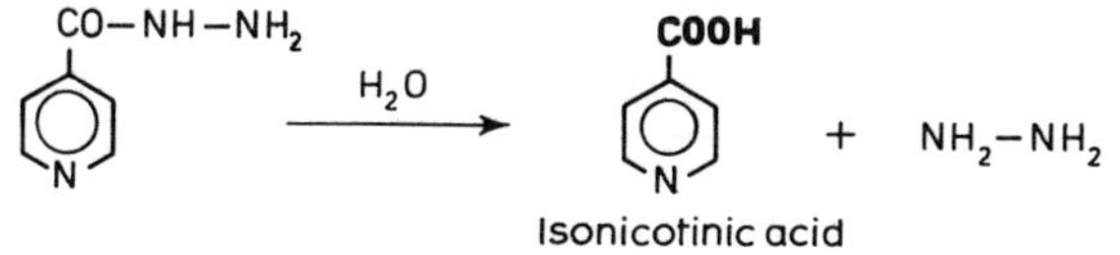

Figure 1.28 Hydrolysis of isoniazid.

The hydrolysis of proteins and peptides by enzymes can also be mentioned here but these enzymes are mainly found in gut secretions and are little involved in drug metabolism except in the further metabolism of glutathione conjugates (discussed later).

1.2.5 HYDRATION

Hydration can be regarded as a specialized form of hydrolysis where water is added to the compound without causing the compound to dissociate into a number of components. Epoxides are particularly prone to hydration by the enzyme, epoxide hydratase, yielding the dihydrodiol. This enzyme is also called epoxide hydrase or hydrolase. The precarcinogenic polycyclic hydrocarbon epoxides in particular undergo this reaction (e.g. benzo[*a*]pyrene 4,5-epoxide (Figure 1.29)). The reaction forms a *trans*-diol.

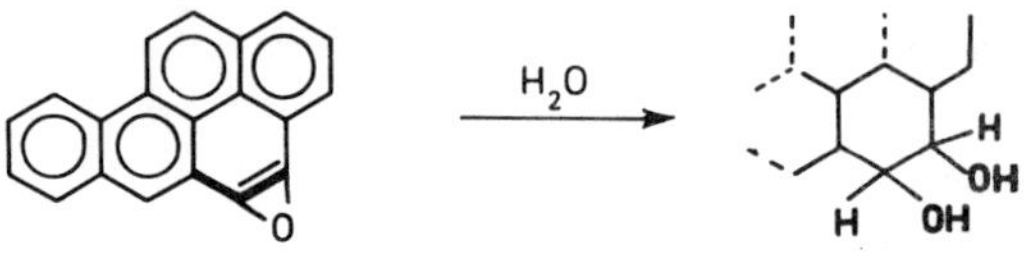

Figure 1.29 Hydration of benzo[*a*]pyrene 4,5-epoxide.

1.2.6 OTHER PHASE I REACTIONS

Many other reactions which cannot be classified into the groups mentioned above have been proposed as possible routes of metabolism for specific drugs. A list of these reactions is given in Table 1.6. Further details of these reactions can be found in the reading list at the end of the chapter.

1.2.7 SUMMARY OF PHASE I METABOLISM

As can be seen from the above, virtually every possible chemical reaction that a compound can undergo can be catalysed by the drug-metabolizing enzyme systems. In most cases the final product contains a chemically reactive functional group, such as −OH, −NH$_2$, −SH, −COOH, etc. and, thus,as we shall see below, is in the correct chemical state to be acted upon by the phase II or conjugative enzymes. Indeed it is recognized that the main function of phase I metabolism is to prepare the compound for phase II metabolism

Table 1.6 Other reactions involved in drug metabolism

Reaction	Compound
Ring cyclization	Proguanil
N-Carboxylation	Tocainide
Dimerization	N-OH-2-Acetylaminofluorene
Transamidation	Propiram
Isomerization	α-Methylfluorene-2-acetic acid
Decarboxylation	L-Dopa
Dethioacetylation	Spironolactone

and not to prepare the drug for excretion. Phase II is the true 'detoxification' of drugs and gives products that are generally water-soluble and easily excreted.

It will also be appreciated that many drugs can undergo a number of the reactions listed; indeed some drugs can pass along many of the routes of metabolism described above. The importance of a particular pathway varies with many factors (most of which are described in Chapters 4 and 5) and it is obviously very difficult to predict the metabolism or a drug from the data given above. Various computer prediction methods for routes of drug metabolism are available and are making useful advances in this field but it is not yet possible to accurately predict qualitatively and quantitatively the metabolism of a particular drug.

1.3 Phase II metabolism

Phase II metabolism or conjugation involves a diverse group of enzymes acting on diverse types of compounds, generally leading to a water-soluble product which can be excreted in bile or urine. Table 1.7 lists the types of conjugation, enzyme involved and major types of drug conjugated.

Table 1.7 Conjugation reactions

Reaction	Enzyme	Functional group
Glucuronidation	UDP–Glucuronyltransferase	$-OH$ $-COOH$ $-NH_2$ $-SH$
Glycosidation	UDP–Glycosyltransferase	$-OH$ $-COOH$ $-SH$
Sulfation	Sulfotransferase	$-NH_2$ $-SO_2NH_2$ $-OH$
Methylation	Methyltransferase	$-OH$ $-NH_2$
Acetylation	Acetyltransferase	$-NH_2$ $-SO_2NH_2$ $-OH$
Amino acid conjugation		$-COOH$
Glutathione conjugation	Glutathione-*S*-transferase	Epoxide Organic halide
Fatty acid conjugation		$-OH$
Condensation		Various

1.3.1 CONJUGATION WITH SUGARS

The major route of sugar conjugation is glucuronidation (conjugation with α-D-glucuronic acid) although conjugation with glucose, xylose and ribose are also possible.

(a) GLUCURONIDATION

The widespread occurrence of glucuronidation (found in all tissues of the mammalian body) is probably due to the co-factor required, UDP–glucuronic acid, being part of intermediary metabolism and closely related to glycogen synthesis (Figure 1.30). The enzymes involved are located in the cytosol.

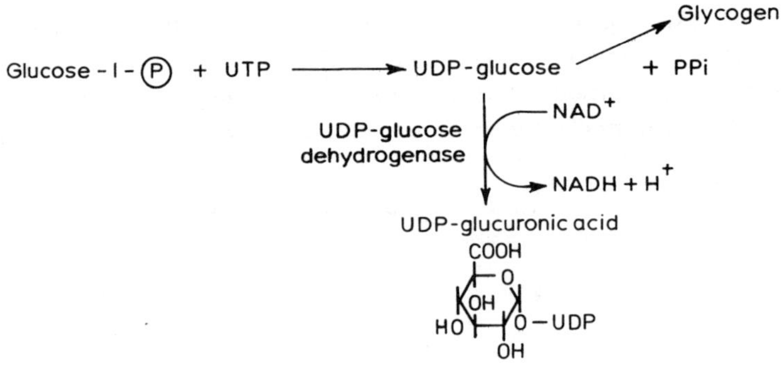

Figure 1.30 Synthesis of UDP–glucuronic acid.

Glucuronide formation is quantitatively the most important form of conjugation for drugs and endogenous compounds (for a discussion of this latter point, see the section on endogenous compound metabolism) and can be found for alcohols, phenols, hydroxylamines, carboxylic acids, amines, sulfonamides and thiols. C-Glucuronides of phenylbutazone and sulfinpyrazone have also been seen (see later).

(i) *O-Glucuronides*

These form from phenols, alcohols and carboxylic acids – the carboxylic acids forming 'ester' glucuronides and the others 'ether' glucuronides. Examples of each of these are shown in Figure 1.31.

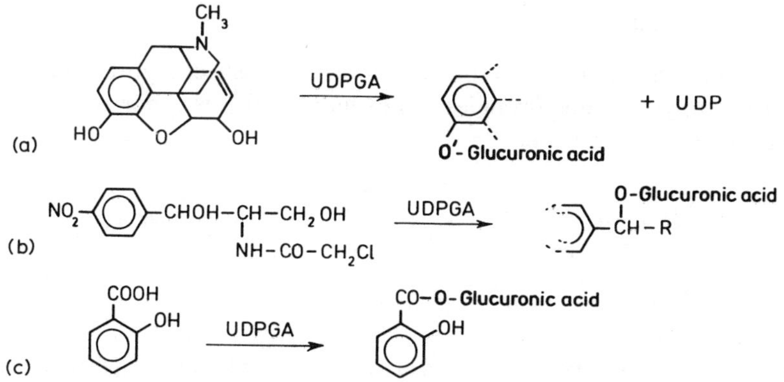

Figure 1.31 The glucuronidation of (a) morphine, (b) chloramphenicol and (c) salicyclic acid.

The reaction is the same in each case requiring the microsomal enzyme, UDP–glucuronyltransferase. It is interesting to note that inversion takes place during the reaction with the α-glucuronic acid forming a β-glucuronide. The formed O-glucuronides are often excreted in bile and thus released into the gut where they can be broken down to the parent compound by β-glucuronidase and possibly reabsorbed. This is the basis of the 'enterohepatic circulation' of drugs discussed in more detail in Chapter 7.

(ii) N-Glucuronides

N-Glucuronides form from amines (mainly aromatic), amides and sulfonamides. It has also been suggested that tertiary amines can form glucuronides giving quaternary nitrogen conjugates. N-Glucuronides may form spontaneously, i.e. without the presence of enzyme. Figure 1.32 shows some examples of N-glucuronide formation.

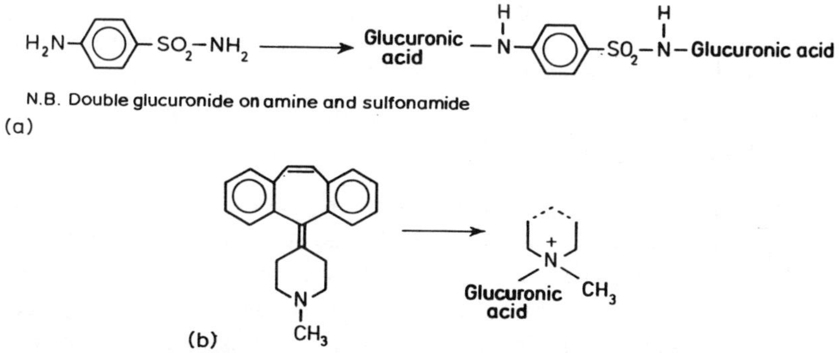

Figure 1.32 The glucuronidation of (a) sulfanilamide and (b) cyproheptidine.

(iii) *S-Glucuronides*

Thiol groups can react with UDPGA in the presence of UDP-glucuronyl-transferase to yield *S*-glucuronides. An example of this is given in Figure 1.33 with antabuse as substrate.

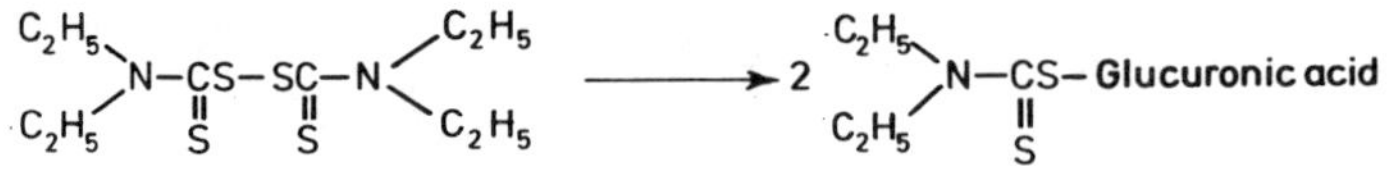

Figure 1.33 The glucuronidation of antabuse.

Direct attachment of glucuronic acid to the carbon skeleton of drugs has also been reported (i.e. *C*-glucuronidation).

(b) OTHER SUGARS

In most species conjugation with glucuronic acid is by far the most important sugar conjugation but in insects conjugation with glucose is more prevalent. The reaction is exactly analogous to glucuronide formation but UDP–glucose is used instead of UDPGA and glucosides are formed. Similar O–, N– and S–glucosides can be formed. Such reactions are also of importance in plants and have been found in mammals to a limited extent.

In certain circumstances UDP–xylose or UDP–ribose can be used giving the corresponding xyloside or riboside. N-Ribosides seem to be the most common and may form non-enzymically but O-xylosides of bilirubin have been found and require a microsomal transferase for formation. An example of a N-riboside formation is shown in Figure 1.34.

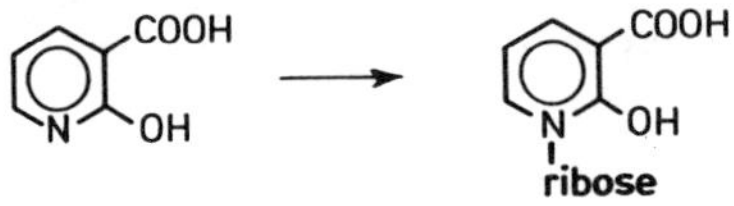

Figure 1.34 The N-ribosylation of 2-hydroxynicotinic acid.

1.3.2 SULFATION

Sulfation is a major conjugation pathway for phenols but can also occur for alcohols, amines and, to a lesser extent, thiols. As with sugar conjugation an 'active' donor is required – being in this case 3'-phosphoadenosine-5'-phosphosulfate (PAPS, Figure 1.35). PAPS is produced by a two-stage reaction from ATP and sulfate as illustrated in Figure 1.36. These reactions occur in the cytosol.

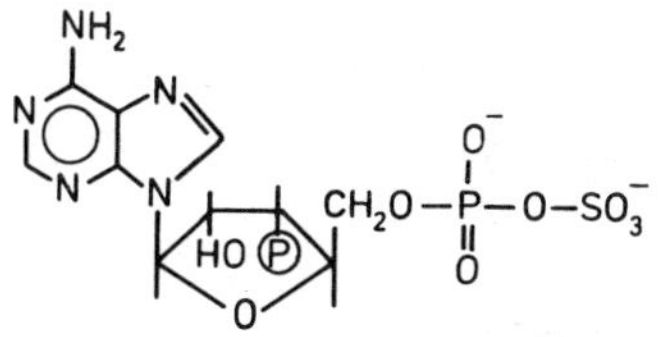

Figure 1.35 The structure of PAPS.

$$SO_4^{2-} + ATP \xrightarrow{\text{ATP-sulfurylase}} \text{Adenosine-5'-phosphosulfate (APS)} + PP_i$$

$$APS + ATP \xrightarrow{\text{APS-kinase}} \text{3'-Phosphoadenosine-5'-phosphosulfate (PAPS)} + ADP$$

Figure 1.36 The formation of PAPS.

Sulfation occurs by interaction of the drug and PAPS in the presence of the cytosolic enzyme, sulfotransferase. Various isoenzymes have been described, named after their preferred substrates; a list of these is given in Table 1.8.

Table 1.8 Sulfotransferases and their substrates

Isoenzyme	Substrate	Site
Phenol sulfotransferase	Isoprenaline	Liver Kidney Gut
Alcohol sulfotransferase	Dimetranidazole	Liver
Steroid sulfotransferase	Oestrone	Liver
Arylamine sulfotransferase	Paracetamol	Liver

The phenol, alcohol and arylamine sulfotransferases are fairly non-specific and will metabolize a wide range of drugs and xenobiotics but the steroid sulfotransferases are specific for a single steroid or a number of steroids of a particular type. For example oestrone sulfotransferase will sulfate oestrone and, to a lesser extent, other oestrogens while testosterone is sulfated by another sulfotransferase. Some examples of sulfate conjugation are shown in Figure 1.37.

As is seen most drugs and endogenous compounds that can be glucuronidated can also be sulfated and this leads to the possibility of competition for the substrate between the two pathways. In general sulfate conjugation predominates at low substrate conjugation and glucuronide conjugation at high

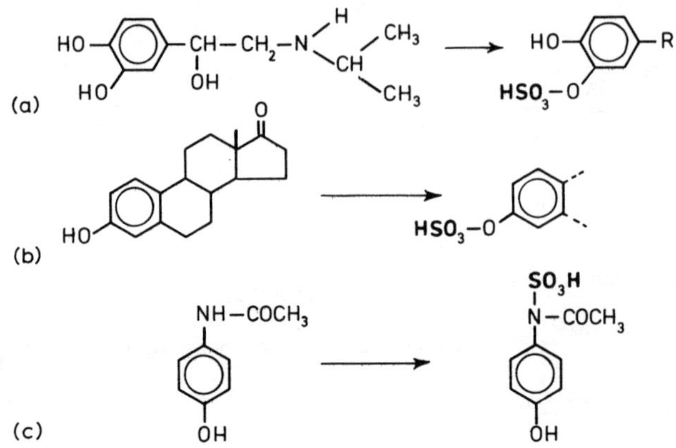

Figure 1.37 Sulfate conjugation of (a) isoprenaline, (b) oestrone and (c) paracetamol.

concentration due to the kinetics of the two reactions and the limited supply of PAPS in the cell compared to UDPGA.

1.3.3 METHYLATION

Methylation reactions are mainly involved with endogenous compound metabolism but some drugs may be methylated by non-specific methyltransferases found in lung, and by the physiological methyltransferases. A list of the methyltransferases and their substrates. is given in Table 1.9.

Table 1.9 The methyltransferases

Enzyme	Substrate	Site
Phenylethanolamine N-methyltransferase	Noradrenaline	Adrenals
Non-specific N-methyltransferase	Various (desmethylimipramine)	Lung
Imidazole N-methyltransferase	Histamine	Liver
Catechol O-methyltransferase	Catechols	Liver Kidney Skin Nerve tissue
Hydroxyindole O-methyltransferase	N-Acetylserotonin	Pineal gland
S-Methyltransferase	Thiols	Liver Kidney Lung

The co-factor, S-adenosylmethionine (SAM), is required to form methyl conjugates and is produced from L-methionine and ATP under the influence of the enzyme, L-methionine adenosyltransferase (Figure 1.38).

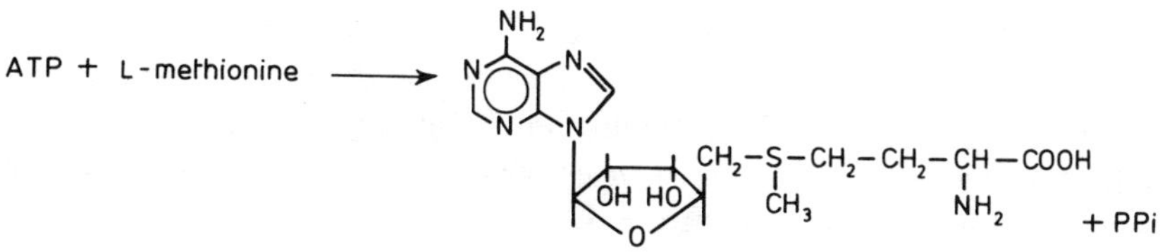

ATP + L-methionine ⟶

Figure 1.38 The formation of *S*-adenosylmethionine.

The non-specific *N*-methyltransferase found in the lung can reverse the *N*-demethylation reactions of phase I metabolism (see Figure 1.39) but most of the other methyltransferases are specific for endogenous compounds (see the section on endogenous metabolism) except the *S*-methyltransferase that is found in the microsomal fraction and which will methylate many thiols (see Figure 1.40) such as thiouracil.

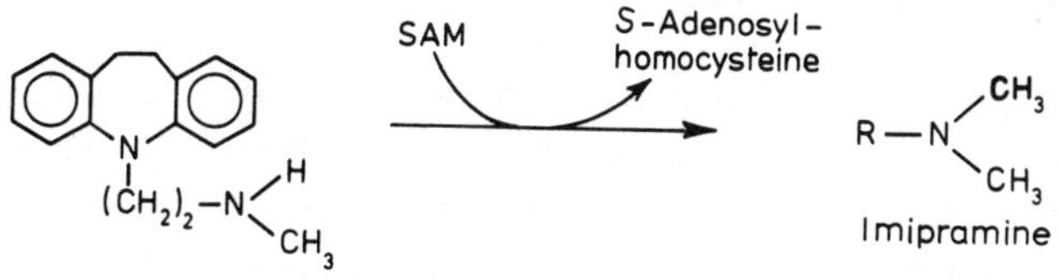

Figure 1.39 The *N*-methylation of desmethylimipramine.

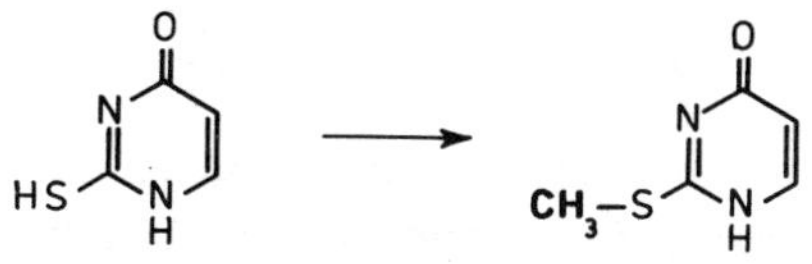

Figure 1.40 The *S*-methylation of thiouracil.

In general, unlike other conjugation reactions, methylation leads to a less polar product and thus hinders excretion of the drug.

1.3.4 ACETYLATION

Acetylation reactions are common for aromatic amines and sulfonamides and require the co-factor, acetyl-CoA, which may be obtained from the glycolysis pathway or via direct interaction of acetate and coenzyme A (Figure 1.41).

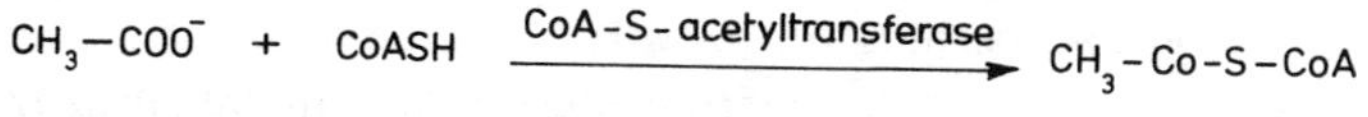

$$CH_3-COO^- \; + \; CoASH \quad \xrightarrow{\text{CoA-S-acetyltransferase}} \quad CH_3-Co-S-CoA$$

Figure 1.41 The formation of acetyl-CoA.

Acetylation takes place mainly in the liver and, interestingly, is found in the Kupffer cells and not in the more usual location of the hepatocytes. Acetylation can also take place in the reticuloendothelial cells of the spleen, lung and gut, and the enzyme is referred to as N-acetyltransferase. Some examples of acetylation are shown in Figure 1.42.

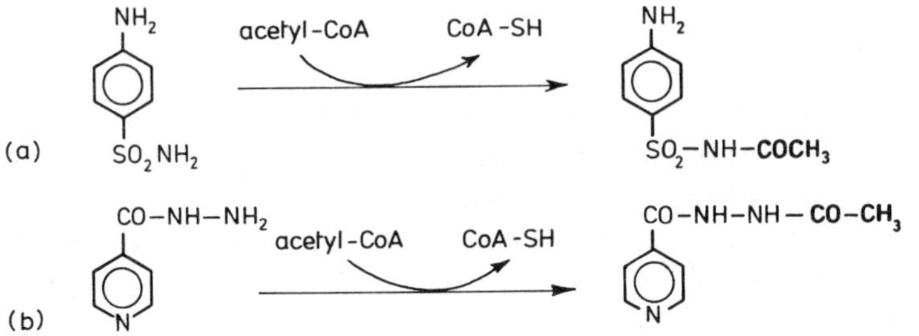

Figure 1.42 The N-acetylation of (a) sulfanilamide and (b) isoniazid.

Sulfanilamide can also be acetylated on the amine nitrogen to give a diacetylated product. The acetylsulfonamides are of particular interest as they are appreciably less soluble in water than the parent drug; the renal toxicity of the earlier sulfonamides has been attributed to precipitation of these conjugates in the kidney.

1.3.5 AMINO ACID CONJUGATION

Exogenous carboxylic acids, in common with acetate noted above, can form CoA derivatives in the body and can then react with endogenous amines, such as amino acids to form conjugates. Amino acid conjugation is, thus, a special form of N-acylation, where the drug and not the endogenous co-factor is activated. The usual amino acids involved are glycine, glutamine, ornithine, arginine and taurine. The generalized reaction is given in Figure 1.43.

$$R-COOH + ATP \longrightarrow R-CO-AMP + PPi$$

$$R-CO-AMP + CoASH \longrightarrow R-CO-S-CoA + AMP$$

$$R-CO-S-CoA + R'-NH_2 \longrightarrow R-CO-NH-R' + CoASH$$

Figure 1.43 The amino acid conjugation of carboxylic acids.

This pathway was implicated in the first described production of a drug metabolite by Keller in 1842 when hippuric acid was found as a urinary excretion product of benzoic acid (Figure 1.44).

The chosen amino acid is related to the intermediary metabolism of the species under study such that ureotelic animals (those excreting urea) tend to use glycine while uricotelic species (those excreting uric acid) use predominantly

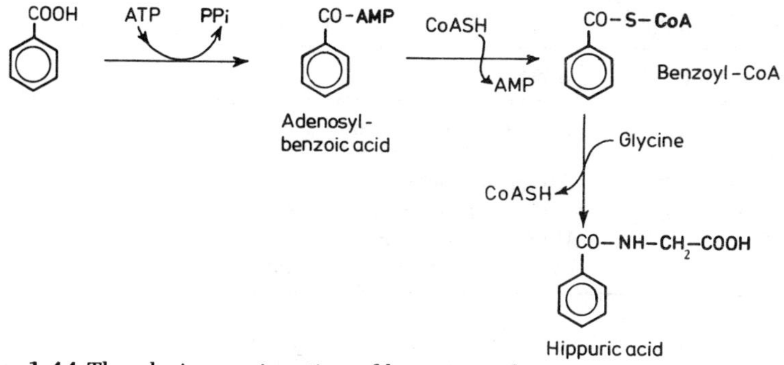

Figure 1.44 The glycine conjugation of benzoic acid.

ornithine. The enzymes involved are not well understood and have been little studied.

Amino acid conjugates of the bile acids will be discussed in a later section.

1.3.6 GLUTATHIONE CONJUGATION

Glutathione is recognized as a protective device within the body for the removal of potentially toxic electrophilic compounds. Many drugs either are, or can be metabolized by phase I reactions to, strong electrophiles, and these can react with glutathione to form (in general) non-toxic conjugates. The list of compounds conjugated to glutathione include epoxides, haloalkanes, nitro-alkanes, alkenes and aromatic halo- and nitro-compounds. Examples of these are given in Figure 1.45.

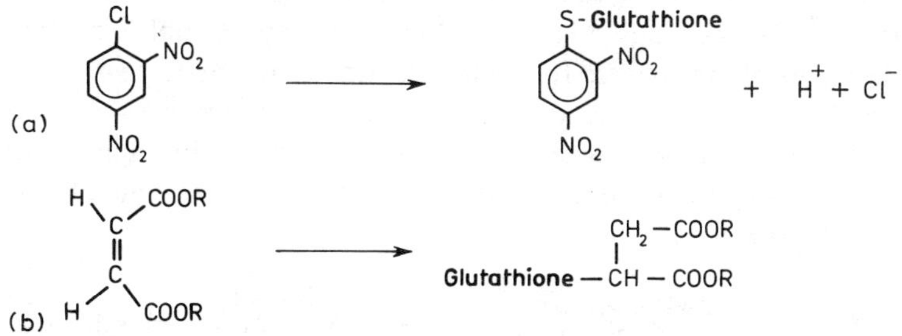

Figure 1.45 Glutathione conjugation of (a) 2,4-dinitro-1-chlorobenzene and (b) esters of maleic acid.

The enzymes catalysing the reactions above are the glutathione-S-trans-ferases which are located in the cytosol of liver, kidney, gut and other tissues. At least six isoenzymes are known with differing substrate specificity as shown in Table 1.10. The interested reader is referred to a recent article by Jakoby (see 1.7 Further reading) which discusses the nomenclature of the glutathione-S-transferases in more detail.

Table 1.10 The isoenzymes of glutathione-*S*-transferase

Isoenzyme	Substrate
L2	4-Nitrophenyl acetate
LB	Mixture of L2 and B2
B2	Ethacrynic acid
A2	1,2-Dichloro-4-nitrobenzene
AC	Mixture of A2 and C2
C2	*trans*-4-Phenyl-3-buten-2-one

The glutathione conjugates may be excreted directly in urine, or more usually bile, but more often further metabolism of the conjugate takes place as illustrated in Figure 1.46.

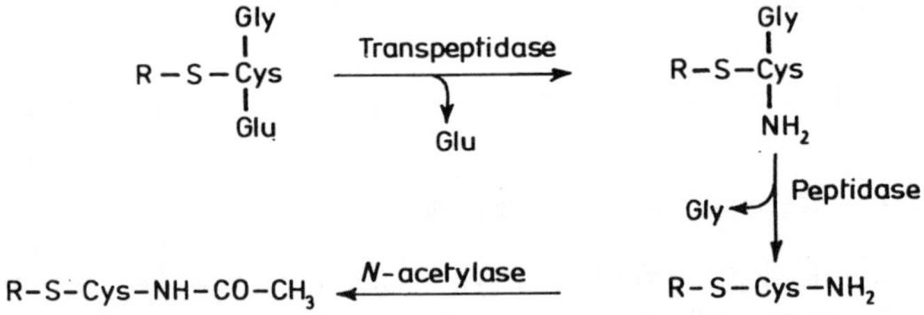

Figure 1.46 The further metabolism of a glutathione conjugate.

The tripeptide glutathione (Gly–Cys–Glu) once attached to the acceptor molecule can be attacked by a glutamyltranspeptidase, which removes the glutamate, and a peptidase, which removes the glycine to yield the cysteine conjugate. These enzymes are found in the liver and kidney cytosol. *N*-Acetylation of the cysteine conjugate can then occur via the normal *N*-acetylation pathway described above to yield the *N*-acetylcysteine conjugate or mercapturic acid. The glycylcysteine, cysteine conjugates and mercapturic acids are all found as excretion products depending on the substrate and species under study. One example of this complete process is found for the metabolism of naphthalene (Figure 1.47).

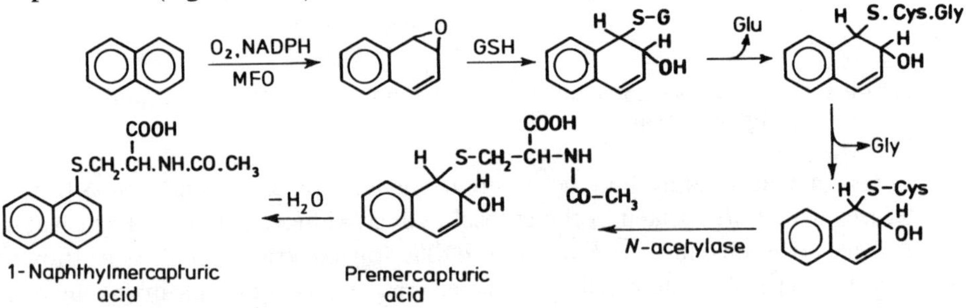

Figure 1.47 The phase I and II metabolism of naphthalene.

1.3.7 FATTY ACID CONJUGATION

Fatty acid conjugation has been shown to occur for 11-hydroxy-Δ^9-tetrahydro-cannabinol. The fatty acids involved are stearic and palmitic acid (Figure 1.48). The microsomal fraction from liver catalyses this reaction. Little is known, however, of the mechanism or whether other compounds can be conjugated in this way.

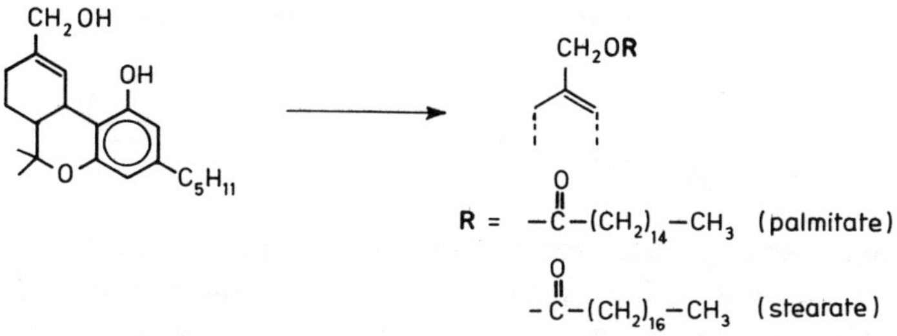

$$R = \quad -\overset{O}{\underset{\|}{C}}-(CH_2)_{14}-CH_3 \quad (palmitate)$$

$$-\overset{O}{\underset{\|}{C}}-(CH_2)_{16}-CH_3 \quad (stearate)$$

Figure 1.48 The conjugation of 11-hydroxy-Δ^9-THC to palmitic and stearic acids.

1.3.8 CONDENSATION REACTIONS

These recently discovered reactions may not be enzymatic but purely chemical (cf. N-glucuronide formation) and have been found for amines and aldehydes. One example is the condensation of dopamine and its own metabolite, 3,4-dihydroxyphenylacetaldehyde, to yield the alkaloid, tetrahydropapaveroline, which is a potent dopamine antagonist (Figure 1.49). As this is a new line of research in drug metabolism it can be expected that more reactions of this type will be discovered.

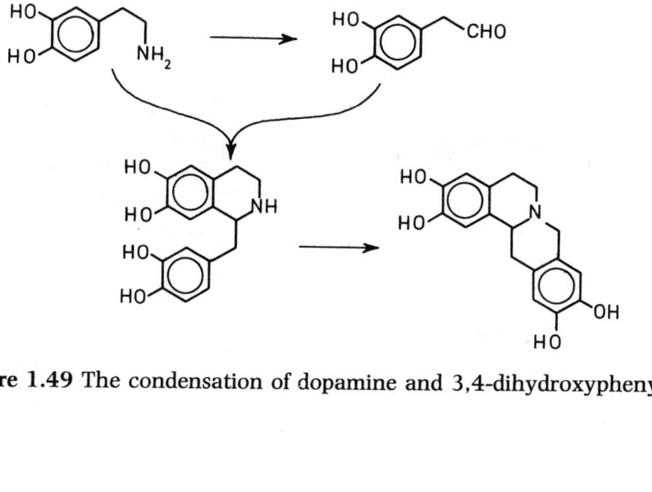

Figure 1.49 The condensation of dopamine and 3,4-dihydroxyphenylacetaldehyde.

1.3.9 SUMMARY OF PHASE II METABOLISM

The above brief description of phase II reactions shows the immense range of possible products of metabolism which, unlike many of the phase I metabolites, have no common link. The one generally common feature is the requirement for some form of energy-rich or 'activated' intermediate whether it be an activated co-factor (e.g. UDPGA, PAPS, SAM, acetyl-CoA) or activated drug. In the main, phase II metabolites are more water-soluble (cf. N-methylation) and conjugation reactions prepare the drug for excretion by one pathway or another.

1.4 Phase III metabolism

A number of workers consider the further metabolism of glutathione conjugates described above (yielding cysteine conjugates and mercapturic acids) as being a third phase of metabolism. This idea has been further expanded when dealing with certain sulfur-containing compounds or compounds that form sulfur-containing conjugates, such as 2-acetamido-4-chloromethylthiazole, caffeine and propachlor.

In these cases the methylthio-derivatives found as excretion products have been postulated to arise as shown in Figure 1.50. The breakdown of the glutathione conjugate is performed by a C–S lyase in the intestinal microflora transferring the –SH group from glutathione to the substrate, where subsequent S-methylation and reabsorption take place. The S-methylated compound is oxidized in the liver to a methylthio-derivative and then excreted.

The series of reactions for the anti-inflammatory drug, 2-acetamido-4-chloromethylthiazole is shown in Figure 1.51.

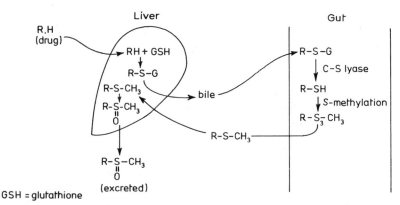

Figure 1.50 Phase III metabolism.

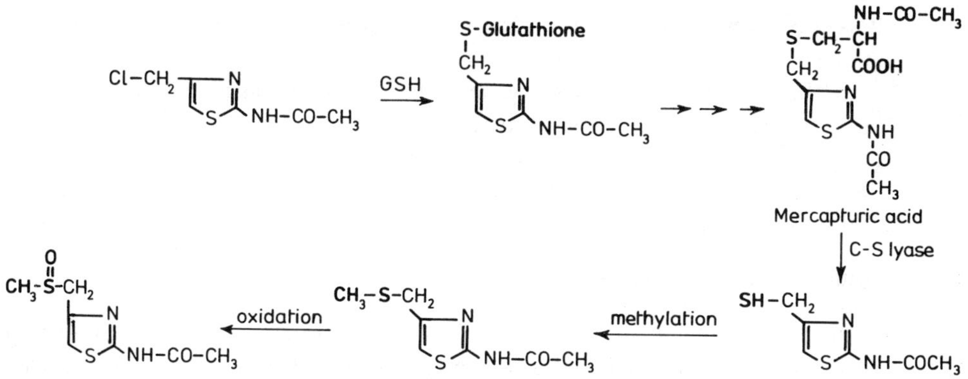

Figure 1.51 The metabolism of 2-acetamido-4-chloromethylthiazole.

Whether this can be considered a further phase of metabolism or simply an unusual form of drug cycling is open to debate but such pathways of metabolism are obviously of importance and should be remembered when trying to predict the likely excretion products of drugs which may form glutathione conjugates.

1.4.1 SUMMARY

In the preceding pages the various reactions that drugs can undergo have been described and the relative importance of the reactions discussed. It will be seen that very many different reactions can be found depending on the drug under study; and a book of this type cannot hope to cover all of these reactions. It is hoped, however, that this chapter has given some insight into the complexity of drug metabolism and the interactions of the complementary, sequential and competing pathways.

The final section of this chapter deals with the interrelationship of drug and endogenous compound metabolism in an attempt to indicate the overlap between the two and how interactions may occur.

1.5 Endogenous metabolism related to drug metabolism

The enzymes discussed above, the 'drug-metabolizing' enzymes, are a diverse group performing a multitude of different reactions. As well as biotransforming many drugs, the majority of the enzymes also metabolize endogenous compounds. It has been suggested that the true function of these enzymes is in endogenous metabolism, and that it is purely fortuitous they also metabolize drugs and other xenobiotics. The greater affinity for the 'natural' substrate in many cases would seem to support this idea but this evidence is not conclusive.

It is, however, accepted that the same enzymes metabolize exogenous and endogenous compounds in many cases.

In this section we will look at endogenous metabolism catalysed by the 'drug-metabolizing' enzymes discussed above. As with the bulk of this chapter, the section will be split into phase I and phase II reactions.

1.5.1 PHASE I

(a) MIXED-FUNCTION OXIDASE

Phase I metabolism is dominated by the mixed-function oxidase system and this is known to be involved in the metabolism of steroid hormones, thyroid hormones, fatty acids and prostaglandins and derivatives.

The metabolism of steroids is intimately linked to that of drugs as can be seen from the common developmental patterns and physiological control, indeed steroid biosynthesis is dependent on cytochrome *P*-450 at many stages. This may be the microsomal or the mitochondrial type of mixed-function oxidase (see Chapter 2) depending on the reaction being studied. The importance of this enzyme is best illustrated by looking at the biosynthesis of steroids from cholesterol.

The rate-limiting step in steroid biosynthesis is the conversion of cholesterol to pregnenolone and this is a multi-stage reaction referred to as side-chain cleavage (Fig. 1.52). A specific form of cytochrome *P*-450 has been isolated from the mitochondria of steroid-producing tissues that performs the above reaction. It is seen that the first two steps are simple aliphatic hydroxylations and require NADPH and molecular oxygen as co-factors (cf. drug metabolism).

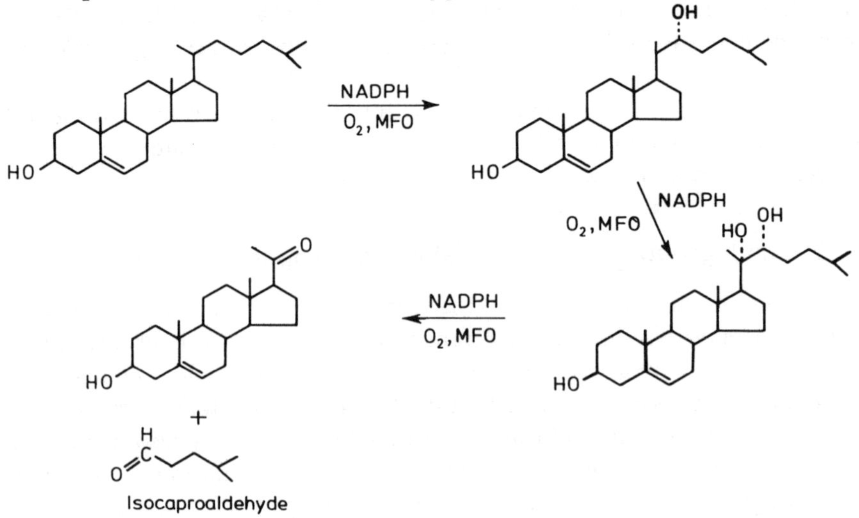

Isocaproaldehyde

Figure 1.52 The conversion of cholesterol to pregnenolone.

The further metabolism of pregnenolone also involves the mixed-function oxidase at many stages (Figure 1.53) some of which are found in the microsomal fraction and some in the mitochondria. Most of the reactions are found predominantly in the steroid-synthesizing tissues but may also be seen elsewhere.

Thus we have cholesterol side-chain cleavage, 11β-, 17α-, and 21-hydroxylations and aromatization of androgens all dependent on cytochrome P-450.

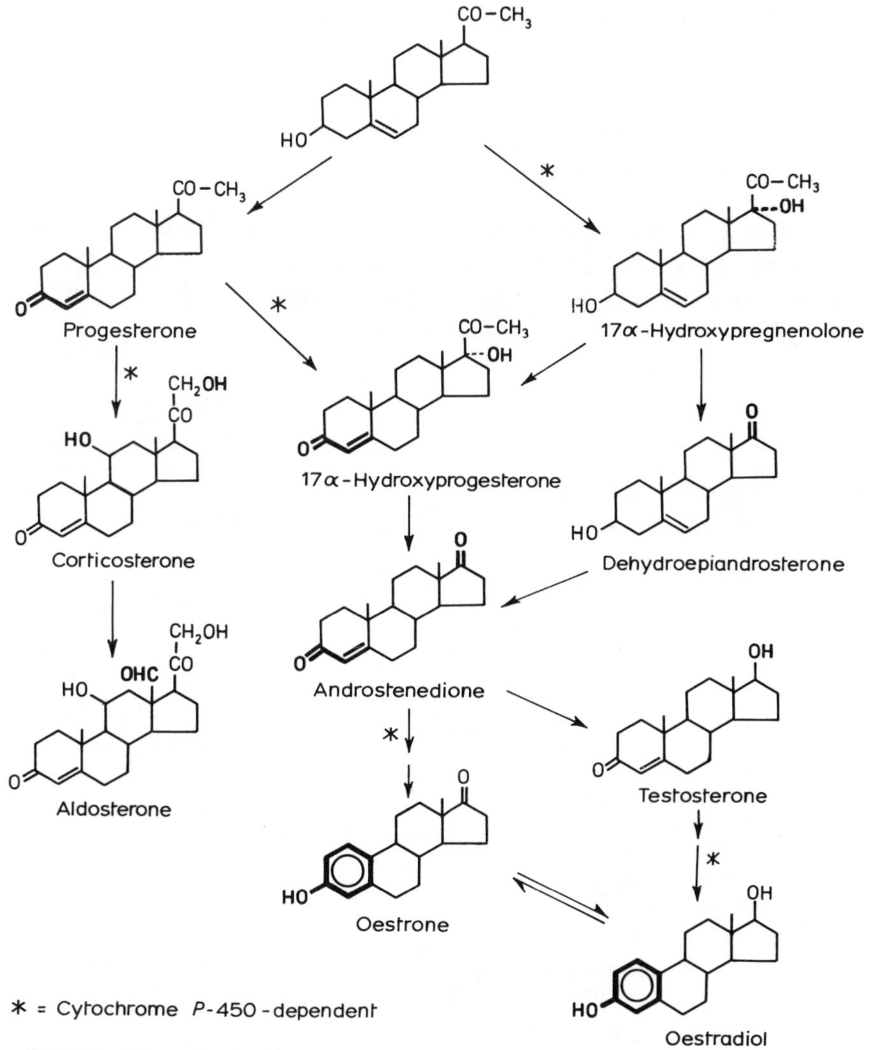

∗ = Cytochrome P-450-dependent

Figure 1.53 The biosynthesis of steroid hormones from pregnenolone.

The breakdown of steroids by the liver and other tissues is also, to a great extent, dependent on the mixed-function oxidase system. All steroids are hydroxylated in various positions by this enzyme and, in most cases, are made less active. One such example is androst-4-ene-3,17-dione which is hydroxylated in the 6β-, 7α- and 16α- positions preferentially (Figure 1.54). The enzymes in this case are located in the microsomal fraction of the liver and are exactly the same enzymes that metabolize drugs. Other steroids are hydroxylated in different positions by the same enzymes.

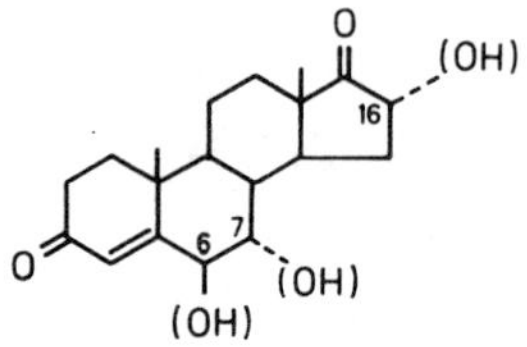

Figure 1.54 The hydroxylation of androst-4-ene-3,17-dione.

A somewhat different scheme is seen for vitamin D (Figure 1.55). After ring opening by UV light of 7-dehydrocholesterol to yield vitamin D$_3$, the vitamin is converted to its active form by 25-hydroxylation in the liver and subsequent 1-hydroxylation by the kidney mitochondria.

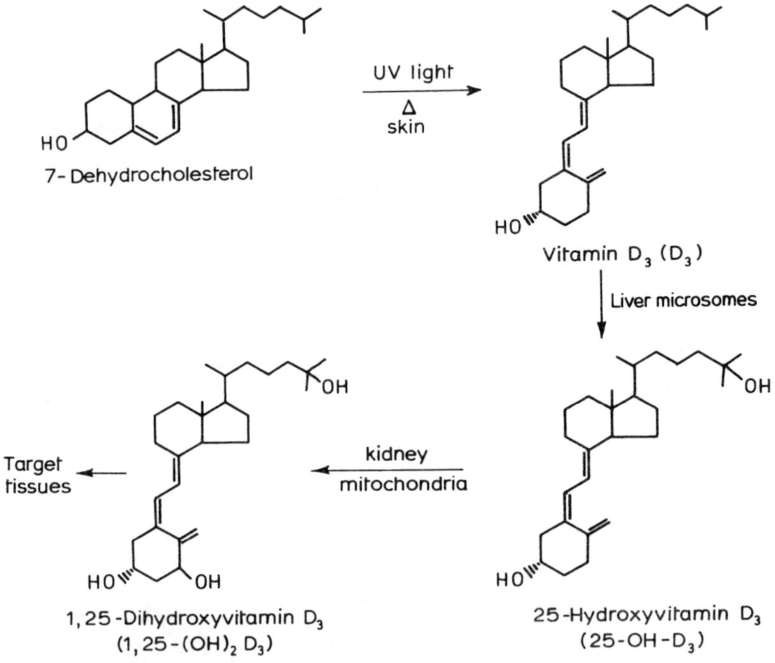

Figure 1.55 The activation of vitamin D$_3$.

The mixed-function oxidase system also metabolizes thyroid hormones by de-iodination (a mechanism for saving the body's store of iodine) and fatty acids. Fatty acids are metabolized by hydroxylation in the ω- and ($\omega - 1$)-positions and can also be converted to the epoxide and thus to the dihydroxy acid (Figure 1.56).

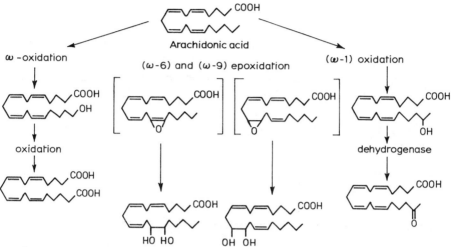

Figure 1.56 The oxidation of fatty acids.

It has been postulated that the biosynthesis of prostaglandins and thromboxanes is also related to the mixed-function oxidase system in requiring cytochrome P-450. The prostaglandin synthetase enzyme is closely related to the mixed-function oxidase (Figure 1.57).

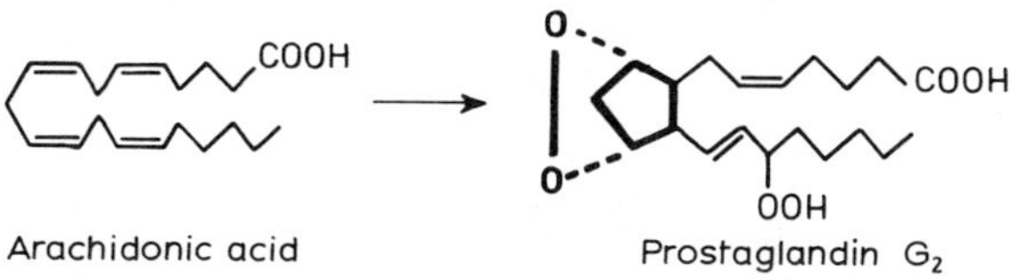

Figure 1.57 The prostaglandin synthetase reaction.

The breakdown of prostaglandins by hydroxylation is also a cytochrome P-450-dependent process.

(b) OTHER OXIDATIONS

Other oxidation reactions occur with endogenous compounds which are not cytochrome P-450-dependent but are related to drug metabolism. The hydroxy

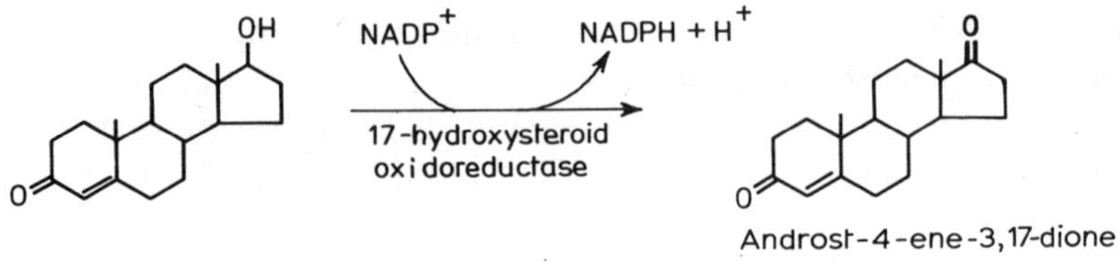

Figure 1.58 The oxidation of testosterone.

steroid oxidoreductases for instance are able to oxidize alcohols to ketones but their physiological function is in steroid metabolism (Figure 1.58).

The monoamine oxidase is primarily an enzyme to break down endogenous neurotransmitters, e.g. noradrenaline (Figure 1.59), but it can also metabolize exogenous amines of similar structure (cf. drug metabolism, earlier in this chapter) whereas diamine oxidase deaminates the endogenous amines, histamine, putrescine and cadaverine.

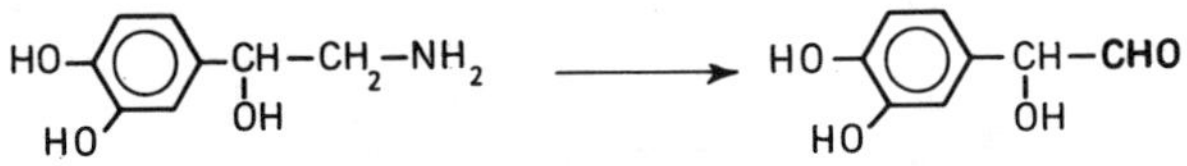

Figure 1.59 The oxidation of noradrenaline.

The xanthine oxidases are primarily related to breakdown of endogenous purines to uric acid via xanthine (Figure 1.60).

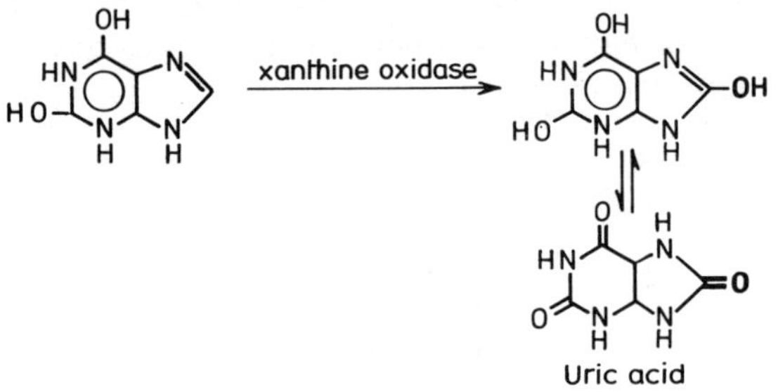

Figure 1.60 The oxidation of xanthine.

(c) OTHER PHASE I REACTIONS

Of the other phase I reactions noted above, hydrolysis is the one which shows most overlap between endogenous and exogenous metabolism. The plasma esterases are closely related to acetylcholinesterase, the enzyme which inactivates acetylcholine (Figure 1.61).

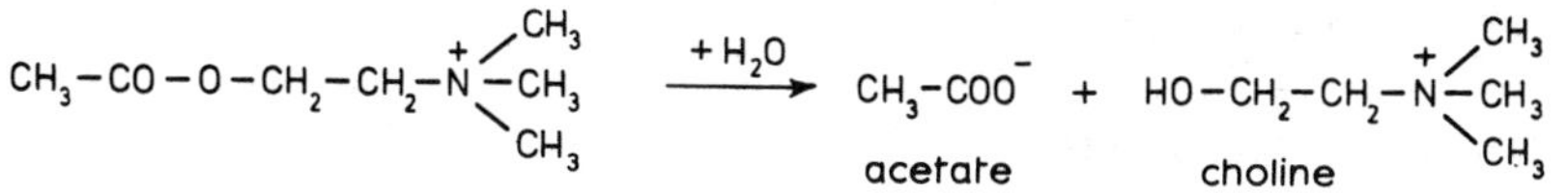

Figure 1.61 The hydrolysis of acetylcholine.

Certain reduction reactions are also seen in the metabolism of endogenous compounds such as the conversion of androst-4-ene-3,17-dione to testo-sterone (see Figure 1.53) and to 5α-androstane-3,17-dione (Figure 1.62) but the relationship of these reactions to reduction of drug substrates is un-clear.

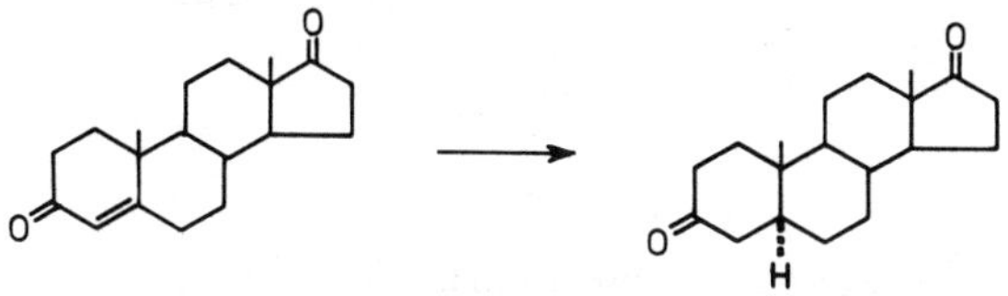

Figure 1.62 The 5α-reduction of androst-4-ene-3,17-dione.

A summary of phase I reactions related to endogenous metabolism is given in Table 1.11.

Table 1.11 Endogenous metabolism by phase I enzymes

Enzyme	Endogenous substrates
Mixed-function oxidase	Steroids Sterols Thyroid hormones Fatty acids Prostaglandins Vitamin D Leukotrienes
Monoamine oxidase	Monoamine neurotransmitters
Diamine oxidase	Histamine Putrescine Cadaverine
Xanthine oxidase	Xanthine
Hydroxysteroid oxidoreductase	Steroids
Acetylcholinesterase	Acetylcholine
Reductases	Steroids

1.5.2 PHASE II

(a) GLUCURONIDATION

Glucuronidation is a common pathway of metabolism for many endogenous compounds including steroid hormones, catecholamines, bilirubin and thyroxine. As with glucuronidation of drugs, this process is a preparation for excretion of the compound; many steroids are excreted as glucuronides into the bile and thus in the faeces. The excretion of bilirubin is dependent on glucuronide formation, and the liver contains a specific form of UDP–glucuronyltransferase for bilirubin.

An example of steroid glucuronide formation is shown in Figure 1.63.

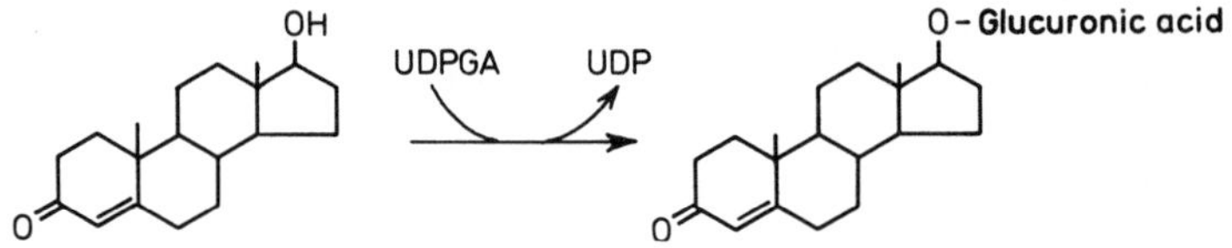

Figure 1.63 The formation of testosterone 17-glucuronide.

(b) SULFATE

Sulfate formation is involved in the biosynthesis of steroids and heparin, each of which have specific sulfotransferases and do not interfere to any great extent with drug metabolism.

(c) METHYLATION

Methylation as stated previously is predominantly a reaction involving endogenous compounds although certain exogenous compounds may also be metabolized (see above). The methyltransferases are listed in Table 1.9 and include phenylethanolamine N-methyltransferase (PNMT) which converts noradrenaline to adrenaline in the adrenal gland; imidazole N-methyltransferase (IMT) which inactivates histamine in the liver; catechol O-methyltransferase (COMT) which inactivates catecholamines mainly in nerve cells and liver; and hydroxyindole O-methyltransferase (HIOMT) which synthesizes melatonin in the pineal gland (Figure 1.64).

(d) OTHER PHASE II REACTIONS

Acetylation and amino acid conjugation reactions are seen for endogenous compounds but are not widespread – the acetylation of serotonin in the biosynthesis of melatonin is one example, and the amino acid conjugation of bile acids is another (Figure 1.65).

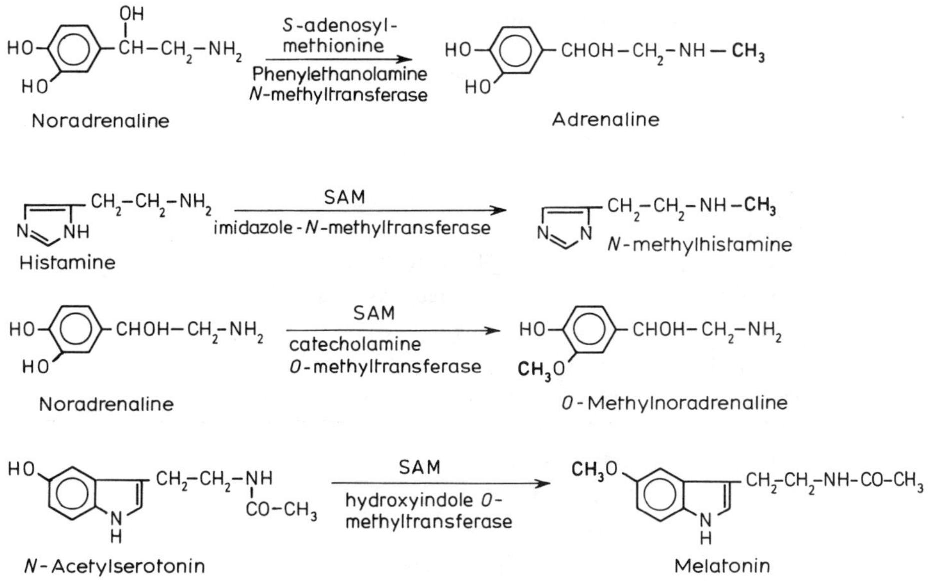

Figure 1.64 Examples of endogenous methyltransferases.

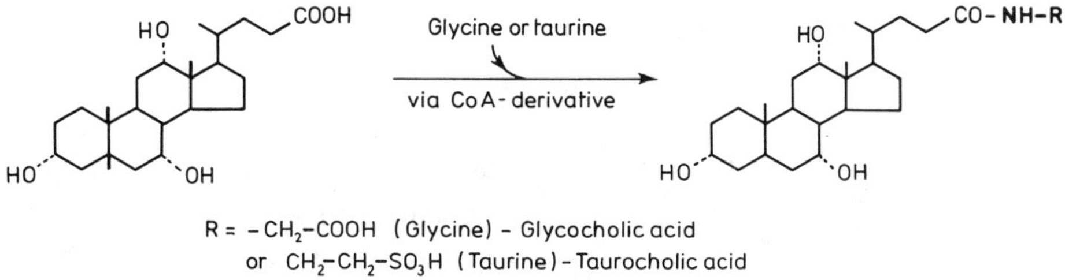

R = –CH$_2$–COOH (Glycine) – Glycocholic acid
or CH$_2$–CH$_2$–SO$_3$H (Taurine) – Taurocholic acid

Figure 1.65 The amino acid conjugation of bile acids.

Glutathione conjugation, however, has recently been shown to be of major importance in the biosynthesis of the novel prostaglandin-like compounds, the leukotrienes. In fact, leukotriene synthesis involves phase I and II metabolism and chemically is very similar to the metabolism of naphthalene (see Figure 1.47) involving epoxide formation, glutathione conjugation and break-down of the conjugate to yield, finally, the cysteine conjugate and perhaps the mercapturic acid (Figure 1.66).

A summary of phase II reactions involving endogenous compounds is given in Table 1.12.

Table 1.12 Phase II metabolism of endogenous compounds

Reaction	Substrates
Glucuronidation	Steroids
	Thyroxine
	Bilirubin
	Catecholamines
Sulfation	Steroids
	Carbohydrates
Methylation	Biogenic amines
Acetylation	Serotonin
Amino acid conjugation	Bile acids
Glutathione conjugation	Arachidonic acid metabolites (leukotrienes)

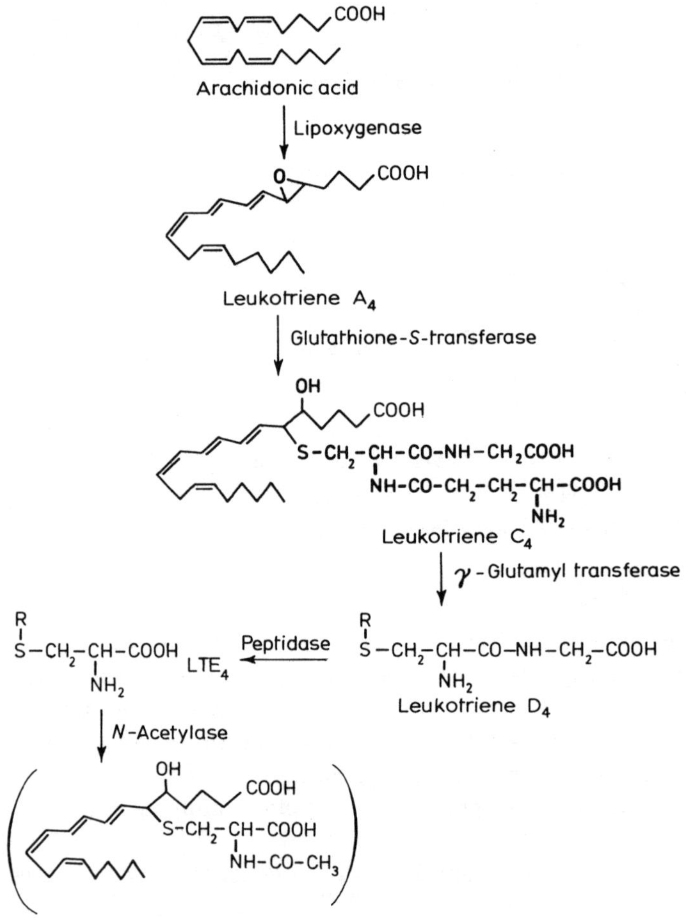

Figure 1.66 The biosynthesis of the leukotrienes.

1.6 General summary

It is apparent from this chapter that there are a large number of enzymes capable of metabolizing drugs to many different products. Many of these enzymes have overlapping substrate specificities and will also metabolize endogenous compounds. There is, therefore, a great probability of competition between drugs and endogenous compounds for the same enzyme; between different enzymes for the same substrate; and between two drugs for the same enzyme. These interactions are often the basis for the toxic or pharmacological actions of drugs. This is discussed in more detail in Chapters 6 and 7.

It should also be emphasized, as stated before, that the reactions noted here are not a complete list of possible reactions but are those of general application. It would be impossible to give all reactions for all drugs, but a general appreciation of the most likely drug metabolic pathways has been given.

1.7 Further reading

TEXTBOOKS AND SYMPOSIA

Aitio, A. (1978) *Conjugation reactions in drug biotransformation*, Elsevier/North Holland, Amsterdam.
Anders, M. W. (ed) (1985) *Bioactivation of foreign compounds*, Academic Press, New York.
Bacq, Z. M. (1975) *Fundamentals of biochemical pharmacology*, Pergamon, Oxford.
Boobis, A. R. *et al.* (1985) *Microsomes and Drug Oxidations*, Taylor and Francis, London.
Creasey, W. A. (1979) *Drug disposition in humans*, Oxford University Press, Oxford, p. 55.
Estabrook, R. W. *et al.* (1972) *Microsomes and drug oxidations*, Williams and Wilkins, Baltimore.
Fishman, W. H. (1961) *Chemistry of drug metabolism*, Thomas, Springfield.
Gorrod, J. W. and Beckett, A. H. (1978) *Drug metabolism in man*, Taylor and Francis, London.
Jenner, P. and Testa, B. (1980) *Concepts in drug metabolism*, Marcel Dekker, New York.
La Du, B. N. *et al.* (1971) *Fundamentals of drug metabolism and drug disposition*, Williams and Wilkins, Baltimore.
Lamble, J. W. (1983) *Drug metabolism and distribution*, Elsevier, Amsterdam.
Pace-Asciak, C. and Granström, E. (1983) *Prostaglandins and related substances*, Elsevier, Amsterdam.
Parke, D. V. (1968) *The biochemistry of foreign compounds*, Pergamon, Oxford.
Parke, D. V. and Smith, R. L. (1977) *Drug metabolism from microbe to man*, Taylor and Francis, London.
Schulster, D. *et al.* (1976) *Molecular endocrinology of the steroid hormones*, Wiley, London.
Siest, G. (ed) (1985) *Drug metabolism: molecular approaches and pharmacological implications*, Pergamon Press, London.
Williams, R. T. (1959) *Detoxification mechanisms*, Chapman and Hall, London.

REVIEWS AND ORIGINAL ARTICLES

Bakke, J. and Gustafsson, J. A. (1984) Mercapturic acid pathway for metabolites or xenobiotics: generation of potentially toxic metabolites during enterohepatic circulation. *TIPS*, **5**, 517–521.

Brenner, R. R. (1977) Metabolism of endogenous substrates by microsomes. *Drug Metab. Rev.*, **6**, 155–212.

Brooks, S. C. *et al.* (1978) Role of sulphate conjugation in estrogen metabolism and activity. *J. Toxicol. Environ. Health*, **4** 283–300.

Cho, A. and Wright, J. (1978) Pathways of metabolism of amphetamine and related compounds. *Life Sci.*, **22** 363–72.

Connelly, J. C. and Bridges, J. W. (1980) The distribution and role of cytochrome P-450 in extrahepatic tissues. *Prog. in Drug Metab.*, **5** 1–109.

Conti, A. and Bickel, M. (1977) History of drug metabolism: discoveries of the major pathways in the 19th century. *Drug Metab. Rev.*, **6** 1–50.

DeLuca, H. F. (1980) Some new concepts emanating from the study of the metabolism and function of vitamin D. *Nutrition Rev.*, **38** 169–82.

Gorrod, J. W. (1978) On the multiplicity of microsomal N-oxidase systems. In *Mechanisms of oxidizing enzymes* (T. P. Singer and R. N. Ondarza), Elsevier/North Holland, New York, 189–97.

Hawkins, D. R. (1981) Novel biotransformation pathways. *Prog. Drug Metab.*, **6** 111–96.

Jakoby, W. B., Ketterer, B. and Mannervik, B. (1984) Glutathione transferases: nomenclature. *Biochem. Pharmacol.*, **23** 2539–2540.

Jenner, P. and Testa, B. (1978) Novel pathways in drug metabolism. *Xenobiotica*, **8** 1–25.

Kumar, R. (1984) Metabolism of 1,25-dihydroxy vitamin D_3. *Physiol. Rev.*, **64** 478–504.

Kupfer, D. (1980) Endogenous substrates of monooxygenases: fatty acids and prostaglandins. *Pharmac. Ther.*, **11** 469–96.

Rafter, J. R. *et al.* (1983) Role of the intestinal microflora in the formation of sulphur-containing conjugates of xenobiotics. *Rev. Biochem. Toxicol.*, **5** 387–408.

Takemori, S. and Kominami, S. (1984) The role of cytochrome P-450 in adrenal steroidogenesis. *TIPS*, **9** 393–6.

Testa, B. and Jenner, P. (1978) Novel drug metabolites produced by functionalization reactions: chemistry and toxicology. *Drug Metab. Rev.*, **7** 325–70.

2

Enzymology and molecular mechanisms of drug metabolism reactions

2.1 Introduction

As described in Chapter 1, drugs and xenobiotics are transformed by a variety of pathways in two distinct stages. The phase I (or functionalization) reactions serve to introduce a suitable functional group into the drug molecule, thereby changing the drug in most cases to a more polar form and hence a more readily excretable form. In addition, the product of phase I drug metabolism may then act as the substrate for phase II metabolism, resulting in conjugation with endogenous substrates, increased water solubility and polarity and drug elimination or excretion from the body. In a quantitative sense, the liver is the main organ responsible for phase I and II drug metabolism reactions, although this is by no means the only organ involved. Drug localization, and hence probably metabolism, in a given tissue is dependent on many factors including the physico-chemical properties of the drug (pK_a, lipid solubility and molecular weight), chemical composition of the organ and the presence of uptake mechanisms which allows the drug to be 'trapped'. As drugs are often given several times per day in high doses for long periods, it is not surprising that the drug-binding and metabolism sites become saturated in a given organ. This would then lead to drug diffusion to other sites in the body and may well explain extra-hepatic drug metabolism and some bizarre side effects observed after prolonged drug treatment. Other organs where drug metabolism reactions

Table 2.1 Morphological and biochemical characteristics of the hepatic endoplasmic
reticulum (ER)

Membranes are 50–80 Å in transverse plane.

ER occupies approximately 15% of total hepatocyte volume.

Volume of ER is 250% of nuclear and 65% of mitochondrial volumes.

Surface area of ER is 37 times that of plasma membrane and 9 times that of outer
mitochondrial membrane.

ER of one hepatocyte has approximately 13×10^6 attached ribosomes.

ER contains 19% total protein, 48% total phospholipid and 58% of total RNA of rat
hepatocyte.

ER membrane consists of 70% protein, 30% lipid, the majority of which is phospholipid,
i.e. approximately 23 molecules of phospholipid per protein molecule.

Phospholipid of ER comprises 55% phosphatidylcholine, 20–25% phosphatidylethanolamine, 5–10% phosphatidylserine, 5–10% phosphatidylinositol and 4–7% sphingo-
myelin.

The fatty acid content of above phospholipids mainly consists of: palmitic ($C_{16:0}$), palmito-
leic ($C_{16:1}$), stearic ($C_{18:0}$), oleic ($C_{18:1}$), linoleic ($C_{18:2}$) and arachidonic acid ($C_{20:4}$).

ER also contains cholesterol ($0.6 \, \mathrm{mg \, g^{-1}}$ liver), triglycerides ($0.5 \, \mathrm{mg \, g^{-1}}$ liver) and
small amounts of cholesterol esters, free fatty acids and vitamin K.

ER contains proteins that are 2% carbohydrate by weight, containing the neutral sugars
mannose and galactose.

ER can be induced by many drugs including phenobarbitone resulting in proliferation
of protein and phospholipid.

---

have been observed include skin, gastro-intestinal tract, gastro-intestinal flora,
lung, blood, brain, kidney and placenta.

Most of our fundamental knowledge regarding the molecular mechanisms of
drug metabolism have been derived from studies on the liver. Although the
molecular mechanisms of drug metabolism reactions can be studied at many
levels of integration including the intact organism, liver perfusion, liver slices
and hepatocyte cell cultures, most of our current knowledge has been derived
from studies on isolated sub-cellular hepatocyte organelles. The morphological
integrity of the hepatocyte can be disrupted by physical means and sub-cellular
organelles may be isolated by consecutive differential centrifugation. With
respect to drug metabolism reactions, two sub-cellular organelles are qualitatively the most important, namely the endoplasmic reticulum and the cytosol
(or soluble cell sap fraction). The phase I oxidative enzymes are almost
exclusively localized in the endoplasmic reticulum, along with the phase II
enzyme, glucuronyltransferase. In addition, other phase II enzymes including

Table 2.2 Enzymatic activities observed in hepatic endoplasmic reticulum

Synthesis of triglycerides, phosphatides, glycolipids and plasmalogens.

Metabolism of plasmalogens.

Fatty acid metabolism including oxidation, elongation and desaturation.

Cholesterol and steroid biosynthesis and metabolism.

Cytochrome *P*-450-dependent drug oxidations, including hydroxylations, side-chain oxidations, deamination, *N*- and *S*-oxidation and desulfuration.

L-Ascorbic acid synthesis.

Aryl- and steroid-sulfatases.

Epoxide hydrolase.

Cytochrome b_5.

NADH–cytochrome b_5 reductase.

NADPH–cytochrome c (*P*-450) reductase.

Glucose-6-phosphatase.

UDP-glucuronyltransferase.

L-Amino acid oxidase.

Azo reductase.

Cholesterol esterase.

5′-Nucleotidase.

Lipid peroxidase.

11β- and 17β-hydroxysteroid dehydrogenases.

the glutathione-*S*-transferases are found predominantly in the cytoplasm. In the intact cell, the endoplasmic reticulum consists of a continuous network of filamentous membrane-bound channels and, on physical disruption, results in the formation of 'microsomes' (literally 'small bodies'). The microsomal fraction of liver cells is an operational term used to describe the 'pinched-off' and vesiculated fragments of the original endoplasmic reticulum, that retain most of their enzymatic activity. As shown in Tables 2.1 and 2.2, the hepatic endoplasmic reticulum serves many important functional roles including drug metabolism reactions. Thus, drug metabolism reactions should not be considered in isolation, but rather as part of an integrated system.

Based on information gained from studies on both intact microsomal membranes, cytosolic fractions and purified enzyme components, it is the purpose of this chapter to clarify, on a molecular level, many of the enzyme-catalysed reactions of drug metabolism. This has been the subject of intense scientific research in recent years, and the interested reader is referred to the further reading section for more detailed information.

2.2 Cytochrome *P*-450-dependent mixed-function oxidation reactions

The most intensively studied drug metabolism reaction is the cytochrome *P*-450-catalysed mixed-function oxidation (MFO) reaction. This reaction catalyses the hydroxylation of literally hundreds of structurally diverse drugs, whose only common feature appears to be a degree of lipophilicity. The MFO reaction conforms to the following stoichiometry:

$$\text{NADPH} + \text{H}^+ + \text{O}_2 + \text{RH} \xrightarrow{\text{cytochrome } P\text{-450}} \text{NADP}^+ + \text{H}_2\text{O} + \text{ROH}$$

where RH represents an oxidizable drug substrate and ROH the hydroxylated metabolite, the overall reaction being catalysed by the enzyme cytochrome *P*-450. During the MFO reaction, reducing equivalents derived from NADPH + H$^+$ are consumed, and one atom of molecular oxygen is incorporated into the substrate whereas the other oxygen atom is reduced to the level of water. Studies using $^{18}\text{O}_2$ have unequivocally shown that the oxygen in the metabolite is derived from air and not from water. In addition to hydroxylation reactions, cytochrome *P*-450 catalyses the *N*-, *O*- and *S*-dealkylation of many drugs (see Chapter 1). These heteroatom dealkylation reactions can be considered as a specialized form of hydroxylation reaction in that the initial event is α-carbon hydroxylation as described in Chapter 1.

2.2.1 COMPONENTS OF THE MFO SYSTEM

(a) CYTOCHROME *P*-450

Cytochrome *P*-450 is the terminal oxidase component of an electron transfer system present in the endoplasmic reticulum responsible for many drug oxidation reactions, and is classified as a haem-containing enzyme (a haemoprotein), with iron protoporphyrin IX as the prosthetic group (Figure 2.1). The enzyme consists of a family of closely-related isoenzymes imbedded in the membrane of the endoplasmic reticulum, and it exists in multiple forms of monomeric molecular weight of approximately 45 000–55 000 (see Chapter 3). The haem is non-covalently bound to the apoprotein and the name cytochrome *P*-450 is derived from the fact that the cytochrome (or pigment) exhibits a spectral absorbance maximum at 450 nm when reduced and complexed with carbon monoxide. The haemoprotein serves as both the oxygen- and substrate-binding locus for the MFO reaction; and in conjunction

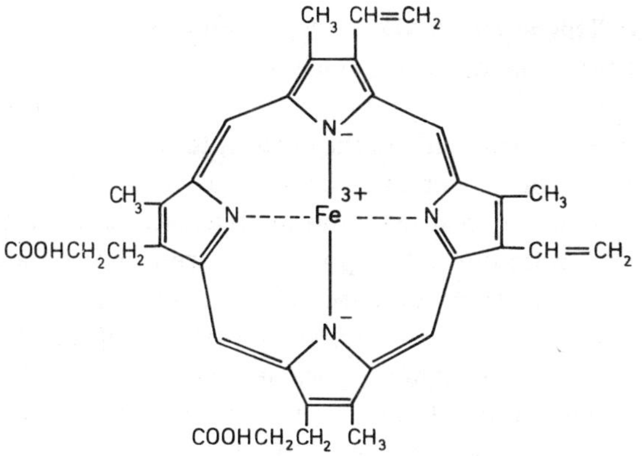

Figure 2.1 Structure of ferric protoporphyrin IX, the prosthetic group of cytochrome
P-450.

with the associated flavoprotein reductase, NADPH–cytochrome P-450 reductase, (see below), it undergoes cyclic oxidation/reduction of the haem iron that
is mandatory for its catalytic function.

(b) NADPH–CYTOCHROME P-450 REDUCTASE

NADPH–cytochrome P-450 reductase is a flavin-containing enzyme (a flavoprotein) consisting of one mole of flavin adenine dinucleotide (FAD) and one
mole of flavin mononucleotide (FMN) per mole of apoprotein (see Figure 2.2 for

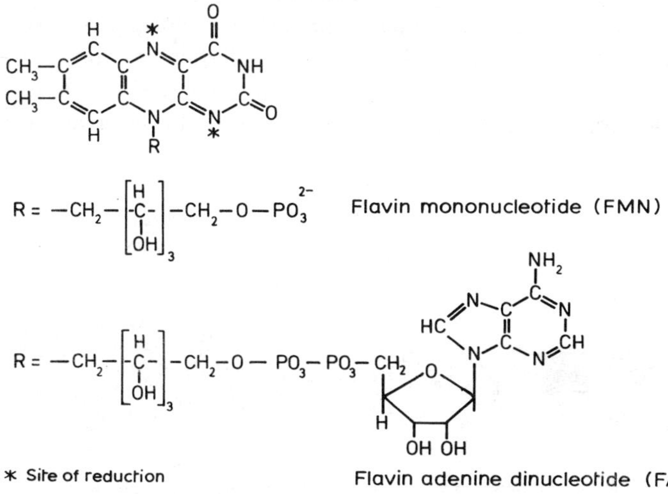

$R = -CH_2-\begin{bmatrix} H \\ -C- \\ OH \end{bmatrix}_3 -CH_2-O-PO_3^{2-}$ Flavin mononucleotide (FMN)

$R = -CH_2-\begin{bmatrix} H \\ -C- \\ OH \end{bmatrix}_3 -CH_2-O - PO_3-PO_3-CH_2$

* Site of reduction   Flavin adenine dinucleotide (FAD)

Figure 2.2 Structures of FAD and FMN, the prosthetic groups of NADPH–cytochrome
P-450 reductase.

structures of these flavins). This makes NADPH–cytochrome P-450 reductase relatively unique, as most other flavoproteins have only FAD *or* FMN as their prosthetic group. The flavoprotein is sometimes termed NADPH–cytochrome c reductase because of the well-known ability of the enzyme to reduce exogenous cytochrome c (an artificial electron acceptor) in the presence of NADPH + H$^+$. However, because cytochrome c is a mitochondrial haemoprotein and not present in the endoplasmic reticulum, the preferred terminology for this enzyme is NADPH–cytochrome P-450 reductase in that cytochrome P-450 is the endogenous acceptor of reducing equivalents from the flavoprotein. The enzyme has a monomeric molecular weight of approximately 78 000 and exists in close association with cytochrome P-450 in the endoplasmic reticulum membrane. In addition to cytochrome P-450, NADPH–cytochrome P-450 reductase is an essential component of the MFO system responsible for drug oxidations in that the flavoprotein transfers reducing equivalents from NADPH + H$^+$ to cytochrome P-450 as:

$$\text{NADPH} + \text{H}^+ \longrightarrow (\text{FAD} \xrightarrow[\text{P-450 reductase}]{\text{NADPH-cytochrome}} \text{FMN}) \longrightarrow \text{Cytochrome P-450}$$

The need for an intermediary electron transfer flavoprotein is readily appreciated in light of the fact that NADPH + H$^+$ is a 2-electron donor and cytochrome P-450 is a 1-electron acceptor. Accordingly, NADPH–cytochrome P-450 reductase is thought to act as a 'transducer' of reducing equivalents by accepting electrons from NADPH and transferring them sequentially to cytochrome P-450 (see above). The precise oxidation/reduction states of NADPH–cytochrome P-450 reductase during cytochrome P-450-dependent drug oxidations are not fully understood, as the redox biochemistry of the two flavins is complex (Figure 2.3 and Table 2.3), although there is strong evidence to support the role of FAD as the acceptor flavin from NADPH + H$^+$ and FMN as the donating flavin to cytochrome P-450 in the electron transfer events.

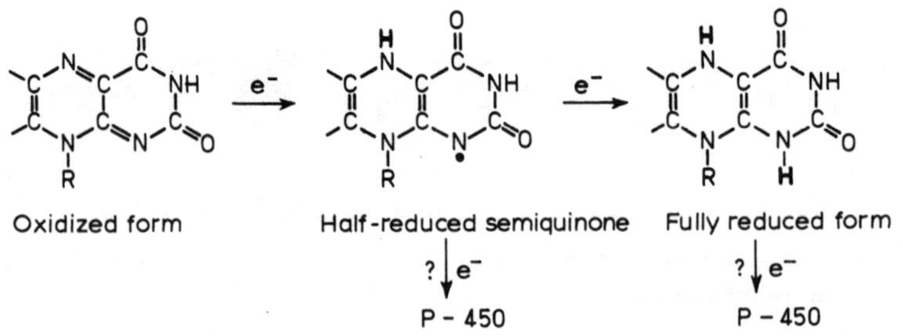

Figure 2.3 Flavin reduction.

Table 2.3 Redox biochemistry of the two flavin prosthetic groups present in NADPH–cytochrome P-450 reductase

$F_1 + H^. \rightleftharpoons F_1H^.$, $E_m = -110 \, mV$		
$F_1H^. + H^. \rightleftharpoons F_1H_2$, $E_m = -270 \, mV$	$E_m = -190 \, mV$	
$F_2 + H^. \rightleftharpoons F_2H^.$, $E_m = -290 \, mV$		
$F_2H^. + H^. \rightleftharpoons F_2H_2$, $E_m = -365 \, mV$	$E_m = -320 \, mV$	

Abbreviations used are: F_1, high-potential flavin (probably FMN); F_2, low-potential flavin (probably FAD); E_m, mid-point redox potential.

(c) LIPID

Early studies on the resolution and reconstitution of MFO activity in drug oxidations have shown the requirement of a heat-stable, lipid component. This component was originally identified as phosphatidylcholine, and later studies showed the fatty acid composition to be critical in determining functional reconstitution of MFO activity. The precise mode of action of lipids is still unknown but it has been suggested that lipid may be required for substrate binding, facilitation of electron transfer or providing a 'template' for the interaction of cytochrome P-450 and NADPH–cytochrome P-450 reductase molecules.

2.2.2 CATALYTIC CYCLE OF CYTOCHROME P-450

As mentioned above, cytochrome P-450 is both the substrate- and oxygen-binding locus of the MFO reaction. The central features of the cytochrome P-450 catalytic cycle is the ability of the haem iron to undergo cyclic oxidation/reduction reactions in conjunction with substrate binding and oxygen activation, as outlined in Figure 2.4. The precise molecular details of this catalytic cycle have not all been fully elucidated and as the reaction cycle proceeds from step 1 to step 6, less information is known.

(a) STEP 1

This is a relatively well-characterized step and involves drug binding to the oxidized (ferric) form of cytochrome P-450. Early experiments in the late 1960s categorized drug binding to cytochrome P-450 into three types, namely type I, type II and modified type II. At the time, these classifications were arbitrarily made on the basis of observed changes in the absorbance spectrum of cytochrome P-450 and subsequently many drugs and xenobiotics have been shown to bind to cytochrome P-450, resulting in characteristic spectral

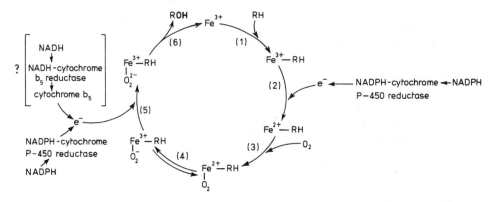

Figure 2.4 Catalytic cycle of cytochrome *P*-450. RH represents the drug substrate, and ROH the corresponding hydroxylated metabolite. (Adapted from White, R. and Coon, M. J. (1980) *Ann. Rev. Biochem.*, **49**, 315–56.)

perturbations of the haemoprotein (see Table 2.4). These spectral perturbations are the result of the ability of various drug substrates to perturb the spin equilibrium of cytochrome *P*-450, which are best understood by considering haem ligation in cytochrome *P*-450.

Table 2.4 Spectral interaction of drugs and other xenobiotics with cytochrome *P*-450[†]

Type I	Type II	Reverse type I
Aldrin	Aniline	Acetanilide
Aminopyrine	Amphetamine	Butanol
Benzphetamine	Cyanide	Diallylbarbituric acid
Caffeine	Dapsone	Ethanol
Chlorpromazine	Desdimethylimipramine	Lidocaine
Cocaine	Imidazole	Methanol
DDT	Metyrapone	Phenacetin
Diphenylhydantoin	Nicotinamide	Rotenone
Ethylmorphine	Nicotine	Theophylline
Halothane	*p*-Phenetidine	Warfarin
Hexobarbital	Pyridine	
Imipramine		
Phenobarbital		
Propranolol		
Testosterone		

[†]Spectral changes of cytochrome *P*-450 induced by xenobiotics have the following UV/visible characteristics in difference spectrum:

Type I, absorption peak at 385–390 nm, and trough at approximately 420 nm;
Type II, absorption peak at 425–435 nm, and trough at 390–405 nm;
Reverse type I (sometimes termed modified type II), absorption peak at 420 nm and trough at 388–390 nm.
(Derived from Schenkman *et al.*, 1981)

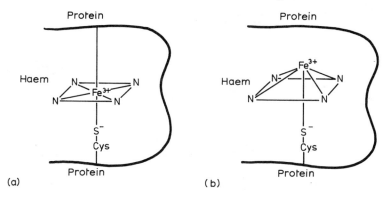

Figure 2.5 Haem iron co-ordination in cytochrome P-450. (a) Hexa-co-ordinated, low-spin P-450 with in-plane iron. (b) Penta-co-ordinated, high-spin P-450 with out-of-plane iron. Note that the fifth ligand is a cysteine residue from the apoprotein and that cytochrome P-450 exists as an equilibrium mixture of low-spin (6-co-ordinated) and high-spin (5-co-ordinated) forms. See text for a detailed discussion of ligation and spin states.

The bonding of the haem iron of cytochrome P-450 to the four pyrrole nitrogen atoms of protoporphyrin IX and the two axial ligands (usually amino acid side chains) laying normal to the porphyrin plane (Figure 2.5) may be aptly described by ligand field theory. Thus, upon co-ordination of the ferric haem iron with these six ligands in an octahedral complex, the electrons occupying the d-orbitals of the ferric iron (which are energetically degenerate in the free ion) are, as a result of differences in their spatial arrangement, subject to differential electron repulsion by the lone-pair electrons of the ligands. Thus, the electrons occupying the d_{z^2} and $d_{x^2-y^2}$ orbitals (the lobes of which collectively exhibit octahedral symmetry and are oriented along the ligand bond axes) experience a greater electron repulsion than electrons occupying the d_{xy}, d_{yz} and d_{xz} orbitals (lying between the bond axes). This results in a splitting in the energy levels of the ferric ion d-orbitals as shown in Figure 2.6.

The magnitude of the energy separation between the two higher-energy orbitals (e_g) and the three lower-energy orbitals (t_{2g}) is called the crystal field splitting (or stabilization) energy, termed ΔE, and is a function of the strength of the ligand to ferric d-orbital repulsion forces and thus the ligand field strength. The magnitude of ΔE has profound effects upon the distribution of the ferric d-electrons. Thus if ΔE is greater than the energetic instability (C) resulting from electron–electron repulsion in a spin-paired d-orbital, then a low-spin d-electron configuration of net spin $S = \frac{1}{2}$ (one unpaired d-electron) is predicted. Conversely, if C is greater than ΔE, a maximal paramagnetic configuration of $S = \frac{5}{2}$ (5 unpaired d-electrons) is predicted, as shown in Figure 2.6.

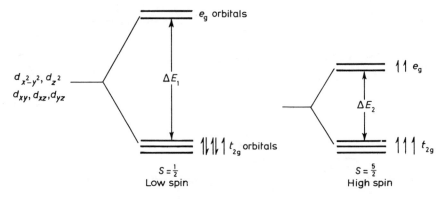

Figure 2.6 *d*-Orbital electron distribution in the low- and high-spin states of cytochrome
    P-450.

From this simplistic description, it is easily seen that a change in the spin
state of the ferric haem iron is associated with a change in ΔE which could be
envisaged as arising due to quantitative or qualitative alterations in the ligands
co-ordinating to the haem iron. Since it is absolutely required that the four
equatorial iron-to-pyrrole nitrogen bonds remain intact, the substrate-induced
spin state changes in cytochrome *P*-450 may arise due to changes in *axial*
ligand co-ordination.

Much effort has been spent by synthetic chemists in an attempt to understand the relationship between the spin state and geometric configuration of
synthetic metal–porphyrin model complexes. It has generally been observed in
such studies that most penta-co-ordinate haem models are high spin with an
out-of-plane displacement of the haem iron, whereas hexa-co-ordinate complexes exhibit an in-plane, low-spin iron (Figure 2.5). These observations
therefore give support to the dogma of haemoprotein biochemistry that all
high- and low-spin haemoproteins are penta- and hexa-co-ordinate respectively.

From such considerations, it is clear that an understanding of the immediate
haem environment of cytochrome *P*-450, and in particular the nature of the
axial ligands, is crucial in understanding its mechanism of catalysis. The
importance of the axial ligands as determinants of haemoprotein *function* is
further substantiated when one considers that cytochrome *P*-450 (a mixed-
function oxidase), haemoglobin (an oxygen carrier), peroxidases and catalase
all contain protoporphyrin IX as their prosthetic group, yet all of them perform
vastly different biological functions.

Most cytochrome *P*-450s exist in substantially the low-spin configuration
with a ferric soret absorption at around 418 nm. When certain drug substrates
(termed type I substrates, including hexobarbitone and benzphetamine) bind to
low-spin cytochrome *P*-450, they usually bind to the protein part of the

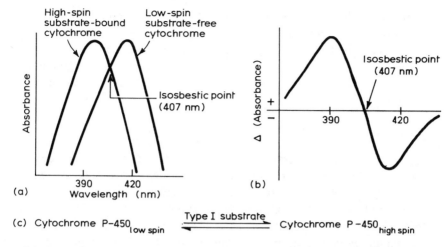

Figure 2.7 Spectral interaction of a type I substrate with cytochrome *P*-450. (a) Influence of substrate on the *absolute* spectrum of cytochrome *P*-450; note the increase in absorbance at 390 nm and decrease in absorbance at 420 nm upon substrate addition. (b) Substrate-induced type I *difference* spectrum; note that the spectral change results from the absorbance changes in (a). (c) Influence of substrate on the spin equilibrium of cytochrome *P*-450; note that type I substrates shift the spin equilibrium to the high-spin form.

molecule and change the conformation and hence the ligation of the haem prosthetic group with the protein. This results in a high spin configuration, and the change from a low spin to high spin configuration results in a characteristic spectral change (type I spectral change), with an absorption maximum at around 390 nm and minimum around 420 nm in the difference spectrum (Figure 2.7). This difference spectrum arises due to the increase in absorbance at 390 nm (high-spin form) and decrease in absorbance at 420 nm on binding of a type I substrate. Thus type I substrates can be considered as those that modulate the spin equilibrium of cytochrome *P*-450 from a low-spin to a high-spin form (Figure 2.7).

In contrast to type I substrates, type II substrates are mainly nitrogenous bases and are thought to ligate to the haem iron of cytochrome *P*-450, resulting in a 6-co-ordinated, low-spin haemoprotein.

An interesting concept related to the drug-induced spin state modulation of cytochrome *P*-450 is that the spin state shift is associated with changes in the mid-point redox potential of the haemoprotein. For example, a shift in the spin state of both bacterial and mammalian cytochrome *P*-450 towards the high-spin form is associated with a shift in the mid-point redox potential of the haemoprotein to a more positive value. The spin–redox coupling phenomenon may well be of functional significance when one considers that the first electron reduction of ferric cytochrome *P*-450 (step 2; see Figure 2.4) by NADPH–cytochrome *P*-450 reductase represents the committed step in cytochrome *P*-450-dependent catalysis. A substrate-induced shift in the haemoprotein mid-point redox potential to a more positive value results in a greater electro-motive force for subsequent facile electron transfer between the flavoprotein and the cytochrome.

(b) STEP 2

This involves the first electron reduction of substrate-bound ferric cytochrome *P*-450 to the ferrous form of the haemoprotein. The reducing equivalent necessary for this reduction is originally derived from NADPH + H^+ and is transferred by the flavoprotein, NADPH–cytochrome *P*-450 reductase. In terms of the electron transfer proteins, there is a substantial difference between the mammalian microsomal system on the one hand and adrenal mito-chondrial systems on the other. In the microsomal system, electron transfer occurs in the sequence NADPH + H^+/NADPH–cytochrome *P*-450 reductase/ cytochrome *P*-450 as described above whereas there is an additional require-ment for an iron–sulphur protein in the adrenal system, namely adrenodoxin.

In the adrenal mitochondrial system electron transfer occurs in the sequence:

$$NADPH + H^+ \rightarrow NADPH\text{-adrenodoxin reductase} \rightarrow adrenodoxin \rightarrow cytochrome\ P\text{-}450$$

It should be noted that unlike microsomal NADPH–cytochrome *P*-450 reductase, adrenal mitochondrial NADPH–adrenodoxin reductase contains only FAD as the sole prosthetic group. In addition, the adrenal mitochondrial cytochrome *P*-450 is different from its microsomal counterpart in that the former haemoprotein does not readily catalyse the oxidation of drugs. To date, two isoenzymes of adrenal mitochondrial cytochrome *P*-450 have been charac-terized, one termed cytochrome $P\text{-}450_{scc}$ which catalyses the side chain cleav-age of cholesterol, and the other termed cytochrome $P\text{-}450_{11\beta}$, active in the 11β-hydroxylation of corticosterone. The endogenous roles for cytochrome *P*-450 have previously been discussed in Chapter 1, and a more extensive consideration of cytochrome *P*-450 isoenzymes is presented in Chapter 3.

As mentioned above, the high-spin/low-spin equilibrium of cytochrome *P*-450 may well be important in this first electron reduction step. However, a full understanding of the spin–redox coupling in steps 1 and 2 of the catalytic cycle is not yet complete because of the inherent complexities associated with the redox biochemistry of the electron donor flavoprotein which con-tains both FAD and FMN as prosthetic groups, and is therefore a potential 4-electron carrier (see Table 2.3). Although the precise redox state of the donor flavoprotein involved in this electron transfer step is not known with any degree of certainty, recent work indicates the fully-reduced state of the low potential flavin as the electron-donating species. Although existing experimental data are strongly supportive of a spin–redox coupling event (with respect to haemoprotein reduction), extrapolations from thermodynamic data (spin state equilibrium) to the kinetic situation (1-electron reduction rate) have to be treated with caution. This is primarily because the electromotive force for a redox reaction is a function of both the forward and backward rate constants for the electron transfer event.

(c) STEP 3

This step involves the binding of molecular oxygen to the binary ferrous cytochrome P-450-substrate adduct. This reaction is not well characterized in the mammalian system due to the unstable nature of the oxy–ferrous–substrate complex, but has been spectrally characterized in the adrenal system and the soluble bacterial system of *Pseudomonas putida* (P-450$_{cam}$, so termed because the bacterium grows on camphor as a sole source of carbon and catalyses the 5-exo-hydroxylation of camphor).

(d) STEPS 4, 5 AND 6

These steps involve putative electron rearrangement, introduction of the second electron and subsequent oxygen insertion and product release. The precise oxidation states of iron and oxygen in these intermediates are far from clear. Step 5 involves the input of a second electron, derived from NADPH–cytochrome P-450 reductase, and possibly also derived from cytochrome b_5, although the precise role of cytochrome b_5 in cytochrome P-450-catalysed drug oxidations remains the subject of much controversy. Similarly step 6 is not well understood and primarily concerns the actual chemical mechanism of oxygen insertion into the carbon substrate, resulting in product formation. A detailed discussion of the inorganic and organic chemistry involved in this reaction is outside the scope of this chapter; the interested reader is referred to the further reading section at the end of the chapter for more detailed information.

It should be pointed out that under certain conditions in the presence of particular drug substrates, the catalytic cycle of cytochrome P-450 becomes 'uncoupled'. The uncoupling involves dissociation between the utilization of reducing equivalents and product formation, resulting in the formation of reduced oxygen species instead of stoichiometric product formation as dictated by the MFO equation described earlier. Accordingly, in producing hydrogen peroxide in an uncoupled system, cytochrome P-450 functions as an NADPH-oxidase as:

$$O_2 + NADPH + H^+ \xrightarrow{P\text{-}450} H_2O_2 + NADP^+$$

Although the precise source of hydrogen peroxide is not known, it is most likely that it arises from dismutation of one of the oxygenated cytochrome *P-450* intermediates occurring during the catalytic cycle.

2.3 Microsomal flavin-containing monooxygenase

This enzyme was originally designated by the name 'microsomal mixed-function amine oxidase' in view of the fact that many tertiary amines were N-oxidized by this enzyme. However, more recent work has shown that the

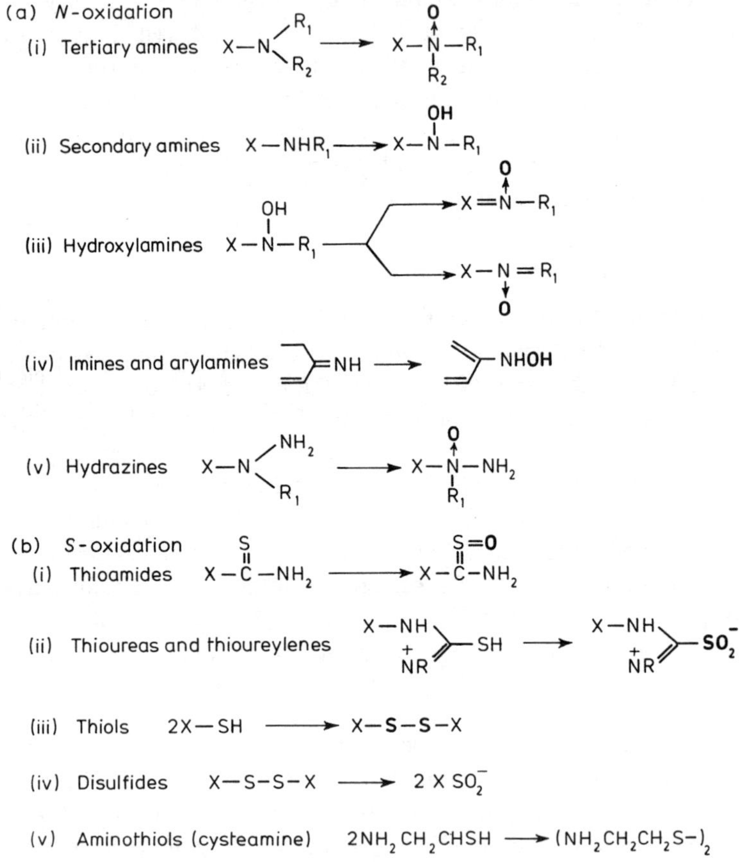

Figure 2.8 Substrates of the microsomal flavin-containing monooxygenase.

enzyme additionally catalyses the S-oxidation of organic compounds (Figure 2.8). Accordingly the enzyme is more appropriately termed the microsomal

FAD-containing monooxygenase (MFMO). Using N,N-dimethylaniline as a representative substrate, the MFMO catalyses the following reaction

$$\text{NADPH} + \text{H}^+ + \text{O}_2 + \text{C}_6\text{H}_5-\text{N}(\text{CH}_3)_2 \xrightarrow{\text{MFMO}} \text{NADP}^+ + \text{H}_2\text{O} + \text{C}_6\text{H}_5-\text{N}(\text{CH}_3)_2 \rightarrow \text{O}$$

The MFMO enzyme is a polymeric protein exhibiting a monomeric molecular weight of 65 000 and containing one mole of FAD per protein monomer. The enzyme is found in many tissues with highest concentrations being found in the microsomal fraction of the liver, and is present in substantial amounts in both man and hog, although lower amounts are present in smaller mammals such as the rat. The flavin monooxygenase uses either NADH or NADPH as a source of reducing equivalents in the above reaction, although the K_m for NADH is approximately ten times higher than that for NADPH; (i.e. NADPH saturates the enzyme at one-tenth the concentration of NADH, and the former is therefore the preferred co-factor). As mentioned above, the MFMO catalyses the oxygenation of many nucleophilic organic nitrogen and sulfur compounds, including many drugs and xenobiotics such as the phenothiazines, ephedrine, N-methylamphetamine, norcocaine and the thioether- and carbamate-containing pesticides (Phorate and Thiofanox). This broad substrate specificity coupled with the wide tissue distribution of the enzyme suggests that the MFMO plays a major role in the oxidative metabolism of drugs and xenobiotics.

Based on kinetic and spectral studies, the mechanism of flavin-dependent monooxygenation is thought to occur as shown in Figure 2.9(a). The reaction involves flavin reduction (step 1), oxygen binding (step 2), internal electron transfer to oxygen forming the peroxy–flavin complex (step 3), substrate binding (step 4), oxygenated product release (step 5) and dissociation of NADP$^+$ yielding the oxidized enzyme (step 6). In the absence of an oxidizable substrate, the peroxy–flavin intermediate slowly decomposes yielding H_2O_2 (step 7). The ordered reaction sequence is summarized in Figure 2.9(b). The peroxy–flavin intermediate is a strong electrophile and should therefore be capable of oxygenating any nucleophilic compound (such as N- and S-containing xenobiotics). As already seen in Figure 2.8 this is indeed the case; however, nucleophilic compounds containing an anionic group are effectively excluded from the active site of the enzyme, and it has been suggested that this structural feature serves to exclude the futile oxidation of normal cellular components, since most endogenous nucleophiles contain one or more negatively charged groups.

It should be emphasized that this flavin monooxygenase is the only known *mammalian* flavoprotein hydroxylase, although many bacterial examples are known. In addition, the reaction mechanism described in Figure 2.8 dictates that substrate binding occurs *after* pyridine nucleotide reduction, again an unusual feature of this enzyme.

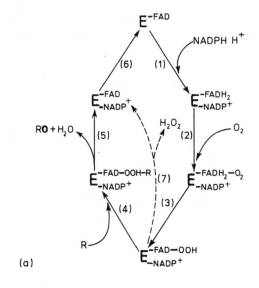

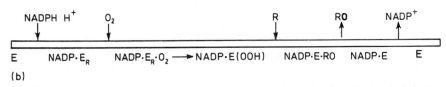

(b)

Figure 2.9 Oxidation of *N*- and *S*-containing xenobiotics by the microsomal flavin-containing monooxygenase. Abbreviations used are (a) E-FAD, oxidized enzyme; E-FADH$_2$, reduced enzyme; R, oxidizable substrate; RO, monooxygenated product; (b) E, oxidized enzyme; E$_R$, reduced enzyme. (Derived from Ziegler, D. M. *et al.* (1980) *Microsomes, drug oxidations and chemical carcinogenesis*, Vol. 2, p. 637 (eds. M. J. Coon *et al.*), Academic Press; and Poulsen, L. L. (1981) *Reviews in Biochemical Toxicology*, Vol. 3, p. 33 (eds. E. Hodgson *et al.*), Elsevier.)

2.4 Prostaglandin synthetase-dependent co-oxidation of drugs

Prostaglandin synthetase is an enzyme present in almost all mammalian cell types and catalyses the oxidation of arachidonic acid to prostaglandin H$_2$, the precursor to other important prostaglandins, thromboxane and prostacyclin. The enzyme has two distinct catalytic functions, namely fatty acid cyclo-oxygenase activity forming prostaglandin G$_2$, and hydroperoxidase activity reducing prostaglandin G$_2$ to prostaglandin H$_2$. As shown in Figure 2.10(a), drugs and xenobiotics are co-oxidized during arachidonic acid metabolism by prostaglandin synthetase, a biotransformation that is related to the hydroper-oxidase component of prostaglandin synthetase. Several drugs are capable of

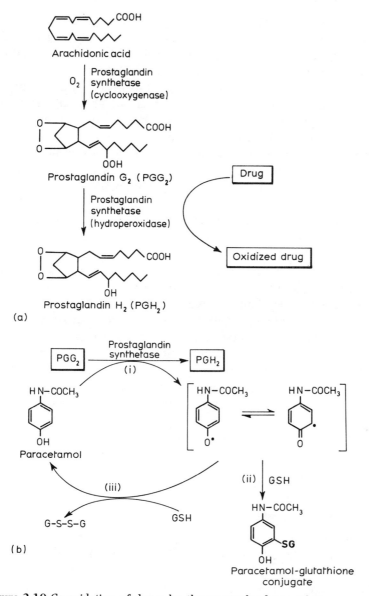

Figure 2.10 Co-oxidation of drugs by the prostaglandin synthetase enzyme system. (a) Role of prostaglandin synthetase in drug oxidations. (b) Postulated mechanism for the prostaglandin synthetase-mediated metabolism of paracetamol. Abbreviation used: GSH, glutathione. (Adapted from Moldéus, P. *et al.* (1982) *Biochemical Pharmacology*, **31**, 1363–8.)

undergoing this co-oxidation reaction including aminopyrine, benzphetamine, oxyphenbutazone and paracetamol as well as chemical carcinogens such as benzidine, benzo[*a*]pyrene, benzo[*a*]pyrene-7,8-dihydrodiol, 7,12-dimethyl-benzanthracene and *N*-(4-(5-nitro-2-furyl)-2-thiazolyl)formamide.

The precise molecular mechanisms of the drug co-oxidation reactions are not clear at present, although some substrates such as the polycyclic aromatic hydrocarbons (benzo[*a*]pyrene and its diol metabolite) can incorporate oxygen into their carbon framework during the course of the reaction. In addition, several *N*-alkyl xenobiotics (including aminopyrine) are actively metabolized by an *N*-demethylation reaction. Furthermore, other xenobiotics such as paracetamol appear to undergo a radical-mediated mechanism resulting in the formation of a glutathione conjugate of the drug (Figure 2.10(b)). This reaction probably involves a 1-electron oxidation resulting in hydrogen abstraction, yielding the phenoxy radical of paracetamol (step (i)). This radical may then have one of two fates. First, the phenoxy radical may tautomerize forming the carbon-centred quinone radical which can then react with cellular glutathione, forming the glutathione conjugate of paracetamol (step (ii)). Alternatively, the phenoxy radical may be reduced with glutathione, re-forming paracetamol (step (iii)). Support is given to this reaction mechanism by the rapid utilization (oxidation) of glutathione during the reaction.

It should be pointed out that paracetamol also undergoes substantial metabolism by the cytochrome *P*-450-dependent MFO system described earlier, although the relative contributions made by these two enzyme systems to the overall metabolism of paracetamol and related compounds is at present not known. Certainly, the prostaglandin synthetase-dependent co-oxidation of certain drugs is a significant metabolic pathway and could conceivably play a major role in drug biotransformation, particularly in those tissues that are rich in prostaglandin synthetase and lacking in MFO activity.

2.5 Reductive drug metabolism

As with the oxidative drug metabolism reactions described above, the microsomal mixed-function oxidase system makes a significant contribution to reductive drug metabolism pathways, and, as shown in Table 2.5, many different chemical groups are susceptible to enzymatic reduction. Although our knowledge of reductive drug metabolism is not as developed as oxidation reactions, some reactions have been relatively well-characterized. For example, tertiary amine oxides are extensively reduced by a cytochrome *P*-450-dependent mechanism whereby amine formation is catalysed by the sequential 2-electron reduction of the haemoprotein in a manner similar to mixed-function amine oxidase activity as described above.

Table 2.5 Examples of reductive drug metabolism

Chemical group reduced	Reaction	Example(s)
Nitro	$-NO_2 \longrightarrow -NH-OH$	Nitrofurantoin Chloramphenicol
Nitroso	$-N{=}O \longrightarrow -NH-OH$	Nitroso-amantadine
Tertiary amine oxide	$-N \rightarrow O \longrightarrow {>}N-OH$	N-Oxides of imipramine Tiaramide Indicine
Hydroxylamine	$-NH-OH \longrightarrow -NH_2$	N-Hydroxyphentermine
Azo	$R_1-N{=}N-R_2 \longrightarrow R_1-NH_2 + R_2-NH_2$	Protosil Amaranth
Quinone	Quinone $\longrightarrow$ semiquinone	Adriamycin Mitomycin C
Nitroso	Denitrosation	CCNU (1-(2-chloroethyl)-3-(cyclohexyl)-1-nitrosourea)
Alkyl halide	$R-X \longrightarrow R^\cdot + X^-$ (X = halogen substituent)	Halothane Chloramphenicol

In addition hydroxylamine reduction is catalysed by two separate enzyme systems. One involves cytochrome *P*-450, and the other involves an NADH H$^+$-dependent system as:

$$\text{NADH + H}^+ \longrightarrow \text{NADH-cytochrome } b_5 \text{ reductase} \rightarrow \text{cytochrome } b_5 \rightarrow F_p \rightarrow \begin{cases} \text{R-NH-OH} \\ \text{R-NH}_2 \end{cases}$$

In this latter system, NADH H$^+$ serves as the preferred source of the necessary reducing equivalents that are then transferred by the cytochrome b_5 system to a terminal flavoprotein (F_p). This latter flavoprotein has been partially characterized from liver microsomes and actively catalyses the reduction of hydroxylamines, although the precise substrate specificity and hence overall contribution to drug metabolism still remains to be clarified. Similarly, although nitro reduction and azo reduction pathways have been recognized for many years, a full understanding of the enzymes involved is still developing. For example, the reduction of azo compounds such as amaranth and other food colorants/dyes is catalysed by several enzyme systems including cytosolic DT–diaphorase, NADPH–cytochrome *P*-450 reductase and cytochrome *P*-450. The latter two enzymes either act in concert or separately catalysing azo reduction, depending on the substrate under consideration.

From the above discussion of the metabolism of amine-containing drugs it is clear that metabolic oxidation/reduction cycling of drugs may occur. This represents an interesting concept in drug biotransformation reactions, as the balance between oxidative and reductive pathways is important in determining both the overall pharmacological and toxicological profile of the drug. For example many drugs are active *per se* whereas others require metabolic activation to express their toxicity as is seen with many *N*-oxidized metabolites of drug xenobiotics.

Many anti-cancer drugs such as adriamycin and mitomycin C undergo reductive metabolism of the quinone moiety, a metabolic pathway that is thought to be a prerequisite for the anti-tumour properties of this class of compounds. As shown in Figure 2.11, the quinone undergoes a 1-electron reduction reaction catalysed by the microsomal flavoprotein NADPH–cytochrome *P*-450 reductase, resulting in the formation of the semiquinone free radical species. This semiquinone metabolite is unstable in the presence of air and is rapidly re-oxidized to form the parent quinone and the superoxide anion radical. This latter reduction product is central to the mode of action of these compounds and is involved in binding to nucleic acids, DNA strand scission and oxygen-dependent cytotoxicity. In addition, the anti-cancer quinone drugs are also metabolized by other enzymes such as cytosolic DT–diaphorase, mitochrondrial NADPH–dehydrogenase and xanthine oxidase, although the relative contributions made by these enzymes still remains to be clarified. Furthermore, it has recently been shown that NADPH–cytochrome

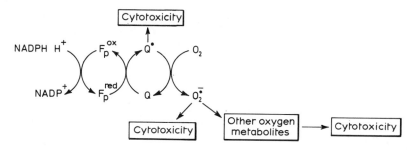

Figure 2.11 Role of NADPH–cytochrome P-450 reductase in the activation of quinone anti-cancer drugs. Abbreviations used: F_p^{ox} and F_p^{red}, oxidized and reduced forms of NADPH–cytochrome P-450 reductase respectively; Q and $Q^{\cdot}$, quinone and semiquinone forms respectively.

P-450 reductase also is responsible for the reductive denitrosation of the nitrosourea anti-tumour drugs such as CCNU. This reductive metabolism results in the formation of nitric oxide and the inactive, denitrosated parent urea and therefore represents a deactivation pathway.

The above two examples highlight the versatility of the enzyme NADPH–cytochrome P-450 reductase. In addition to functioning as an intrinsic component of the mixed-function oxidase system, this flavoprotein can independently catalyse the NADPH H^+-dependent 1-electron reduction of quinones and nitrosoureas, thus utilizing exogenous drugs as electron acceptors instead of the physiological acceptor, cytochrome P-450.

Halothane is a widely-used, volatile anaesthetic, and this halogenated hydrocarbon is metabolized in both oxidative and reductive pathways in the liver. Whereas oxidative metabolism of halothane by the mixed-function oxidase system is generally considered to be a detoxication pathway, reductive metabolism of this anaesthetic has been implicated in the well-documented toxicity of the drug. As shown in Figure 2.12(a), halothane is reductively metabolized by two successive dehalogenation reactions (debromination and defluorination), metabolic pathways that are stimulated by enzyme induction with phenobarbitone, thus implicating the cytochrome P-450-dependent mono-oxygenase system in the biotransformation process. Further induction and inhibition studies pointed to a central role of cytochrome P-450 in the reductive dehalogenation of halothane; the proposed participation of the haemoprotein is shown in Figure 2.12(b). This proposed mechanism has many features in common with the previously described mixed-function oxidase reaction of cytochrome P-450 in that the scheme proposes substrate binding and two 1-electron reduction steps (perhaps involving cytochrome b_5). However, the reaction mechanisms diverge in that during the *anaerobic* reduction of halothane, no oxygen is present and hence the reducing equivalents are not

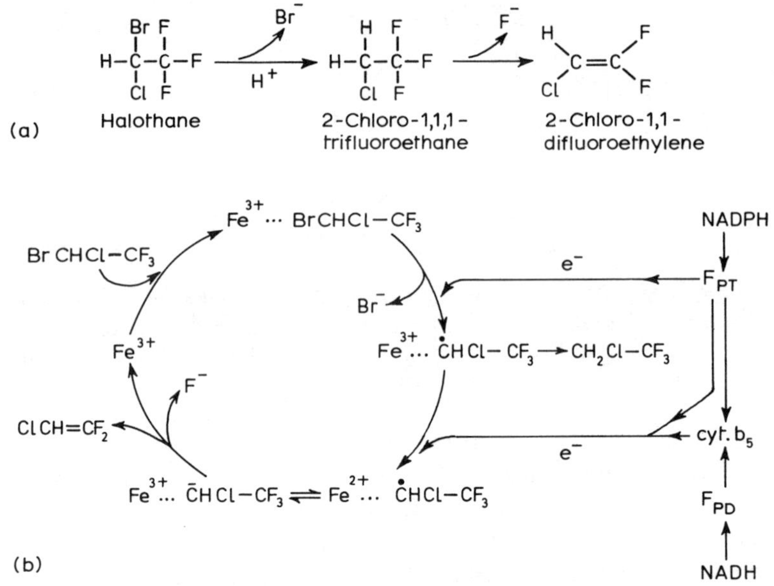

(a)

(b)

Figure 2.12 Reductive dehalogenation of halothane. (a) Halothane metabolism forming 2-chloro-1,1,1-trifluoroethane and 2-chloro-1,1-difluoroethylene.
(b) Proposed reaction scheme of cytochrome P-450 in the dehalogenation
of halothane. Abbreviations used: Fe^{3+} and Fe^{2+}, the oxidized and reduced
haem of cytochrome P-450; F_{PT}, NADPH–cytochrome P-450 reductase;
cyt. b_5, cytochrome b_5; F_{PD}, NADH–cytochrome b_5 reductase. (Derived
from Ahr, W. *et al.* (1982) *Biochemical Pharmacology*, **31**, 383–90.)

used to activate molecular oxygen, but rather are contributory to the formation
of the radical and carbanion complexes of halothane, themselves the probable
precursors of the dehalogenated metabolites. This reaction scheme may be
superficially surprising in light of the high affinity of cytochrome P-450 for
oxygen, and it may be predicted that oxygen would actively compete for the
available reducing equivalents. However, certain cells have a very low oxygen
tension, particularly in the centre of liver lobules; under these almost anaerobic
conditions, it is plausible that cytochrome P-450 would function in a reductive
mode as described. Accordingly, the prevailing tissue oxygen tension may very
well be an important determinant of whether oxidative or reductive drug
metabolism occurs.

2.6 Epoxide hydrolase

Among the many reactions catalysed by the microsomal mixed-function
oxidase system is the oxidation of a number of olefins and aromatic compounds

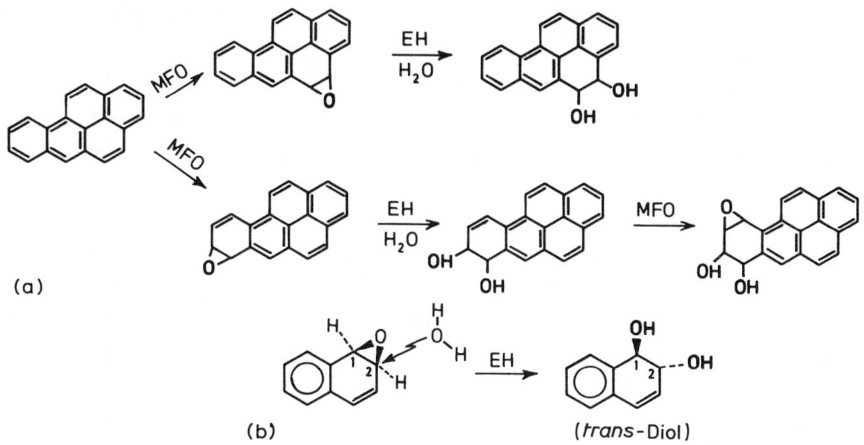

Figure 2.13 Epoxide formation and metabolism. (a) Scheme for the metabolism of the polycyclic aromatic hydrocarbon, benzo[a]pyrene resulting in the formation of epoxides, diols and diol–epoxides. (b) Stereospecific hydration of 1,2-naphthalene oxide by epoxide hydrolase. Abbreviations used: MFO, mixed-function oxidase enzymes; EH, epoxide hydrolase.

to form epoxide (or oxirane) metabolites. These epoxides are formed as metabolites of drugs such as carbamazepine, cyproheptadine, protiptyline and other xenobiotics, including environmental pollutants of the polycyclic aromatic hydrocarbon class of compounds. The epoxides thus formed have several biological fates including: direct excretion *in vivo*; non-enzymatic rearrangement to form phenols; irreversible binding to cellular nucleic acids and proteins; conjugation with endogenous glutathione; enzymatic hydration by epoxide hydrolase to form dihydrodiol metabolites; or further oxidation to diol–epoxides. As shown in Figure 2.13(a), epoxidation can occur at various sites within the same molecule and resultant oxirane ring opening by epoxide hydrolase leads to the formation of both diol and diol–epoxide metabolites.

Epoxides are reactive electrophilic species, and epoxide hydrolase (sometimes termed epoxide hydratase) catalyses the nucleophilic attack of a water molecule on one of the two electron-deficient carbon atoms of the oxirane ring. As shown in Figure 2.13(b), epoxide hydration of certain epoxide substrates can be highly stereoselective with respect to product formation, resulting in predominant formation of the *trans*-diol isomer. However, the degree of stereospecific epoxide hydration is variable from one substrate to another and is governed by both steric and electronic characteristics of the substrate itself. In addition, it appears that the hydration reaction is also regioselective in that the less sterically hindered carbon in the 2-position (Figure 2.13(b)) incorporates water-derived oxygen far more readily than the 1-position.

Epoxide hydrolase is widely distributed throughout the animal kingdom (including Man). In the male rat it occurs in almost every tissue examined, with highest activities being found in the liver, and smaller, although significant, amounts being found in the testes, kidney, lung and adrenal gland. Hepatic epoxide hydrolase has been found to be non-uniformly distributed across the liver lobule. Similar amounts are present in mid-zonal and periportal hepatocytes with significantly more enzyme present in centrilobular hepatocytes in uninduced rat liver, a distribution that is in accord with the distribution of cytochrome P-450. Thus, centrilobular hepatocytes appear to have the greatest capacity for both generating and hydrating epoxides. In the liver, epoxide hydrolase occurs predominantly in the endoplasmic reticulum fraction; recent studies have indicated the enzyme to be present in nuclear membranes and the cytosol of the hepatocyte, and absent in peroxisomes, lysosomes and mitochrondria. The concentration of epoxide hydrolase is induced by most of the xenobiotic inducers of the mixed-function oxidase system (Chapter 3) and there is some evidence to suggest that the enzyme exists in multiple forms, with different substrate specificities. The highly purified enzyme derived from experimental animals exhibits a monomeric molecular weight of approximately 48 000–54 000. The absorption spectrum indicates that the enzyme is devoid of both haem and flavin chromophore prosthetic groups. It is of interest that human liver microsomes contain relatively high levels of epoxide hydrolase activity, and enzyme from this source has been purified and characterized. There is a substantial variation in the enzyme activity within the human population, suggesting that xenobiotic induction observed in animal studies may be relevant to the human situation. Furthermore, it has been proposed that human liver contains more than one form of epoxide hydrolase, some of which are immunochemically distinct from the rat liver enzyme.

In addition to metabolizing epoxides of drugs and xenobiotics, it should be noted that epoxide hydrolase also catalyses the hydration of endogenous epoxides. These include $(16\alpha,17\alpha)$-epoxyandrosten-3-one (androstene oxide) and $(16\alpha,17\alpha)$-epoxyestratrienol (estroxide) at much higher rates than exogenous epoxides, suggesting a substantial role for this enzyme in endogenous metabolic reactions.

Much attention has focused on epoxide hydrolase, primarily because of the role played by the enzyme in the formation of chemical carcinogens from otherwise innocuous xenobiotics (see Chapter 6 for a fuller discussion). In addition, epoxide hydrolase has been postulated to be a preneoplastic antigen, and therefore may prove useful as an early marker of liver cancer. The interested reader is referred to the bibliography at the end of this chapter for a fuller discussion of this latter phenomenon.

Table 2.6 Types of functional groups undergoing conjugation reactions with glucuronic acid

Functional group	Type	Example
Hydroxyl	Primary, secondary and tertiary alcohols, phenols, hydroxylamines	Indomethacin Paracetamol 4-Hydroxy-coumarin Aspirin Chloromphen Morphine
Carboxyl	Aromatic, arylalkyl	Nicotinic acid Aminosalicylic acid Clofibrate
Amino	Aromatic amines, sulfonamides, aliphatic tertiary amines	Meprobamate Dapsone Sulfafurazole
Sulfhydryl	Thiols, dithioic acids	2-Mercapto-benzothiazole

2.7 Glucuronide conjugation reactions

As indicated previously, phase I drug metabolism pathways represent a 'functionalization' reaction in that the drug is chemically primed by oxidation to facilitate subsequent conjugation reactions with endogenous compounds, thus enhancing their excretion. One of the most important conjugation reactions (phase II) is that of glucuronide conjugation, and many drugs are metabolized through this pathway. As shown in Table 2.6, many functional groups have the potential to be glucuronidated, and it should be emphasized that the versatility of this pathway dictates that certain drugs can be *directly* conjugated with glucuronic acid, thus bypassing the usual requirement for phase I metabolism. In a similar fashion to the mixed-function oxidase enzymes, many endogenous compounds serve as substrates for the glucuronidation reaction, including bilirubin, many steroid hormones, thyroxine, triiodothyronine and catechols derived from catecholamine metabolism. This latter observation raises the intriguing question of whether glucuronidation reactions of drugs represents a late development by the organism and that the 'natural' role of this pathway is for physiological compounds.

The reaction mechanism for glucuronide formation and fate of the conjugates is shown in Figure 2.14. The early stages of this reaction are clearly involved in glycogen synthesis through the common intermediate of UDP–glucose – again highlighting the intimate relationship between drug metabolism reactions and endogenous metabolic pathways. The readily available UDP–glucose may well explain the major role played by glucuronidation in drug metabolism. The key enzyme in glucuronidation reactions is

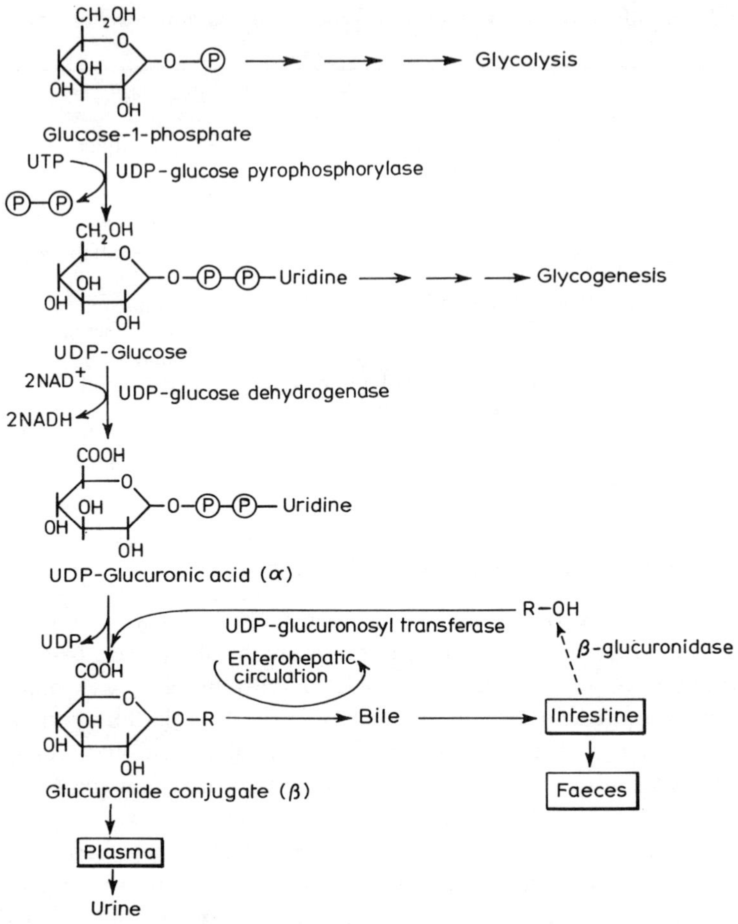

Figure 2.14 Enzymes involved in glucuronide formation and biological fate of the conjugates. (From Bowman, W. C., and Rand, M. J. (1980) *Textbook of pharmacology*, 2nd edn, Blackwell.)

UDP–glucuronosyltransferase (EC 2.4.1.17, sometimes abbreviated to glucuronyl transferase); this enzyme catalyses the transfer of glucuronic acid to a suitable drug acceptor molecule, forming the glucuronide conjugate. It should be emphasized that the C1 atom of glucuronic acid in UDP–glucuronic acid is on the α-configuration, and during transfer to an acceptor drug substrate, inversion occurs resulting in formation of the β-configuration. The resulting drug conjugate is then excreted either in the urine or faeces (Figure 2.14) and it appears that the molecular weight of the drug is a critical determinant in dictating the route of excretion. For example, in the rat glucuronide conjugates of molecular weight greater than 400 are excreted predominantly in the bile (i.e. drugs with molecular weight greater than approximately 200), whereas lower molecular weight conjugates primarily undergo urinary excretion. Thus high molecular weight drugs – such as morphine, chloramphenicol and glutethimide and glucuronide conjugates of both endogenous and exogenous steroids – are excreted in the bile and hence into the intestine. However, the intestine contains significant amounts of the enzyme β-glucuronidase, an enzyme that catalyses the hydrolysis of the glucuronide conjugate resulting in the formation of free drug which may then be re-absorbed, transported to the liver and then undergo re-conjugation and re-excretion. This behaviour is termed *enterohepatic recirculation* and may make a significant contribution, prolonging the half-life of the drug in the body, with the obvious result of potentiating the pharmacological action of the drug.

The enzyme UDP–glucuronosyltransferase is found in almost all mammalian species with the notable exceptions of the cat and a mutant strain of rat called the Gunn rat. In the cat, this species is particularly susceptible to the pharmacological actions of morphine, an observation that is readily rationalized by the fact that the major route of morphine metabolism is by glucuronidation. The Gunn rat is an interesting example of enzyme deficiency in that this strain is completely incapable of forming glucuronide conjugates of bilirubin whereas glucuronosyltransferase activity towards most other substrates is apparently normal. This early observation coupled to the fact that glucuronosyltransferase activity is induced by many drugs and xenobiotics (resulting in altered substrate specificities) has led to the theory that this enzyme exists in multiple forms. Although investigation of the UDP–glucuronosyltransferase isoenzymes has not been as extensively described as for cytochrome P-450, there is much evidence to suggest that multiple forms do exist. The most investigated species has been the rat and recently a *tentative* classification has been proposed based on substrate specificities (see Table 2.7).

UDP–glucuronosyltransferase enzymes are present in many tissues, mostly in the liver but also in kidney, small intestine, lung, skin, adrenals and spleen. The enzyme is mainly localized in the membrane of hepatic endoplasmic reticulum fractions and is therefore ideally positioned to glucuronidate the products of the mixed-function oxidase reactions. The enzyme has no prosthetic group, and the monomeric molecular weight of highly purified enzyme preparations varies from approximately 50 000 to 60 000. The catalytic activity of the glucuronosyltransferases is substantially influenced by the presence of lipids, and although the specific mode of action of lipids has not been elucidated, this may well be an important observation with respect to the existence of proposed multiple forms of the enzyme. An interesting feature of UDP–glucuronosyltransferase activity is that the microsomal,

Table 2.7 Substrate specificities of hepatic microsomal UDP–glucuronosyltransferase in the rat

Form of enzyme	Substrate glucuronidated
A	2-Aminobenzoate
	2-Aminophenol
	3-Hydroxybenzo(α)pyrene
	N-Hydroxy-2-naphthylamine
	Morphine
	1-Naphthol
	4-Nitrophenol
	Testosterone
B	Bilirubin
	Morphine
C	Oestrone
	4-Nitrophenol
D	Chloramphenicol
	4-Hydroxybiphenyl
	Morphine

(Derived from Burchell, 1981)

membrane-bound enzyme exhibits 'latency', i.e. full enzyme activity is only expressed in the presence of membrane perturbants such as detergents. The physiological and pharmacological significance (if any) of this enzyme latency has not been fully elucidated as yet.

2.8 Glutathione-S-transferase

The glutathione-S-transferase family of enzymes are soluble proteins predominantly found in the cytosol of hepatocytes; they catalyse the conjugation of a variety of compounds with the endogenous tripeptide glutathione (glutamylcysteinylglycine, abbreviated to GSH) as follows

$$R-CH_2-X \xrightarrow[\text{glutathione } S\text{-transferase}]{\text{GSH}} R-CH_2-SG$$

where $R-CH_2-X$ represents hundreds of electrophilic substrates. In addition to their ability to catalyse the above conjugation reaction, certain glutathione-S-transferases (such as glutathione-S-transferase B or ligandin) have the ability to *bind* a variety of endogenous and exogenous substrates without metabolism. Examples of these two distinct roles of glutathione-S-transferase are given in Table 2.8. It should be emphasized that glutathione conjugation is possible with either unchanged drugs or their electrophilic metabolites, the only apparent chemical prerequisite being the presence of a suitably electrophilic

Table 2.8 Role of glutathione-*S*-transferases in the conjugation and binding of endogenous and exogenous compounds

Binding function	Conjugation function
Bilirubin	Vitamin K$_3$
Oestradiol	Oestradiol-17β
Cortisol	Paracetamol
Testosterone	Sulfobromophthalein
Tetracyclin	Parathion
Penicillin	Urethane
Ethacrynic acid	1-Chloro-2,4-dinitrobenzene

centre enabling reactivity with the nucleophilic glutathione. In this respect, glutathione conjugation significantly differs from both glucuronide and sulfate conjugation, in that in the latter two reactions both the glucuronide and sulfate moieties must first be 'activated' in the form of UDP–glucuronic acid and 3'-phosphoadenosine-5'-phosphosulfate respectively, prior to conjugation. Such chemical reactivity of glutathione and electrophiles can, in some cases, allow the conjugation reaction to proceed non-enzymatically. As with the high molecular weight glucuronide conjugates, glutathione metabolites are rarely removed from the body by urinary excretion; preferential elimination occurs in the bile.

Many glutathione conjugates are not excreted *per se* but rather undergo further enzymatic modification of the peptide moiety, resulting in the urinary or biliary excretion of cysteinyl–sulfur substituted *N*-acetylcysteines, more commonly referred to as mercapturic acids. As shown in Figure 2.15 for an arene oxide metabolite, mercapturic acid formation is initiated by glutathione conjugation, followed by removal of the glutamate moiety by glutathionase and subsequent removal of glycine by a peptidase enzyme, the latter two enzymes being present in both liver and kidney. In the final step, the amino group of cysteine is acetylated by a hepatic *N*-acetylase resulting in formation of the mercapturic acid derivative.

From the above discussion it is clear that glutathione conjugation serves as a protective mechanism whereby potentially toxic, electrophilic metabolites are 'mopped-up' either as glutathione conjugates or mercapturic acids. As will be discussed in Chapter 6, cellular levels of glutathione are an important determinant of xenobiotic toxicity.

The glutathione-*S*-transferase enzymes exist in multiple forms, and the original nomenclature of A, B, C, etc. in rat liver based on substrate specificities and α, β, γ, etc. in human liver based on isoelectric points has proved confusing. More recently it has been shown that the glutathione-*S*-transferases are

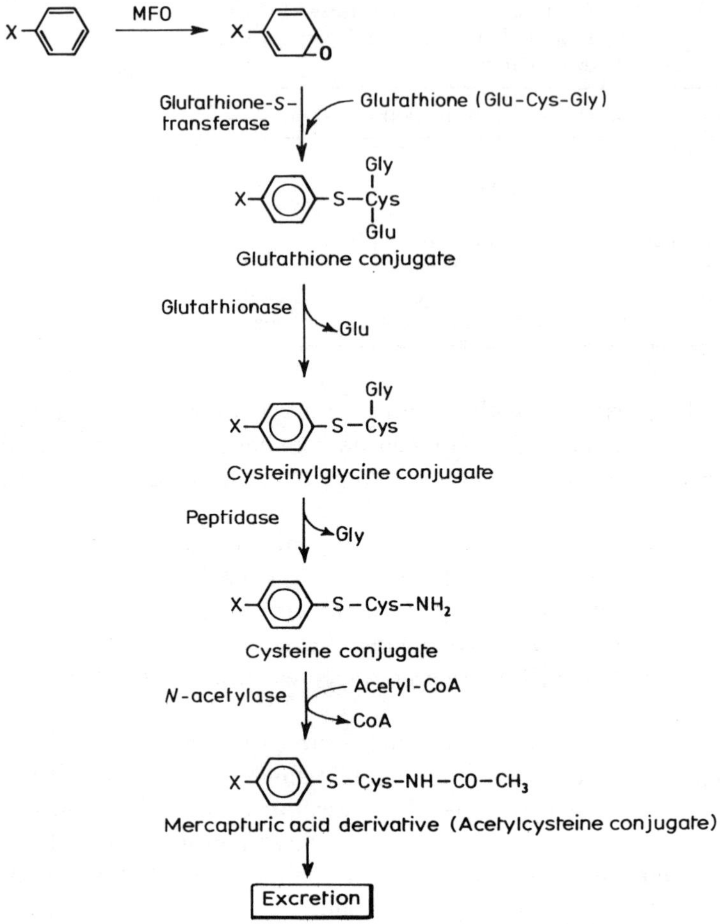

Figure 2.15 Role of glutathione in mercapturic acid biosynthesis. Abbreviations used: MFO, mixed function oxidase; Glu, glutamate; Cys, cysteine; Gly, glycine; CoA, Coenzyme A.

composed of two similar, but non-identical, sub-units. For example, the glutathione transferase B consists of two protein sub-units (termed Y_a and Y_c) of monomeric molecular weights 22 000 and 25 000 respectively. The Y_a and Y_c sub-units are found as binary combinations resulting in two homodimers and one heterodimer, providing a rationalization for the existence of three multiple forms. Ligandin, the major protein involved in binding of both exogenous and endogenous substrates (Table 2.8), is a homodimer consisting of identical Y_a sub-units; it would therefore appear that the high-affinity binding function of glutathione-*S*-transferases is associated with the Y_a

sub-unit. Furthermore, heterodimers containing the Y_a sub-unit have associated binding capabilities. Recently, another sub-unit (termed Y_b, of approximate monomeric molecular weight equal to 23 500) has been identified, thus extending the number of known isoenzymes. A new nomenclature system has recently been proposed for the glutathione-S-transferase isoenzymes (see 2.12 Further reading, Jakoby *et al.*, 1984).

The glutathione-S-transferases are inducible by various xenobiotics including phenobarbitone, and it has been shown that acute administration of phenobarbitone results in a rapid elevation of functional mRNA specific for glutathione transferase B. In addition, the mRNA directing the synthesis of the Y_a sub-unit is selectively elevated by phenobarbitone, whereas the Y_c is relatively unaffected. Thus the mRNAs coding for each sub-unit are subjected to different control mechanisms. Similarly, induction of glutathione-S-transferase B has been observed with the polycyclic aromatic hydrocarbon, 3-methylcholanthrene, and probably is a reflection of increased synthesis of the Y_a sub-unit. It has been hypothesized that the Y_c sub-unit (larger molecular weight) is the primary gene transcript, and that the Y_a sub-unit is a post-translational modification of the Y_c sub-unit. However, in light of the above induction data, it would appear that this hypothesis is incorrect and that the Y_a and Y_c sub-units are encoded by different mRNAs.

2.9 Sulfate conjugation

Many drugs are oxidized to a variety of phenols, alcohols or hydroxylamines which can then serve as excellent substrates for subsequent sulfate conjugation, forming the readily excretable sulfate esters. However, inorganic sulfate is relatively inert and must first be 'activated' by ATP in the following mechanism:

$$\text{ATP} + \text{SO}_4^{2-} \xrightarrow{\text{ATP-sulfurylase}} \text{Adenosine-5'-phosphosulfate and pyrophosphate}$$
$$\text{(APS)}$$

$$\text{APS} + \text{ATP} \xrightarrow{\text{APS-phosphokinase}} \text{3'-Phosphoadenosine -5'-phosphosulfate + ADP}$$
$$\text{(PAPS)}$$

$$\text{PAPS} + \text{R-OH} \xrightarrow{\text{Sulfotransferase}} \text{R-O-SO}_3^- + \text{3'-phosphoadenosine-5'-phosphate}$$

For phenolic metabolites, the key enzyme in this sequence is sulfotransferase (phenol–sulfotransferase, EC 2.8.2.1). The sulfotransferase enzymes are soluble enzymes found in many tissues including liver, kidney, gut and platelets; they catalyse the sulfation of drugs such as paracetamol, isoprenaline, salicylamide and many steroids. It appears that the sulfotransferases exist in multiple enzyme forms with the steroid-sulfating enzymes being distinct from the sulfotransferases responsible for drug conjugation reactions. It should be emphasized that sulfate conjugation reactions are not as widespread, or of as quantitative importance, as glucuronide conjugation reactions, due in part to the limited bioavailability of inorganic sulfate, and hence of PAPS. This is particularly true when a drug is actively metabolized to phenolic products, or when high body burdens of phenolic drugs are reached, resulting in effective saturation of this metabolic pathway.

2.10 Amino acid conjugation

Many classes of drugs including anti-inflammatory, hypolipidaemic, diuretic and analgesic agents have a carboxylic acid as part of their structure and as such are susceptible to conjugation with endogenous amino acids prior to excretion. In a similar manner to both glucuronide and sulfate conjugation, amino acid conjugation of free carboxylic acid groups in drugs requires metabolic activation, according to the following scheme:

$$R-COOH + ATP \longrightarrow R-CO-AMP + H_2O + PP_i$$

$$R-CO-AMP + CoASH \longrightarrow R-CO-SCoA + AMP$$

$$R-CO-SCoA + NH_2-R'-COOH \longrightarrow R-CONH-R'-COOH + CoASH$$

where R—COOH represents the drug, CoASH is coenzyme A and $NH_2-R'-COOH$ is a donor amino acid. In this scheme, the inert carboxyl group is activated to its acyl-coenzyme A derivative, prior to amide formation with the amino function of the donating amino acid. As shown in Table 2.9, this conjugation reaction occurs in many species, utilizing a variety of amino acids, and appears to be a complementary pathway to glucuronidation of carboxyl groups.

Table 2.9 Amino acids utilized in the conjugation of carboxylic acids

Amino acid	Species	Acid
Glycine	Mammals	Aromatic, heterocyclic and acrylic acids
	Non-primate mammals	Arylacetic acids
Glutamine	Primates	Arylacetic acids
	Rat, rabbit, ferret	2-Naphthylacetic acid
Taurine	Mammals, pigeon	Arylacetic acids
Ornithine	Birds	Aromatic and arylacetic acids
Glutamic acid	Fruit bats	Benzoic acid
Aspartic acid	Rat	o, p'-DDA (DDT metabolite)
Alanine	Mouse, hamster	p, p'-DDA (DDT metabolite)
Histidine	African bats	Benzoic acid

(Derived from Caldwell, J. (1980) in *Concepts in drug metabolism*, Part A, (eds. P. Jenner and B. Testa), Marcel Dekker, New York, p. 221.)

This conjugation reaction occurs extensively in hepatic mitochondria and has been used to advantage in chemical tests of liver function. Benzoic acid is conjugated with glycine, resulting in excretion of the benzylglycine conjugate, sometimes referred to as hippuric acid. Under conditions of normal liver function, a specified amount of hippuric acid is excreted within a few hours after either oral administration or slow intravenous injection. In parenchymal liver disorders such as hepatitis or cirrhosis, the urinary output of hippuric acid is low (assuming normal renal function) and therefore constitutes a useful indicator of hepatic viability.

2.11 Control and interactions of drug metabolism pathways

From the previous chapter and the above discussion, it is clear that ingested drugs can be metabolized by a variety of chemical pathways, catalysed by different enzyme systems (Figure 2.16). As with most biotransformation pathways, drug metabolism reactions do not usually occur at random: specific biological control mechanisms are operative at several stages in the overall process. In addition, a particular drug metabolism pathway does not usually operate in isolation: the activity of one pathway can influence the activity in another. Furthermore, many drug biotransformation pathways are intimately related to endogenous metabolic pathways, both sharing the same source of co-factors, co-substrates, prosthetic groups and even enzyme systems, thereby imposing an additional level of control on drug metabolism. The above concepts will be developed in this section, and, where possible, specific examples will be given.

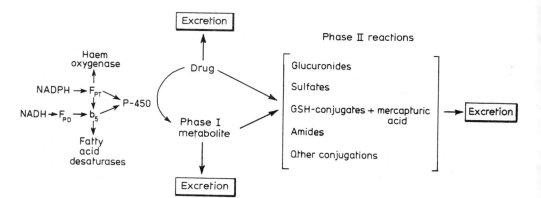

Figure 2.16 Drug metabolism pathways. Abbreviations used: F_{PT}, NADPH–cytochrome P-450 reductase; F_{PD}, NADH–cytochrome b_5 reductase; P-450, cytochrome P-450; b_5, cytochrome b_5.

2.11.1 SUBSTRATE AND OXYGEN AVAILABILITY

The majority of drugs are lipophilic in nature, and therefore metabolism represents an efficient means of clearing the drug from the body. If metabolism is a prominent feature of clearance, then the 'bioavailability' of the drug assumes an important role in that the more readily accessible the drug is to the drug-metabolizing enzymes, then the greater will be its metabolism. Accordingly, the physico-chemical properties of the drug, such as degree of ionization or lipophilicity, are important in dictating the absorption of the drug and access to the membrane-bound and soluble drug-metabolizing enzymes. As most of the phase I oxidation enzymes are located in the lipid-rich, and therefore lipophilic, membrane of the hepatic endoplasmic reticulum, it then follows that a substantial degree of drug lipophilicity is required to ensure adequate substrate availability. Many studies have shown that this is indeed the case, and significant correlations have been repeatedly found between the lipid–water partition coefficient of drugs and their extent of binding to, and metabolism by, the phase I enzymes in general, and cytochrome *P*-450 in particular. Therefore, the physico-chemical nature of the drug itself is an important determinant of drug availability and hence of potential to be metabolized.

As previously discussed, molecular oxygen is an essential requirement for cytochrome *P*-450-dependent monooxygenation of drugs. In most body tissues, oxygen is freely available and in sufficiently high concentrations to ensure adequate drug oxidation. However, tissue concentrations of oxygen may well be very low under certain physiological conditions and in the relatively hypoxic centre of the liver mass, thus placing a possible constraint, and therefore control, on drug oxidations. The availability of oxygen is an important determinant of the route or pathway of drug metabolism. For example, halothane is metabolized by both oxidative and reductive, anaerobic pathways – yielding metabolites which are quite different from each other and, more importantly, which have been postulated to have different toxicities. Although our understanding of the role of tissue levels of oxygen in drug metabolism is still in its infancy, it remains an area of fundamental importance.

2.11.2 NADPH SUPPLY

NADPH is an obligatory requirement for cytochrome *P*-450-dependent drug oxidations, therefore the availability of this reduced pyridine nucleotide is an important control mechanism in drug oxidations. As shown in Figure 2.17, hepatic NADPH is derived from two sources, the major pathway being the pentose phosphate pathway (sometimes referred to as the hexose monophosphate shunt), further augmented by reducing equivalents derived from the

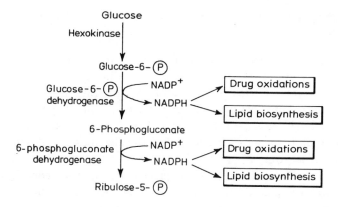

(a)

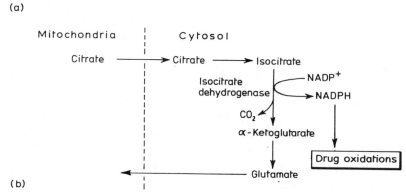

(b)

Figure 2.17 Biosynthesis of NADPH utilized in drug oxidations. (a) Pentose phosphate pathway. (b) $NADP^+$-linked, isocitrate dehydrogenase.

mitochondrial translocation of NADPH. In addition to supplying the necessary reducing equivalents for drug oxidations, NADPH is required in endogenous biosynthetic pathways including fatty acid biosynthesis. For example, during the biosynthesis of palmitic acid starting from acetyl Co-A, 14 moles of NADPH are consumed per mole of palmitic acid formed, thus placing a substantial demand on the availability of cellular NADPH during active lipid biosynthesis. In addition, the availability of NADPH for drug oxidations is critically influenced by the cellular $NADP^+$/NADPH ratio which, in turn, is linked to the activity of the $NADP^+$-linked dehydrogenases such as isocitrate dehydrogenase and glucose-6-phosphate dehydrogenase. Accordingly, the availability of NADPH in drug oxidations is subsequentially influenced by prevailing metabolic conditions forming a coupled, interactive system and therefore constitutes a control point in drug oxidations.

2.11.3 SYNTHESIS AND DEGRADATION OF CYTOCHROME P-450

In any enzyme-catalysed reaction, the absolute amount of active enzyme contributes to the overall reaction, thus the concentration or amount of the drug-metabolizing enzymes is clearly important. As the amount of enzyme present is a dynamic balance between enzyme synthesis and enzyme degradation, factors that alter the steady-state level of the enzymes then make a significant contribution to drug metabolism. Of all the enzymes responsible for drug metabolism, cytochrome P-450 has been the most intensively studied. The biogenesis and catabolism of this haemoprotein will now be considered with particular emphasis placed on the role of haemoprotein turnover as a control mechanism in drug oxidations. It must be emphasized that the following *concepts* are also applicable to the regulation of the other drug-metabolizing enzymes, and that cytochrome P-450 is only being used here as a well-documented example.

(a) SYNTHESIS OF CYTOCHROME P-450

The holoenzyme of cytochrome P-450 consists of both haem and protein moieties, which are therefore subjected to different biosynthetic control mechanisms, both of which contribute to the final, steady-state level of the enzyme. As shown in Figure 2.18, the biosynthesis of intact cytochrome P-450 is a complex, co-ordinated process and involves different sub-cellular compartments of the hepatocyte during assembly of the intact holoenzyme. A major point of control is the utilization of the haem prosthetic group. Not only is haem inserted into cytochrome P-450, but it is also inserted into mitochrondrial cytochromes and other hepatic haemoproteins such as catalase and cytochrome b_5. Accordingly the total hepatic demand for haem is dictated not only by cytochrome P-450 but by other cellular haem-proteins, again illustrating the interrelationship between drug oxidations and normal cellular processes. In addition, many drugs and chemicals have the ability to influence haem biosynthesis by either inducing the enzyme δ-aminolaevulinic acid synthetase – the rate limiting step in haem biosynthesis – or by causing a depletion of existing free haem. This latter point is noteworthy because ∂-aminolaevulinic acid synthetase is subjected to negative feedback inhibition by haem; therefore certain drugs that initiate haem depletion, cause a 'rebound' effect in haem synthesis resulting in acute attacks of porphyria in genetically predisposed subjects.

Synthesis of the apoprotein moiety of cytochrome P-450 is also subjected to control by the ability of drugs (such as the barbiturates) to induce protein

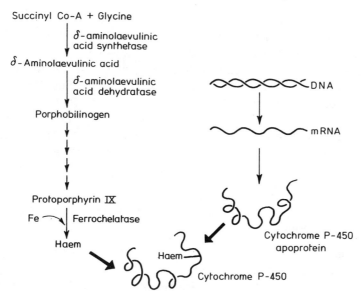

Figure 2.18 Biosynthesis of cytochrome *P*-450.

synthesis. Although drug induction of cytochrome *P*-450 is considered in more detail later on (Chapter 3), it is relevant to point out that not only is cytochrome *P*-450 induced by drugs, but different isoenzymes (or multiple forms) are induced by different drugs. These cytochrome *P*-450 isoenzymes exhibit substantial differences in their respective abilities to catalyse the oxidation of structurally diverse drugs, and it is then quite clear that the isoenzyme complement of individual haemoproteins is an important determinant of the ability of the liver to metabolize a specific drug. In view of the common occurrence of polypharmacy – where patients are exposed to more than one drug (one of which may be an enzyme inducer) – this 'drug-induced control mechanism' has significant ramifications in both clinical pharmacology and toxicology (see Chapters 6 and 7).

(b) DEGRADATION OF CYTOCHROME *P*-450

The major pathway of haem degradation involves an enzyme termed 'haem oxygenase', resulting in the eventual formation of bile pigments such as bilirubin. The complete microsomal haem oxygenase system requires both the haem oxygenase protein and the flavoprotein, NADPH–cytochrome *P*-450 reductase. The participation of this latter flavoprotein is interesting in that NADPH–cytochrome *P*-450 reductase is also a necessary component of the cytochrome *P*-450-dependent drug oxidation system, as previously discussed.

Therefore, during the normal course of drug oxidations, the flow of reducing equivalents through the reductase is not exclusively channelled to cytochrome *P*-450; and, during periods of active hepatic haem oxidation, there is competition exerted on the oxidation reaction by haem oxygenase activity, thus exerting another level of control on drug oxidation. In addition, many drugs and chemicals, especially those with an olefinic moiety, have the ability to covalently bind and inactivate the haem group in cytochrome *P*-450. This would then constitute another control mechanism whereby cytochrome *P*-450 activity (and hence certain drug oxidation reactions) is substantially inhibited by prior or concomitant exposure to this class of drugs.

2.11.4 CONTROL OF DRUG METABOLISM BY ENDOGENOUS CO-SUBSTRATES

As shown in Table 2.10, many of the enzymes of drug metabolism also catalyse the metabolism of a plethora of endogenous substrates. Some of these enzymes are relatively specific for endogenous substrates, such as a variant of cytochrome *P*-450 (termed cytochrome P-450$_{scc}$) responsible for the side chain cleavage of cholesterol in the adrenals, whereas others, such as hepatic cytochrome *P*-450, are less specialized and catalyse steroid, fatty acid and prostaglandin hydroxylation in addition to drug oxidations. For this latter type of drug-metabolizing enzyme, there is therefore competition for available enzyme between the drug and the endogenous substrate. Many factors are important in determining which substrate will be preferentially metabolized, including the tissue levels, the effective local concentration at the active site and the relative affinities of the competing substrates for the enzyme in question. As many endogenous substrates are in a constant state of flux due to synthesis, utilization and degradation reactions, it is obvious that a precise analysis of the role of the endogenous co-substrates as competitors for the enzyme systems *in vivo* is difficult. Nevertheless, it is absolutely clear that competition does occur *in vitro* and therefore represents another mechanism whereby drug metabolism is subjected to a degree of control.

Table 2.10 Endogenous co-substrates of the drug-metabolizing enzymes

Cytochrome *P*-450	Glucuronosyltransferase	Glutathione transferase
Fatty acids	Bilirubin	Bilirubin
Leukotrienes	Serotonin	Cortisol
Prostaglandins	Testosterone	Testosterone
Steroids		Glutathione
Cholesterol		Leukotrienes
Vitamin D$_3$		
Thyroxine		

2.11.5 PARTICIPATION OF CYTOCHOME b_5

As indicated earlier, the precise role of cytochrome b_5 in drug oxidation reactions is far from clear, as no uniform effect has been observed. For example, cytochrome b_5 has been reported to either stimulate, inhibit, have no effect or even be an obligatory component of cytochrome P-450-dependent oxidations, dependent on both the nature of the drug undergoing metabolism and the isoenzyme of cytochrome P-450. In those reactions dependent on cytochrome b_5, electron flow probably occurs as

NADH $\longrightarrow$ NADH-cytochrome b_5 reductase $\longrightarrow$ cytochrome b_5 $\longrightarrow$ cytochrome P-450

It should also be noted that cytochrome b_5 is also reduced by NADPH–cytochrome P-450-reductase, thereby placing another 'drain' on the reducing equivalents of this flavoprotein. The main biological function of hepatic microsomal cytochrome b_5 is to participate in the desaturation of long-chain, fatty acid acyl-CoA derivatives, providing reducing equivalents for the terminal desaturase enzymes. The desaturation of fatty acids in the endoplasmic reticulum is an active process and includes the Δ^5-5-, Δ^5-6- and Δ^5-9-desaturases; it therefore constitutes a potent drain on cytochrome b_5-mediated reducing equivalents and, consequently, significantly influences those drug oxidation reactions mediated by cytochrome b_5. In addition, unlike cytochrome P-450, cytochrome b_5 is relatively insensitive to induction by exogenous drugs and chemicals. In uninduced, liver microsomes, the molar ratio of cytochrome P-450 to cytochrome b_5 is approximately $2:1$ – during induction this can increase to around $6:1$. Therefore the molecular association between these two haemoproteins is almost certainly influenced by induction and may then significantly alter both quantitative and qualitative aspects of drug metabolism.

2.11.6 GLUCURONIDATION

As indicated in Figure 2.14, the conjugation of drugs and their metabolites with glucuronic acid is intimately related to carbohydrate metabolism, via UDP–glucuronic acid (UDPGA) – the donor of the glucuronide moiety. The synthesis of UDPGA is not the sole metabolic pathway for glucose-1-phosphate and UDP–glucose; these two intermediates are important in both glycolysis and glycogenesis pathways. From the viewpoint that glucuronidation is both an extensive and a not-readily saturable reaction, it would appear that, under normal metabolic conditions, the supply of UDPGA is not rate-limiting in conjugation reactions. However, under conditions of excessive utilization of carbohydrate or glycogenesis the flux of UDPGA through glucuronidation mechanisms is impaired, again illustrating the interaction of drug metabolism with normal metabolic processes. In addition, like cytochrome *P*-450, the UDP–glucuronosyltransferases are subjected to induction by clinically used drugs, and are important in the metabolism of endogenous compounds. Therefore the concepts discussed for cytochrome *P*-450 are equally applicable to the UDP–glucuronosyltransferases leading to altered substrate specificity after induction, and subject to competition by endogenous substrates.

2.11.7 CELLULAR COMPETITION FOR GLUTATHIONE

In addition to acting as a co-substrate for the glutathione-*S*-transferase-catalysed conjugation of electrophilic drugs and chemicals, glutathione has other cellular functions. Two molecules of glutathione are oxidized by the enzyme glutathione peroxidase (in the presence of an oxidized substrate such as lipid peroxides) forming the disulfide of glutathione. The glutathione disulfide may then, in turn, be reduced back to glutathione by the enzyme glutathione reductase, thus setting up a cycle of gluathione utilization coupled to the detoxication of cellular peroxides. However, under conditions of oxidative stress when peroxide concentrations are high, the formation of glutathione disulfide exceeds the capacity of the reductase, and high gluta-thione disulfide levels build up, are removed from the hepatocyte and excreted in the bile. The net result of this process is to deplete the hepatocyte of glutathione and thereby reduce the availability of this co-substrate for the glutathione-*S*-transferase-catalysed conjugation of drugs.

Another major cellular utilization of glutathione is in the biosynthesis of the leukotrienes, including leukotrienes LTC_4, LTD_4 and LTE_4. These leukotrienes are derived originally from arachidonic acid, and condensation of leukotriene A_4 (an epoxide of arachidonic acid) with glutathione (catalysed by glutathione-*S*-transferase) results in the formation of LTC_4 and subsequently, LTD_4 and LTE_4. Accordingly, it is clear that when there is a high cellular demand for glutathione in leukotriene biosynthesis, the available levels of glutathione for xenobiotic conjugation are decreased and may become limiting under certain patho-physiological situations.

In conclusion, it must be emphasized that both phase I and phase II drug metabolism pathways cannot be considered in isolation, but rather as part of a coupled, interactive system, interfacing directly with many endogenous metabolic pathways. As our knowledge of the pathways and enzymology of drug metabolism advances, then so too must our knowledge of their control and interaction with other enzyme systems.

2.12 Further reading

BOOKS AND SYMPOSIA

Anders, M. W. (ed.) (1985) *Bioactivation of foreign compounds*, Academic Press, New York.
Arias, I. M. and Jakoby, W. B. (1976) *Glutathione: metabolism and function*, Raven Press, New York.
Boobis, A. R. *et al.* (1985) *Microsomes and drug oxidations*, Taylor and Francis, London.
Caughey, W. S. (1979) *Biochemical and clinical aspects of oxygen*, Academic Press, New York.
Dutton, G. J. (1980) *Glucuronidation of drugs and other compounds*, C.R.C. Press, Florida.
Fawcett, D. W. (1981) *The cell*, 2nd edn, Saunders, Philadelphia.
Jenner, P. and Testa, B. (1980, 1981) *Concepts in drug metabolism*, Parts A and B, Marcel Dekker, New York.
La Du, B. N. (1972) *Fundamentals of drug metabolism and drug disposition*, Williams and Wilkins, Baltimore.
Lamble, J. (1983) *Drug metabolism and distribution*, Elsevier, Amsterdam.
Mulder, G. J. (1982) *Sulphate metabolism and sulphate conjugation*, Taylor and Francis, London.
Nozaki, M. *et al.* (1982) *Oxygenases and oxygen metabolism*, Academic Press, New York.
Rack Paul, K. and Rein, H. (1984) *Cytochrome P-450. Structural and functional relationships: biochemical and physiochemical aspects of mixed function oxidases*, Akademie-Verlag, Berlin.
Sato, R. and Omura, T. (1978) *Cytochrome P-450*, Kodansha, Academic Press, Tokyo.
Schenkman, J. B. and Kupfer, D. (1981) *Hepatic Cytochrome P-450 Monooxygenase System*, Pergamon Press, New York.
Siest, G. (ed.) (1985) *Drug metabolism: molecular approaches and pharmacological implications*, Academic Press, New York.
Vereczkey, L. and Magyar, K. (1985) *Cytochrome P-450, biochemistry, biophysics and induction*, Elsevier/Akademiai kiado, Amsterdam and Budapest.

REVIEWS AND ORIGINAL ARTICLES

Bakke, J. and Gustaffson, J. A. (1984) Mercapturic acid pathway metabolites of xenobiotics: generation of potentially toxic metabolites during enterohepatic circulation. *TIPS*, **5**, 517–521.
Beaty, N. and Ballou, D. (1980) Transient kinetic study of liver microsomal FAD-containing monooxygenase. *J. Biol. Chem.*, **255**, 3817–24.
Björkhem, I. (1977) Rate-limiting step in microsomal cytochrome P-450 catalysed hydroxylations. *Pharmacol. Ther.*, (A) **1**, 327–48.
Burchell, B. (1981) Identification and purification of multiple forms of UDP–glucuronosyltransferase. In *Reviews in biochemical toxicology* (eds E. Hodgson *et al.*), Vol. 3, Elsevier, p. 1–32.
Caldwell, J. (1982) Conjugation reactions in foreign compound metabolism: definition, consequences and species variation. *Drug Metab. Rev.*, **13**, 745–77.

Capdevila, J., Saeki, Y. and Falck, J. R. (1984) The mechanistic plurality of cytochrome P-450 and its biological ramifications. *Xenobiotica*, **14**, 105–18.

Chasseaud, L. (1979) The role of glutathione and glutathione S-transferases in the metabolism of chemical carcinogens and other electrophilic reagents. *Adv. Cancer Res.*, **29**, 175–274.

Coon, M. J. *et al.* (1977) Highly purified liver microsomal cytochrome P-450: properties and catalytic mechanism. *Croat. Chem. Acta*, **49**, 163–77.

DePierre, J. and Dallner, G. (1975) Structural aspects of the membrane of the endoplasmic reticulum. *Biochim. Biophys. Acta*, **415**, 411–72.

Estabrook, R. W., Martin-Wixtrom, C., Saeki, Y., Renneberg, R., Hildebrandt, A. and Werringloer, J. (1984) The peroxidatic function of liver microsomal cytochrome P-450: comparison of hydrogen peroxide and NADPH-catalyzed N-demethylation reactions. *Xenobiotica*, **14**, 87–104.

Gibson, G. G. and Tamburini, P. P. (1984) Cytochrome P-450 spin state: inorganic biochemistry and functional significance. *Xenobiotica*, **14**, 27–47.

Gunsalus, I. C. and Sligar, S. G. (1978) Oxygen reduction by the cytochrome P-450 monooxygenase systems. *Adv. Enzymol.*, **47**, 1–44.

Hajjar, N. P. and Hodgson, E. (1980) Flavin adenine dinucleotide-dependent monooxygenase: its role in the sulfoxidation of pesticides in mammals. *Science*, **209**, 1134–6.

Hlavica, P. (1982) Biological oxidation of nitrogen in organic compounds and disposition of N-oxidised products. *C.R.C. Crit. Rev. Biochem.*, **January**, 39–101.

Holtzman, J. L. (1979) The role of the stimulation of NADPH–cytochrome P-450 reductase activity in hepatic microsomal mixed-function oxidase activity. *Pharmacol. Ther.*, **4**, 601–27.

Jakoby, W. B. (1977) The glutathione S-transferases: a group of multifunctional detoxification proteins. *Adv. Enzymol.*, **46**, 383–414.

Jakoby, W. B. *et al.* (1984) Sulfotransferases active with xenobiotics − comments on mechanism. In *Progress in drug metabolism* (eds. J. W. Bridges and L. F. Chasseaud), Vol. 8, Taylor and Frances, London, p. 11–33.

Jansson, I. and Schenkman, J. B. (1977) Studies on three microsomal electron transfer enzyme systems. Specificity of electron flow pathways. *Arch. Biochem. Biophys.*, **178**, 89–107.

Kaplowitz, N. *et al.* (1985) The regulation of hepatic glutathione. *Ann. Rev. Pharmacol.*, **25**, 715–744.

Ketterer, B. (1982) The role of non-enzymatic reactions of glutathione in xenobiotic metabolism. *Drug Metab. Rev.*, **13**, 161–87.

Kumaki, K. *et al.* (1978) Correlation of type I, type II and reverse type I difference spectra with absolute changes in spin state of hepatic microsomal cytochrome P-450 iron from five mammalian species. *J. Biol. Chem.*, **253**, 1048–58.

Levy, G. *et al.* (1982) Pharmacokinetic consequences and toxicologic implication of endogenous co-substrate depletion. *Drug Metab. Rev.*, **13**, 1009–20.

Lu, A. Y. H. and West, S. B. (1978) Reconstituted mammalian mixed-function oxidases: requirements, specificities and other properties. *Pharmacol. Ther.*, (A) **2**, 337–58.

Masters, B. S. S. and Okita, R. T. (1980) The history, properties and function of NADPH–cytochrome *P*-450 reductase. *Pharmacol. Ther.*, **9**, 227–44.

McLane, K. E. *et al.* (1983) Reductive drug metabolism. *Drug Metab. Rev.*, **14**, 741–99.

Mulder, G. J. (1984) Sulfation-metabolic aspects. In *Progress in drug metabolism* (eds. J. W. Bridges and L. F. Chasseaud), Vol. 8, Taylor and Frances, London, p. 35–100.

Noshiro, M. and Omura, T. (1978) Immunochemical study on the electron pathway from NADH to cytochrome *P*-450 of liver microsomes. *J. Biochem.*, **83**, 61–77.

O'Brien, P. J. (1978) Hydroperoxides and superoxides in microsomal oxidations. *Pharmacol. Ther.*, **(A) 2**, 517–36.

Oesch, F. (1979) Epoxide hydrolase. In *Progress in drug metabolism* (eds. J. W. Bridges and L. F. Chasseaud), Vol. 3, Wiley, p. 253–301.

Oshino, N. (1978) Cytochrome b_5 and its physiological significance. *Pharmacol. Ther.*, **(A) 2**, 477–515.

Poulsen, L. L. (1981) Organic sulfur substrates for the microsomal flavin-containing monooxygenase. In *Reviews in biochemical toxicology* (eds. E. Hodgson *et al.*), Vol. 3, Elsevier, p. 33–49.

Poulsen, L. L. and Ziegler, D. M. (1979) The liver microsomal FAD-containing monooxygenase. Spectral characterization and kinetic studies. *J. Biol. Chem.*, **254**, 6449–57.

Powis, G. and Jansson, I. (1979) Stoichiometry of the mixed-function oxidase. *Pharmacol. Ther.*, **7**, 297–311.

Prough, R. A. and Ziegler, D. M. (1977) The relative participation of liver microsomal amine oxidase and cytochrome *P*-450 in *N*-demethylation reactions. *Arch. Biochem. Biophys.*, **180**, 363–72.

Schenkman, J. B. and Gibson, G. G. (1983) Status of the cytochrome *P*-450 cycle. In *Drug metabolism and distribution* (ed. J. Lamble), Elsevier, p. 7–11.

Schenkman, J. B. *et al.* (1967) Spectral studies of drug interactions with hepatic microsomal cytochrome *P*-450. *Mol. Pharmacol.*, **3**, 113–23.

Schenkman, J. B. *et al.* (1981) Substrate interaction with cytochrome *P*-450. *Pharmacol. Ther.*, **12**, 43–71.

Sligar, S. G. (1976) Coupling of spin, substrate and redox equilibria in cytochrome *P*-450. *Biochem.*, **15**, 5399–406.

Sligar, S. G., Gelb, M. H. and Heimbrook, D. C. (1984) Bio-organic chemistry and cytochrome *P*-450 -dependent catalysis. *Xenobiotica*, **14**, 63–86.

Strobel, H. W. *et al.* (1980) NADPH–cytochrome *P*-450 reductase and its role in the mixed-function oxidase reaction. *Pharmacol. Ther.*, **8**, 525–37.

Vermillion, J. L. *et al.* (1981) Separate roles for FMN and FAD in catalysis by liver microsomal NADPH–cytochrome *P*-450 reductase. *J. Biol. Chem.*, **256**, 266–77.

Weisburger, J. H. and Weisburger, E. K. (1973) Biochemical formation and pharmacological, toxicological and pathological properties of hydroxylamines and hydroxamic acids. *Pharmacol. Rev.*, **25**, 1–52.

Ziegler, D. M. and Poulsen, L. L. (1978) Hepatic microsomal mixed-function amine oxidase. *Method. Enzymol.*, **52**, 142–51.

Ziegler, D. M. *et al.* (1980) Kinetic studies on the mechanism and substrate specificity of the microsomal flavin-containing monooxygenase. In *Microsomes, drug oxidations and chemical carcinogenesis* (eds. M. J. Coon *et al.*), Vol. 2, Academic Press, p. 637–45.

3

Induction and inhibition of drug metabolism

3.1 Introduction

The study of drug metabolism in experimental animals in general and Man in particular is ideally studied under strictly controlled conditions, such that we only observe the influence of the normal physiological and biochemical processes that contribute to the metabolism of the drug in question. However, this ideal situation is rarely achieved, and the metabolism of drugs is substantially influenced by the deliberate or passive intake of many chemical substances that Man is increasingly being exposed to either in his environment, for medical reasons or as a result of his life style. These chemical substances are derived from a variety of sources and include pharmaceutical products, cosmetics, food additives and industrial chemicals. As summarized in Table 3.1, the magnitude of the various chemicals in use today, and hence the potential exposure to Man, is staggering.

While it is clear that the ingestion of drugs, and to a certain extent food additives, is a previously determined, conscious act, many of the chemicals in Table 3.1 enter the body by more subtle means as exemplified by the pollution of food chains by insecticides and the accidental (sometimes intentional) exposure to industrial chemicals and solvents from the environment. The magnitude of this latter problem is clearly seen in a recent study in the USA, where the Environmental Protection Agency reported that 288 different classes of chemical compounds were identified in domestic drinking water supplies.

Table 3.1 Chemicals estimated to be in use today

Classification	Number
Active ingredients of pesticides	1500
Pharmaceutical products (drugs)	6000
Food additives with nutritional value	2500
Food additives to promote product life	3000
Additional chemicals in use (including industrial chemicals)	50 000

From the above considerations, it is clear that Man is either intentionally or accidentally exposed to many chemical substances that have the potential to alter drug metabolism. Accordingly, it is the purpose of this chapter to outline the induction and inhibition of drug metabolism by these chemicals, and to rationalize, wherever possible, their mode(s) of action on a molecular basis. Other factors affecting drug metabolism (including species, genetic, sex, age and dietary factors) are considered in the two following chapters, and the pharmacological, toxicological and clinical implications of altered drug metabolism are considered in subsequent chapters.

3.2 Induction of drug metabolism

3.2.1 INDUCTION OF DRUG METABOLISM IN MAN

Many currently used drugs of diverse pharmacology and chemical structure are well known to induce either their own metabolism or the biotransformation of other drugs in Man. The list of drugs shown in Table 3.2 is by no means complete and only reflect those drugs for which there is a reasonably strong body of evidence for their ability to induce drug metabolism in Man: almost certainly this list is much longer in reality.

As indicated in Chapter 1, the liver is the major organ responsible for drug metabolism in most species, and as far as Man is concerned, a major problem is how to assess the extent of hepatic drug metabolism induction. Several methods have been proposed to study induction in Man and these include (1) increased drug clearance, (2) decreased drug plasma half-life, (3) increased plasma γ-glutamyl transferase, (4) increased urinary excretion of D-glucaric acid, (5) increased urinary 6β-hydroxycortisol and (6) plasma bilirubin levels. Although none of these methods can equivocally substantiate the induction of drug metabolism in Man, taken collectively they provide a reasonable indication of induction (see Park, 1982 for a critique of these assessment techniques; also Chapter 7). Although the mechanism(s) involved in the

Table 3.2 Therapeutic drugs that induce their own metabolism or the biotransformation of other drugs *in Man*

Classification	Examples
Analeptics	Nikethamide
Analgesic, antipyretic and anti-inflammatory drugs	Antipyrine
	Phenylbutazone
Antibiotics	Rifampicin
Anticonvulsants	Carbamazepine
	Phenytoin
Antifungal drugs	Griseofulvin
Antilipidaemics	Halofenate
Antimalarials	Quinine
Diuretics	Spironolactone
Psychotropic drugs	Chlorimipramine
Sedatives and hypnotics	Amylobarbitone
	Barbitone
	Chloral Hydrate
	Cyclobarbitone
	Dichloralphenazone
	Glutethimide
	Hexobarbitone
	Mandrax (a mixture of methaqualone and diphenyhydramine)
	Meprobamate
	Phenobarbitone
Steroids	Testosterone
Vitamins	Vitamin C

(Adapted from Bowman and Rand, 1980.)

induction of drug metabolism in Man are not clearly defined, the induction of specific liver enzymes (particularly the mixed-function oxidase enzymes of the endoplasmic reticulum; see Chapter 1) play a substantial role and have profound implications in clinical pharmacology, as discussed in Chapters 5 and 7.

Clearly then, there are many problems associated with both the assessment and understanding of the basic mechanisms involved in the induction of drug metabolism in Man, not the least of which are the ethical considerations. As a consequence of these limitations, much attention has focused on the use of experimental animals in drug induction studies. Although animal studies have proved extremely useful in characterizing the phenomena of drug metabolism and its induction, it must always be borne in mind that animal experiments only give an *indication* of the situation in Man.

3.2.2 INDUCTION OF DRUG METABOLISM IN EXPERIMENTAL ANIMALS

The duration and intensity of pharmacological action of many drugs is primarily dictated by their rate of metabolism, and, as a corollary, chemical inducers that modify drug metabolism would be expected to radically alter the pharmacological effects of drugs. A good example of this phenomenon is the influence of phenobarbitone and benzo[a]pyrene on the metabolism and duration of action of the muscle relaxant, zoxazolamine. As shown in Figure 3.1, zoxazolamine undergoes metabolic hydroxylation at the 6-position by liver homogenates; also, as shown in Table 3.3, pretreatment of experimental animals with either phenobarbitone or the polycyclic aromatic hydrocarbon, benzo[a]pyrene, results in a substantial increase in zoxazolamine metabolism and, consequently, a significant decrease in the paralysis time elicited by the drug.

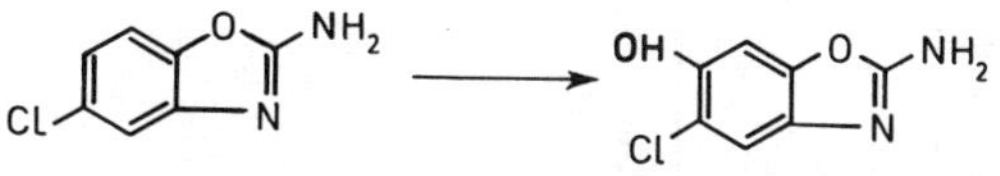

Figure 3.1 Metabolism of zoxazolamine by rat liver homogenates.

Clearly the range of drugs and chemicals that have the ability to induce similar hepatic drug metabolism has been more thoroughly investigated in laboratory animals than in Man, and, as documented in Table 3.4, many structurally diverse drugs and chemicals have been shown to induce liver drug metabolism in various species. There is apparently no structure–activity relationship in the ability of these various inducers to stimulate drug metabolism, and the only common physico-chemical property is that the majority of these compounds are relatively lipophilic in nature. Whereas no general conclusions can be made, it will be shown later that there is a well-defined structure–activity relationship for some of these classes of compounds (see section on mechanisms of induction).

3.2.3 ROLE OF CYTOCHROME P-450 IN THE INDUCTION OF DRUG METABOLISM

In an attempt to localize the site of induction of drug metabolism, significant advances have been made in considering the role of the liver. As outlined in Chapter 1, the liver serves as the main organ responsible for drug metabolism and it was not entirely unexpected that significant hepatic alterations in the drug-metabolizing enzyme systems were noted in response to inducing agents. Of particular importance is the hepatic cytochrome P-450 enzyme system.

Table 3.3 Influence of phenobarbitone or benzo[a]pyrene pretreatment on the metabolism and pharmacological action of zoxazolamine in the rat

Parameter	Control (saline-treated)	Phenobarbitone-treated[†]	Benzo[a]pyrene-treated[*]
Paralysis time (mins)	137 ± 15	62 ± 21	20 ± 12
Whole body decay ($t_{1/2}$, mins)	102	38	12
Zoxazolamine metabolism (nmol per mg protein per hour)	3.4	14	15.3

[†] animals were pretreated with phenobarbitone (30 mg kg⁻¹, i.p.) twice daily for 4 days and killed 24 h after the last injection
[*] animals were pretreated with a single i.p. injection of benzo[a]pyrene (20 mg kg⁻¹) 24 h prior to sacrifice
(Adapted from Trevor, A. (1972) in *Fundamentals of drug metabolism and drug disposition* (eds. B. N. La Du, H. G. Mandel and E. L. Way), Williams and Wilkins, Baltimore.)

Table 3.4 Inducers of hepatic drug metabolism in experimental animals

Classification	Example	Use or occurrence
Drugs	Phenobarbitone and most barbiturates	Sedative/hypnotic
	Phenytoin	Anti-convulsant
	Pregnenolone-16α-carbonitrile	Catatoxic steroid
	Rifampicin	Antibiotic
	Triacetyloleandomycin	Antibiotic
	Clofibrate	Hypolipidaemic
Alcohols	Ethanol	Beverage, skin disinfectant
Flavones	5,6-Benzoflavone	Synthetics, citrus fruits
Food additives and anutrients	Butylated hydroxyanisole (BHA), butylated hydroxytoluene (BHT) and ethoxyquin	Food antioxidants
	Isosafrole	Oils of sassafras, nutmeg and cinnamon
Halogenated hydrocarbons	2,3,7,8-Tetrachlorodibenzo-p-dioxin (TCDD)	Contaminant of herbicides and defoliants (2,4,5-T)
	3,3',4,4'-Tetrachlorobiphenyl	Insulator in capacitors/transformers
	3,3',4,4',5,5'-Hexabromobiphenyl	Flame retardant
Insecticides	DDT (dichlorodiphenyl-trichloroethane)	Agricultural pesticide
	Chlordecone (Kepone)	Organochlorine pesticide
	Piperonyl butoxide	Insecticide synergist
Polycyclic aromatic hydrocarbons	Including 3-methylcholanthrene, phenanthrene, chrysene, 1,2-benzanthracene and benzo[a]pyrene	Environmental pollutants found in industrial and domestic combustion products, cigarette smoke and oil contaminants
Solvents	Toluene and xylenes	Solvents, cleaning agents and degreasers

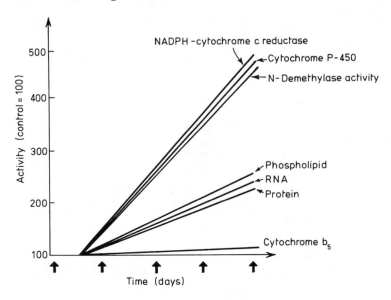

Figure 3.2 Induction of hepatic endoplasmic reticulum enzymes by phenobarbitone. Arrows indicate the daily injection of phenobarbitone. (Adapted from Ernster, L. and Orrenius, S. (1965) *Fed. Proc.*, **24**, 1190.)

Early studies in the mid-1960s clearly showed that both cytochrome *P*-450 and its associated flavoprotein reductase, NADPH–cytochrome *P*-450 reductase, were substantially induced in response to phenobarbitone pretreatment and was paralleled by induction of drug metabolism. This observed inductive effect of phenobarbitone was not, however, confined to the enzymes of drug metabolism: other enzymes of the hepatic endoplasmic reticulum were induced (Figure 3.2), indicative of a general proliferation of this sub-cellular organelle.

Nevertheless it soon became clear that induction of drug metabolism was generally accompanied by increases in liver microsomal cytochrome *P*-450 content. In addition, different inducers did not uniformly increase the metabolism of all drugs to the same extent, i.e. certain inducers did indeed substantially increase drug metabolism; other inducers had little or no effect; and paradoxically, certain 'inducers' actually decreased the metabolism of some drugs investigated. An example of this diversity of drug metabolism responses to various inducers is shown in Table 3.5.

The inducers shown in Table 3.5 are all well known to induce liver microsomal cytochrome *P*-450, and their influence on the rate of drug metabolism depends on the substrate being examined. In addition to exhibiting a certain degree of substrate specificity, inducers are well documented to exhibit

Table 3.5 Influence of various inducers on the metabolism of various model drug substrates

Drug	Inducer[†,*]				
	Control	PB	PCN	MC	ARO
Ethylmorphine	13.7 ± 0.8	16.8 ± 4.3	24.9 ± 3.5	6.4 ± 0.5	9.5 ± 1.2
Aminopyrine	9.9 ± 0.8	13.9 ± 1.7	9.7 ± 1.3	7.6 ± 1.8	13.7 ± 1.2
Benzphetamine	12.5 ± 1.2	45.7 ± 14.0	6.6 ± 0.7	5.7 ± 1.1	15.8 ± 2.7
Caffeine	0.48 ± 0.12	0.65 ± 0.07		0.52 ± 0.06	0.64 ± 0.09
Benzo[a]pyrene	0.14	0.14	0.14	0.33	

[†]abbreviations of inducers used: PB, phenobarbitone; PCN, pregnenolone-16α-carbonitrile; MC, 3-methylcholanthrene; ARO, Arochlor 1254
[*]all drug-metabolizing activities are expressed as nmol product formed per minute per nmol cytochrome P-450 (V_{max} values)
(Adapted from Powis, G., Talcott, R. E. and Schenkman, J. B. (1977) In *Microsomes and Drug Oxidations* (eds. V. Ullrich, A. Roots, A. Hildebrandt, R. W. Estabrook and A. H. Conney), Pergamon Press, pp. 127–35.)

Table 3.6 Influence of cytochrome *P*-450 induction on the *in vitro* metabolism of R- and S-warfarin

Inducer	Hydroxylated warfarin metabolites[†]			
	R-isomer		s-isomer	
	7-OH	8-OH	7-OH	8-OH
Uninduced	0.22	0.04	0.04	0.01
Phenobarbitone	0.36	0.07	0.09	0.02
3-Methylcholanthrene	0.08	0.50	0.04	0.04

[†]metabolism is expressed as nmol warfarin metabolite formed per nmol cytochrome *P*-450 per minute.

both stereo- and regio-selectivity towards the metabolism of several drugs. This is exemplified by the influence of inducers on the metabolism of the R- and s-isomers of warfarin, both isomers of warfarin being hydroxylated at various positions of the molecule by the cytochrome *P*-450-dependent mixed-function oxidase system of the liver endoplasmic reticulum (Table 3.6).

3.2.4 INDUCTION OF MULTIPLE FORMS (ISOENZYMES) OF CYTOCHROME *P*-450

In view of the extremely broad substrate specificity of liver microsomal cytochrome *P*-450 towards the metabolism of drugs, and the diversity of responses to inducers as outlined above, it was initially proposed that these observations could be rationalized by assuming the existence of more than one form of isoenzyme of cytochrome *P*-450. Thus different inducers would have the potential to elevate the levels of a specific sub-population of cytochrome *P*-450, each with a characteristic substrate specificy towards the metabolism of drugs. This concept of cytochrome *P*-450 multiplicity has gained wide acceptance in recent years, and has had a profound influence on drug metabolism studies. Validation of this hypothesis has been achieved largely by the development of techniques enabling the cytochrome *P*-450 isoenzymes to be solubilized and purified from liver endoplasmic reticulum fragments such that structural and functional comparisons of highly purified cytochrome *P*-450 preparations can be assessed and compared.

The exact number of cytochrome *P*-450 isoenzymes is not known with any degree of certainty, but clearly there are strain differences and tissue differences in these isoenzymes, in addition to the presence of more than one form in a given tissue of a given species. The reason for this uncertainty in the exact number of cytochrome *P*-450 variants is that the characterization of the

Table 3.7 Distinctive criteria for the assignment of cytochrome *P*-450 heterogeneity in highly purified preparations

Spectral properties of the ferric, ferrous and carbonmonoxy–ferrous states.

Spectral interactions with drug substrates.

Substrate specificities in reconstituted enzyme systems.

Immunological properties including lack of cross-reactivity of antibodies to heterologous cytochrome *P*-450 antigens.

Monomeric molecular weights.

Amino acid composition.

N- or *C*-Terminal amino acid sequences.

Peptide fragmentation patterns by chemical or enzymatic means.

multiple forms is a relatively recent occurrence, with the first successful (partial) purification being achieved in 1968. Another problem associated with the exact number of cytochrome *P*-450 variants is the different criteria used by different laboratories in assessing cytochrome *P*-450 heterogeneity and a lack of standard techniques in assessing their structural and functional properties. The unequivocal assignment of unique structure to cytochrome *P*-450 isoenzymes is not possible at present because of the difficulty in crystallizing membrane-bound proteins for X-ray crystallography studies. Currently accepted criteria for cytochrome *P*-450 heterogeneity are shown in Table 3.7.

The most intensively studied cytochrome *P*-450s are those derived for the endoplasmic reticulum of rat and rabbit liver. Advantage has been taken of the fact that phenobarbitone and 3-methylcholanthrene (and other polycyclic aromatic hydrocarbons) induce different cytochrome *P*-450 proteins in both of these species; the structural and functional properties of these isoenzymes have been studied in detail. In general, most of the criteria outlined in Table 3.7 have been satisfied for these induced haemoproteins and, therefore on this basis, it is widely believed that phenobarbitone and 3-methylcholanthrene are representative of two distinct classes of inducers of drug metabolism. Apart from the biochemical diversity between these two induced variants of cytochrome *P*-450, there is a substantial pharmacological relevance for the existence of multiple forms in that these two enzyme variants exhibit substantially different substrate specificities with respect to drug metabolism (oxidation) reactions. This pharmacological diversity towards drug oxidations is readily seen in Table 3.8, which shows the substrate specificities of both phenobarbitone- and 3-methylcholanthrene-induced rat liver cytochrome *P*-450s.

Table 3.8 Substrate specificities of two forms of rat liver cytochrome *P-450* induced by either phenobarbitone or 3-methylcholanthrene

Substrate	Form of cytochrome *P-450*	
	Phenobarbitone-induced form	3-Methylcholanthrene-induced form
	(nmol metabolite formed per minute per nmol cytochrome *P-450*)	
Benzphetamine	52.0	2.5
Benzo[*a*]pyrene	0.2	3.9
Ethoxycoumarin	4.1	56.0
Testosterone		
6β-hydroxylation	0.2	0.3
7α-hydroxylation	0.7	1.0
16α-hydroxylation	1.5	0.2

The activities of the two induced cytochrome *P-450* variants shown in the above table were determined in the presence of highly purified forms of each isoenzyme and therefore reflect the catalytic activities of each enzyme variant.

Table 3.8 clearly shows that the nature of the induced cytochrome *P-450* isoenzyme is important in determining the extent of drug oxidation. For example benzphetamine serves as an excellent substrate for the phenobarbitone-induced variant whereas the 3-methylcholanthrene form only poorly metabolizes this substrate. In contrast, ethoxycoumarin is rapidly metabolized by the polycyclic aromatic hydrocarbon-induced isoenzyme whereas the barbiturate-induced variant does not oxidize ethoxycoumarin as efficiently. It should be further emphasized that the liver of a particular species (including Man) usually contains more than one cytochrome *P-450* variant, and therefore the overall ability of the liver to metabolize drugs (i.e. those drugs whose metabolism is cytochrome *P-450*-dependent) is dictated by both the type and amount of the cytochrome *P-450* sub-populations.

Although the scientific evidence is not definitive at present, information is beginning to accumulate indicating that human liver contains similar cytochrome *P-450* isoenzymes as are observed in experimental animals. The purification and characterization of human liver cytochrome *P-450*s is already underway. It has been shown that the hepatic haemoproteins from human and rat share certain features of structural, functional and immunological similarity.

3.2.5 SIGNIFICANCE OF MULTIPLE FORMS OF CYTOCHROME *P-450*

The existence of multiple forms of cytochrome *P-450* is not solely a biochemical curiosity, but has profound ramifications in both pharmacology and toxicology.

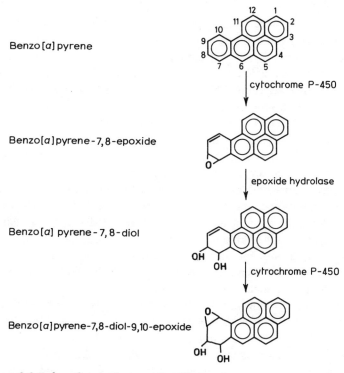

Benzo[a]pyrene

cytochrome P-450

Benzo[a]pyrene-7,8-epoxide

epoxide hydrolase

Benzo[a]pyrene-7,8-diol

cytrochrome P-450

Benzo[a]pyrene-7,8-diol-9,10-epoxide

Figure 3.3 Role of cytochrome P-450 in the activation of the precarcinogen benzo[a]pyrene.

Some of the more important consequences of cytochrome P-450 heterogeneity include:

(1) The existence of cytochrome P-450 isoenzymes may, in part, rationalize the substantial differences in drug metabolism that are observed as a function of sex, species, age, nutritional status and inter-subject variability (discussed in Chapters 4 and 5).

(2) Multiple forms of cytochrome P-450 may provide an explanation of why only certain tissues are susceptible to a chemical carcinogenic challenge from the environment. For example, many chemicals that are known to cause cancer in experimental animals are biologically inert *per se* and require metabolic oxidation by the cytochrome P-450 enzyme system before they can ultimately express their carcinogenicity. An excellent example of the role of cytochrome P-450 on the activation of innocuous chemicals to potent carcinogens is shown in Figure 3.3.

In this example, inert benzo[a]pyrene (a ubiquitous environmental pollutant) is first metabolized by cytochrome P-450 forming the 7,8-epoxide derivative which subsequently serves as the substrate for another microsomal enzyme, epoxide hydrolase, to form the 7,8-diol derivative of benzo[a]pyrene. This latter diol is further metabolized by cytochrome P-450 to the potent, ultimate carcinogen, benzo[a]pyrene 7,8-diol-9,10-epoxide, which can then bind to nucleic acids and initiate the complex series of events of carcinogenesis. Therefore it is clear that any tissue that contains the appropriate cytochrome P-450 isoenzymes to catalyse the two oxidation reactions in Figure 3.3 (and of course epoxide hydrolase) may be susceptible to carcinogenesis by this chemical. In reality, the biological situation is more complex than outlined above, and other factors including, for example, the role of the detoxifying, conjugating (phase II) enzymes and the role of DNA repair mechanisms are important in determining tissue susceptibility to chemical carcinogens. However, it is clear from the above considerations that cytochrome P-450 has a substantial role to play in chemical carcinogenesis.

(3) The induction of cytochrome P-450 isoenzymes by commonly used drugs such as phenobarbital has important ramifications in clinical pharmacology. For example it is not an uncommon clinical practice to use combination drug therapy where a patient is being treated with more than one drug at a time, and many drug–drug interactions have been observed, particularly with enzyme (cytochrome P-450) inducers such as phenobarbitone. A well-documented drug–drug interaction has been observed in patients who are being treated with both phenobarbitone (a sedative) and warfarin derivatives (anti-coagulants). Because phenobarbitone induces the cytochrome P-450 enzymes in the liver that are responsible for the metabolism of warfarin, the effective pharmacological levels of warfarin are thereby reduced and the dose of warfarin has to be substantially increased to maintain effective, therapeutic levels. The problem arises when the phenobarbitone treatment is withdrawn and the metabolism of warfarin is accordingly reduced, resulting in increased, toxic plasma levels of warfarin because of the low therapeutic index of this drug.

(4) As discussed in Chapter 1, cytochrome P-450 is not only responsible for the metabolism of drugs and xenobiotics but actively plays a role in the oxidation of many endogenous compounds such as steroids, prostaglandins, fatty acids and vitamin D_3. Although our understanding of the cytochrome P-450 isoenzymes involved in endogenous compound metabolism is not as well developed as compared to those cytochrome P-450s responsible for drug metabolism, it is clear that a substantial

alteration of the former group of cytochrome P-450 isoenzymes by drug and environmental inducers may well influence many aspects of intermediary metabolism where cytochrome P-450 is involved.

Therefore it is clear that the induction of the drug-metabolizing enzymes is particularly important in the areas of clinical pharmacology and toxicology; the reader is referred to Chapters 6 and 7 for a more detailed discussion of this phenomenon.

3.2.6 INDUCTION OF EXTRAHEPATIC DRUG METABOLISM

Although the liver is the main organ responsible for drug metabolism in most species, significant activities are present in extrahepatic tissues including lung, kidney, skin and intestinal mucosa. Whereas the liver appears to be a particularly sensitive target organ for the induction of drug-metabolizing enzymes in general and cytochrome P-450 in particular, the inductive response in extrahepatic tissues is more variable. Extrahepatic enzyme induction depends not only on the nature of the inducing agent and the extrahepatic tissue – it also depends on the particular drug substrate under investigation. For example, Table 3.9 shows that cigarette smoke (containing polycyclic aromatic hydrocarbon inducing agents) substantially increases the hydroxylation of benzo[a]pyrene in lung and placenta and is a less effective inducing agent in the intestine. Similarly, induction of phenacetin metabolism in the lung is only 5% of that observed with benzo[a]pyrene metabolism in the same tissue.

Table 3.9 Induction of phenacetin and benzo[a]pyrene metabolism by cigarette smoke in extrahepatic tissues of the rat

Enzyme activity	Induction (as percentage of control value)			
	Liver	Intestine	Lung	Placenta
Phenacetin de-ethylation	20	100	60	
Benzo[a]pyrene hydroxylation	120	120	1200	500

3.2.7 MECHANISMS OF CYTOCHROME P-450 INDUCTION

Although the precise molecular mechanisms of cytochrome P-450 induction are not fully understood at present, much effort has been expended in trying to rationalize the inductive response of the drug-metabolizing enzymes in hepatic tissue. Figure 3.4 shows the functional components of the hepatic mixed-function oxidase system responsible for cytochrome P-450-dependent drug metabolism.

Accordingly, induction of drug metabolism may arise as a consequence of

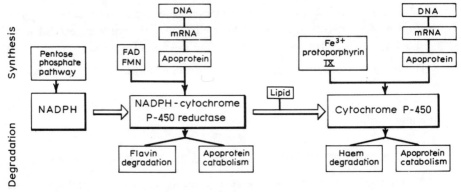

Figure 3.4 Synthesis and degradation of the functional components of the hepatic mixed-function oxidase system.

increased synthesis, decreased degradation, activation of pre-existing components or a combination of these three processes. More specifically, Table 3.10 summarizes the biochemical effects noted on response to enzyme inducers such as phenobarbitone. From this table, it is clear that enzyme inducers have a variety of effects on the functional components of the mixed-function oxidase system, particularly on the terminal haemoprotein, cytochrome P-450. Current evidence suggests that the mechanism of induction of cytochrome P-450 falls into one of two types, dependent on the inducer used. The two types of inducers that have been most extensively studied are the phenobarbitone and the polycyclic aromatic hydrocarbon classes.

Table 3.10 Possible mechanisms of induction of the hepatic microsomal drug oxidizing system

(1) Increased synthesis or stability of nuclear 45S precursor rRNA.
(2) Enhancement of DNA-dependent RNA polymerase.
(3) Increased nucleocytoplasmic transport of ribonucleoprotein.
(4) Increased synthesis or stability of mRNA coding for NADPH–cytochrome P-450 reductase or cytochrome P-450.
(5) Induction of phospholipid biosynthesis.
(6) Increased haem or flavin biosynthesis.
(7) Decreased apoprotein or haem/flavin degradation.

Treatment of experimental animals with phenobarbitone results in a substantial increase in the hepatic levels of translatable polysomal mRNA for cytochrome P-450. Specific complementary DNA probes (cDNA) to cytochrome P-450 mRNA have been synthesized, and, using cDNA-mRNA hybridization techniques, it has conclusively been shown that 4 h after phenobarbitone pretreatment, a fourteen-fold increase in the level of mRNA coding for cytochrome P-450 was observed. This mRNA induction was accompanied by increases in

Hepatocyte

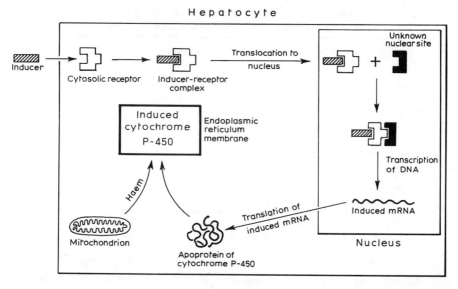

Figure 3.5 Receptor-mediated induction of cytochrome *P*-450 by polycyclic aromatic hydrocarbons. (Adapted from Nebert, D. W. *et al.* (1984) in *Extrahepatic Drug Metabolism and Chemical Carcinogenesis* (eds. J. Rydström *et al.*), Elsevier, Amsterdam, pp. 379–88.)

intranuclear RNAs that represent precursors to cytochrome *P*-450 mRNA. Accordingly, it would appear that the major inductive effect of phenobarbitone in the liver is to increase specific mRNA levels by augmenting transcription, rather than by stabilizing pre-existing levels of protein precursors or increased translational efficiency. At present, no specific cytoplasmic or nuclear receptors for phenobarbitone have been identified.

In contrast to phenobarbitone induction of hepatic drug-metabolizing enzymes, induction by environmental polycyclic aromatic hydrocarbons – such as 3-methylcholanthrene, *β*-naphthoflavone, benzo[*a*]pyrene or 2,3,7,8-tetrachlorodibenzo-*p*-dioxin (TCDD) – is thought to be associated with a specific cytosolic receptor. As shown in Figure 3.5, polycyclic aromatic hydrocarbon inducers combine with a specific cytosolic protein receptor in a similar fashion to hormone receptors. The inducer–receptor complex is then translocated to the nucleus of the hepatocyte whereupon induction-specific RNA is transcribed from DNA in an as-yet-unknown manner. Large amounts of newly translated, specific cytochrome *P*-450 are then incorporated into the membrane of the hepatic endoplasmic reticulum, resulting in the observed induction of metabolism of certain drugs and xenobiotics. It should be noted that although the extent of induction of the drug-metabolizing enzymes by polycyclic aromatic hydrocarbons is not as pronounced as observed for phenobarbital, the gross

Table 3.11 Potency of various compounds as competitors of binding of 3-methylcholanthrene to the mouse hepatic cytosolic receptor

Competitor	Competitor concentration giving 50% inhibition of 3-methylcholanthrene binding (M)[†]
2,3,7,8-Tetrachlorodibenzo-*p*-dioxin	0.3×10^{-9}
Dibenz[*a,h*]anthracene	0.1×10^{-8}
Dibenz[*a,c*]anthracene	0.3×10^{-8}
β-Naphthoflavone	0.1×10^{-7}
Benzo[*a*]pyrene	0.1×10^{-7}
Benz[*a*]anthracene	0.5×10^{-7}
6-Aminochrysene	0.8×10^{-7}
Pregnenolone-16α-carbonitrile	0.1×10^{-6}
Anthracene	0.8×10^{-6}

[†] 3-methylcholanthrene concentration was 10 nM.
(Adapted from Okey, A. B. and Vella, L. M. (1982) *Eur. J. Biochem.*, **127**, 39–47.)

levels of cytochrome *P*-450 do not represent the induction of specific forms of cytochrome *P*-450. For example, the specific isoenzyme variant of cytochrome *P*-450 inducible by these environmental pollutants is present in very low amounts in non-induced liver (approximately 5%) and increases approximately 8-to-16-fold on induction. This observation is similar to that seen with phenobarbitone induction, except that the absolute level of cytochrome *P*-450 upon phenobarbitone induction is much larger, due in part to the exaggerated proliferative response of this barbiturate.

Extensive studies have been carried out on the ability of various polycyclic aromatic hydrocarbons to interact with the above cytosolic receptor and hence induce specific cytochrome *P*-450 variants. For example, Table 3.11 shows the rank-order potency of various compounds to inhibit the binding of 3-methylcholanthrene to the cytosolic receptor. From this table is it seen that 2,3,7,8-tetrachlorodibenzo-*p*-dioxin is a potent inhibitor of 3-methylcholanthrene binding to the cytosolic receptor. In general the data in Table 3.11 correlate well with the relative potency of these compounds to induce cytochrome *P*-450. In addition, it should be noted that certain strains of mice are non-responsive to these inducers and are characterized by an absence of the cytosolic receptor. It would appear that phenobarbitone does not react with the proposed receptor, further substantiating the conclusion that the modes of induction of phenobarbitone and polycyclic aromatic hydrocarbons are dissimilar, resulting in the separate induction of at least two distinct isoenzyme variants of cytochrome *P*-450 in response to these inducers. It should be emphasized that both phenobarbitone and the polycyclic aromatic hydrocarbons can each induce more than one specific isoenzyme of cytochrome *P*-450. Current evidence suggests that these inducers (and probably other classes of inducers) elevate the concentration of several isoenzymes with the concomitant decrease in other multiple forms. The precise mechanism(s) whereby these inducers simultaneously turn on and turn off gene expression is not clear and remains an area of active research.

3.2.8 INDUCTION OF NON-CYTOCHROME P-450 DRUG-METABOLIZING ENZYMES

Although cytochrome P-450 is an important enzymatic determinant of drug metabolism, it is by no means the only drug-metabolizing enzyme whose levels are induced in response to a chemical or drug challenge. Indeed, most of the enzymes involved in drug metabolism are induced to various extents by a structurally diverse group of chemicals and drugs; some examples are shown in Table 3.12. In general, the inducers listed in Table 3.12 are relatively non-specific in that they cause a general proliferation of the hepatic endoplasmic reticulum membrane or of the enzymes of drug metabolism. However, it should be pointed out that some of the enzymes shown in Table 3.12 exist in multiple forms (e.g. the glucuronyltransferases) or as homo/heterodimers of two subunits (e.g. the glutathione-S-transferases). Accordingly, the induction of glucuronyltransferase is highly dependent on the nature of the inducer used. Induction of this latter enzyme with phenobarbitone results in the induction of a form of the transferase that preferentially utilizes chloramphenicol as substrate whereas induction with 3-methylcholanthrene results in a transferase that has a specificity for 3-hydroxybenzo[a]pyrene as substrate. In a similar manner, there is evidence to suggest that the different sub-units of glutathione-S-transferase are differentially induced by phenobarbitone. Therefore, the induction of non-cytochrome P-450 enzymes responsible for drug metabolism (particularly the glucuronyltransferases and the glutathione-S-transferases) impose another level of control on the overall metabolic fate of a drug.

3.3 Inhibition of drug metabolism

A major concern of clinical pharmacologists is the area of drug–drug interactions in which two or more drugs are co-administered resulting in either therapeutic incompatibility or toxic reactions. Although the 'blunderbuss' approach of polypharmacy has significantly diminished in recent years, many patients are still treated with a combination of different drugs. For example a recent study of 138 randomly selected IV solutions has shown that 24% of these solutions contained two drugs and 14% contained five or more drugs. Just as one drug can induce the metabolism of a second drug, as discussed in

Table 3.12 Induction of drug metabolizing enzymes

Enzyme	Inducer
Epoxide hydrolase	2-Acetylaminofluorene Aldrin Arochlor 1254 Dieldrin Ethoxyquin Isosafrole 3-Methylcholanthrene Phenobarbitone *trans*-Stilbene oxide
Glucuronyltransferase	Dieldrin Isosafrole 3-Methylcholanthrene Phenobarbitone Polychlorinated biphenyls 2,3,7,8-Tetrachlorodibenzo-*p*-dioxin
NADPH–Cytochrome *P*-450 reductase	2-Acetylaminofluorene Dieldrin Isosafrole Phenobarbitone Polychlorinated biphenyls *trans*-Stilbene oxide
Glutathione-*S*-transferase	2-Acetylaminofluorene 3-Methylcholanthrene Phenobarbitone 2,3,7,8-Tetrachlorodibenzo-*p*-dioxin *trans*-Stilbene oxide
Cytochrome b_5	2-Acetylaminofluorene Butylated hydroxytoluene Griseofulvin

the previous section, the inhibition of drug metabolism by other drugs or xenobiotics is a well-recognized phenomenon. Accordingly, it is the purpose of this section to focus on well-defined examples of the inhibition of drug metabolism, particularly at the level of liver cytochrome P-450. This inhibition of drug metabolism by drugs or xenobiotics can take place in several ways including the destruction of pre-existing enzymes, inhibition of enzyme synthesis or by complexing and thus inactivating the drug-metabolizing enzyme. (The reader is also referred to Chapters 4 and 5 where additional consideration is given to inhibition of drug metabolism, and to Chapters 6 and 7 where the pharmacological, toxicological and clinical implications of this phenomenon are documented.)

3.3.1 INHIBITION OF DRUG METABOLISM BY DESTRUCTION OF HEPATIC CYTOCHROME *P*-450

Many therapeutic drugs and environmental xenobiotics have the ability to destroy cytochrome *P*-450 in the liver by a variety of mechanisms. For example it has been known for several years that xenobiotics containing an olefinic (C=C) or acetylenic (C≡C) function are porphyrinogenic, resulting in the formation of 'green pigments' in the liver. Some representative examples are given in Table 3.13. The chemical natures of these green pigments have recently been identified in most instances as alkylated or substrate–haem adducts derived from cytochrome *P*-450. Interestingly, the majority of these olefinic and acetylenic compounds are relatively inert *per se* and require metabolic activation by cytochrome *P*-450 itself (prior to adduct formation); they are therefore classified as 'suicide substrates' of the haemoprotein. It should be pointed out that the above suicide substrates are relatively selective towards cytochrome *P*-450 in that cytochrome b_5 concentrations (the other haemoprotein of the hepatic endoplasmic reticulum membrane) are usually not affected by these porphyrinogenic xenobiotics.

Table 3.13 Inhibitors of the drug-metabolizing enzymes: drugs and xenobiotics that destroy hepatic cytochrome *P*-450

Olefinic derivatives	Acetylenic derivatives
Allobarbital	Acetylene
Allylisopropylacetamide	Ethchlorvynol
Aprobarbital	Ethinylestradiol
Ethylene	Norethindrone
Fluoroxene	
Secobarbital	
Vinyl chloride	

A major consequence of haem modification by the above compounds is a significant and sustained drop in the levels of functional cytochrome *P*-450, which in turn, results in a reduction in the capacity of the liver to metabolize drugs (Table 3.14). In addition, it would appear likely that the isoenzymes of hepatic cytochrome *P*-450 exhibit differential susceptibilities to destruction by olefinic xenobiotics as exemplified by the pronounced susceptibility of a phenobarbitone-induced variant (Table 3.14). The primary target of olefinic drug-induced loss of functional activity is at the haem locus and is substantiated by the observation that the administration of exogenous haem substantially restored both the hepatic cytochrome *P*-450 content and drug-metabolizing activity after allylisopropylacetamide treatment, a compound well known to destroy cytochrome *P*-450.

Table 3.14 Influence of allylisopropylacetamide (AIA) on hepatic drug metabolism, cytochrome b_5 and cytochrome *P-450*

Parameter	Source of liver microsomes		
	Control	Phenobarbital-induced	3-Methylcholanthrene-induced
	(% of activity in non-AIA-treated animals)		
Cytochrome *P-450*[†]	84	33	74
Cytochrome b_5[†]	n.d.*	113	n.d.*
Ethylmorphine N-demethylase[‡]	62	8	35
p-Chloro-N-methylaniline N-demethylase[‡]	75	51	75
Hexobarbital 3'-hydroxylase[‡]	80	22	62

Male rats were treated with either phenobarbital, 3-methylcholanthrene or without pretreatment (control). After an overnight fast, animals were then injected with allylisopropylacetamide (200 mg kg^{-1}), killed one hour later and hepatic microsomes prepared by ultracentrifugation.
[†] nmol haemoprotein mg^{-1} protein
*not determined
[‡] metabolism is expressed as nmol product formed per mg protein per 15 min.
(Derived from Farrell, H. and Correia, M. A. (1980) *J. Biol. Chem.*, **255**, 10128–33.)

Table 3.15 Influence of allylisopropylacetamide (AIA) on the pharmacological activity of hexobarbitone and zoxazolamine

	Control	AIA-pretreated
Hexobarbitone sleeping time (mins)	37.8 ± 2.0	235.6 ± 27.8
Zoxazolamine paralysis time (mins)	257.6 ± 10.5	477.8 ± 31.5

Rats were given either hexobarbitone ($150 \, \mathrm{mg \, kg^{-1}}$, i.p.) or zoxazolamine ($100 \, \mathrm{mg \, kg^{-1}}$, i.p.) eleven hours after allylisopropylacetamide ($300 \, \mathrm{mg \, kg^{-1}}$, s.c.).
(Adapted from Unseld, B. and De Matteis, F. (1978) *Int. J. Biochem.*, **9**, 865–9.)

The above suicidal activation of olefinic and acetylenic drugs to active metabolites resulting in cytochrome *P*-450 haem destruction has profound pharmacological implications. For example, pretreatment of experimental animals with allylisopropylacetamide results in a significant increase in both hexobarbitone-induced sleeping time and zoxazolamine-induced paralysis time (Table 3.15), both of these drugs undergoing cytochrome *P*-450 metabolism. These results also support the concept that allylisopropylacetamide preferentially destroys the phenobarbitone-inducible cytochrome *P*-450 isoenzyme in that the sleeping time due to hexobarbitone (a preferred substrate of this isoenzyme) was increased 6-fold, whereas the paralysis time due to zoxazolamine (not readily metabolized by this cytochrome *P*-450 variant) was only increased 2-fold.

Accordingly, inhibition of drug metabolism by olefinic and acetylenic drugs and xenobiotics depends not only on the chemical nature of the drug itself but also on the prevailing complement of cytochrome *P*-450 isoenzymes and their substrate specificities. It should be pointed out that although the above examples have highlighted the ability of allylisopropylacetamide to destroy cytochrome *P*-450 and consequently inhibit drug metabolism, many drugs (listed in Table 3.13) have similar properties. In view of the common occurrence of olefinic and acetylenic groups in pharmaceutical products in use today, it is clear that many drug–drug interactions may be rationalized at the level of cytochrome *P*-450 destruction.

3.3.2 METAL IONS AND HEPATIC CYTOCHROME *P*-450

Related to the above inhibitory effects of olefinic and acetylenic compounds on drug metabolism is the ability of metal ions to substantially inhibit mixed-function oxidase activity. The influence of metal ions on drug metabolism activities will be generally considered in Chapter 5; it is informative to concentrate here on the role of cobalt in drug biotransformation reactions. As shown in Table 3.16, cobalt (in the form of cobalt-haem) has a pronounced

Table 3.16 Acute effects of cobalt-haem on hepatic drug metabolism and haem biosynthesis

Activity	Saline control	Cobalt-haem-treated
Ethylmorphine demethylase (μmol HCHO mg^{-1} h^{-1})	0.555 ± 0.06	0.062 ± 0.02
Aniline hydroxylase (nmol p-aminophenol mg^{-1} h^{-1})	89.42 ± 6.90	32.75 ± 3.01
Microsomal haem (nmol mg^{-1})	1.85 ± 0.04	0.89 ± 0.05
Cytochrome P-450 (nmol mg^{-1})	0.80 ± 0.04	0.19 ± 0.03
Cytochrome b$_5$ (nmol mg^{-1})	0.35 ± 0.01	0.23 ± 0.01
Haem oxygenase (nmol bilirubin mg^{-1} h^{-1})	2.65 ± 0.11	15.62 ± 0.09
δ-Aminolaevulinate synthetase (nmol product mg^{-1} h^{-1})	0.201 ± 0.05	0.082 ± 0.01

A single dose of cobalt-haem ($125\,\mu$mol kg^{-1}, s.c.) was given to rats and the above data determined 72 h later.
(Adapted from Drummond, H. and Kappas, A. (1982) *Proc. Nat. Acad. Sci.*, **79**, 2384–8.)

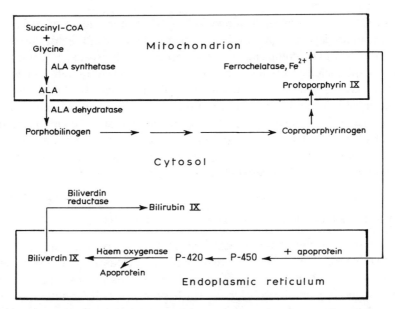

Figure 3.6 Biosynthesis of hepatic cytochrome P-450–haem. Abbreviation: ALA, δ-aminolaevulinic acid. (Adapted from Testa and Jenner, 1981.)

influence on both drug metabolism and the biosynthesis/degradation of hepatic haem. In particular, subsequent to cobalt-pretreatment, drug metabolism is substantially decreased as is the hepatic microsomal content of cytochrome *P*-450 and total haem. These results can be rationalized by the observation that cobalt has a pronounced inhibitory effect on the rate-limiting step of haem biosynthesis (δ-aminolaevulinate synthetase) and additionally causes a substantial increase in haem catabolism, as reflected in the 6-fold increase in haem oxygenase activity. The importance of these latter two enzymes in the synthesis and degradation of cytochrome *P*-450 haem is shown in Figure 3.6. Therefore in contrast to the olefinic and acetylenic drugs described above, that act primarily by modifying *existing* cytochrome *P*-450–haem, metal ions such as cobalt exert their inhibitory influences on drug metabolism by modulating both the *synthesis* and *degradation* of the haem prosthetic group of cytochrome *P*-450.

3.3.3 INHIBITION OF DRUG METABOLISM BY COMPOUNDS FORMING INACTIVE COMPLEXES WITH HEPATIC CYTOCHROME *P*-450

In addition to modulating the synthesis/degradation of hepatic cytochrome *P*-450, certain classes of drugs and xenobiotics can inhibit drug metabolism by totally different means, e.g. by forming spectrally detectable, inactive complexes with the haemoprotein. These compounds are substrates of cytochrome *P*-450 and require metabolism to exert their full inhibitory effects, in a similar manner to the olefinic and acetylenic drugs described earlier. However, unlike the latter group of drugs, the complex-forming inhibitors are metabolized by cytochrome *P*-450 forming a metabolic intermediate (or product) that binds tightly, but reversibly to the haemoprotein, thus preventing its further participation in drug metabolism and forming the basis of the observed inhibition. Examples of this class of inhibitors are shown in Table 3.17.

A direct comparison of the inhibition of drug metabolism by many of the drugs shown in Table 3.17 is complicated by the observation that the parent drugs themselves exhibit some degree of competitive or non-competitive inhibition, however it is clear that pre-incubation of the inhibitor with liver homogenates (i.e. metabolism) results in a substantial increase in the inhibitory action of these drugs. Furthermore, the above observations are reflected *in vivo* where it has been observed that pretreatment of experimental animals with these inhibitors results in a substantial increase in both hexobarbital narcosis and zoxazolamine paralysis time.

Mechanistic studies on the inhibition by the above xenobiotics have mainly been attempted with amphetamine and methylenedioxybenzene compounds.

Table 3.17 Drugs and xenobiotics inhibiting drug metabolism by complexing with cytochrome *P*-450

Nitrogenous compounds	Non-nitrogenous compounds
Amphetamine	Isosafrole
Benactyzine	Piperonal
Cimetidine	Piperonyl butoxide
Dapsone	Safrole
Despramine	Sesamol
2-Diethylaminoethyl-2,2-diphenylvalerate (SKF 525 A)	
2,5-Dimethoxy-4-methylamphetamine (STP)	
Diphenylhydramine	
Fenfluramine	
Isoniazid	
Methadone	
Methamphetamine	
Nortriptyline	
Oleandomycin	
Phenmetrazine	
Propoxyphene	
Sulfanilamide	
Triacetyloleandomycin	

Although the precise nature of the inhibitory, reactive metabolites responsible for the observed inhibition have not been absolutely delineated, there is strong evidence to support the theory that amphetamines act through the nitroso (or nitroxide) metabolite and the methylenedioxybenzene derivatives are activated to a reactive carbene, and subsequent ligation to cytochrome *P*-450 (Figure 3.7). The complexes thus formed exhibit distinctive spectral characteristics and normally absorb maximally at 448–456 nm with the reduced (ferrous) form of cytochrome *P*-450.

An interesting example of the above inhibition of drug metabolism is seen with the antibiotic, triacetyloleandomycin. Triacetyloleandomycin (similar in structure to erythromycin) is widely used in Man to treat patients who are sensitive to penicillin, and several reports have appeared where the administration of this antibiotic produces severe drug–drug reactions. For example, concomitant administration of triacetyloleandomycin with oral contraceptives may produce liver cholestasis, ischemic incidents with ergotamine, neurologic signs of carbamazepine intoxication and theophylline intoxication, suggesting that triacetyloleandomycin may somehow decrease the metabolism of various drugs in humans. Triacetyloleandomycin is interesting in that it induces its own demethylation and subsequent oxidation to a metabolite that forms a stable, 456 nm-absorbing complex with ferrous cytochroeme *P*-450 in the liver.

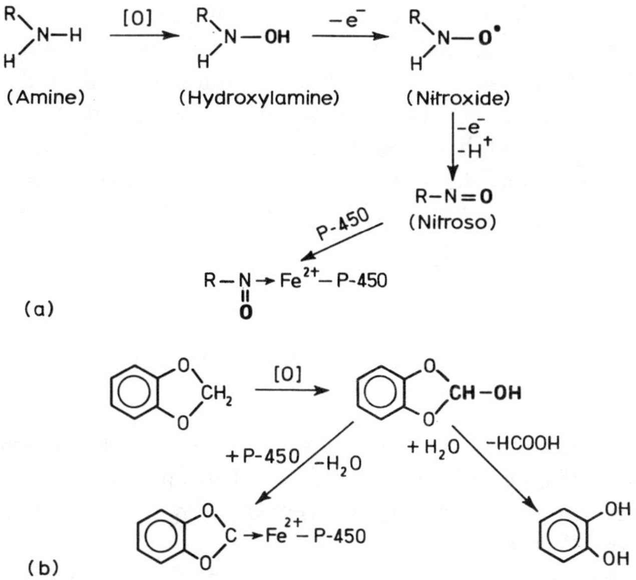

(a)

(b)

Figure 3.7 Proposed scheme for the formation of inhibitory cytochrome P-450 complexes. (a) Amphetamines. (b) Methylenedioxybenzene compounds. (Adapted from Testa and Jenner, 1981.)

Table 3.18 Influence of triacetyloleandomycin on hexobarbitone metabolism and sleeping time

Drug pretreatment	Hexobarbitone hydroxylase ($nmol\,min^{-1}\,mg^{-1}$)	Hexobarbitone sleeping time (mins)
None	1.8 ± 0.7	22 ± 8
1 h after TAO[†], $1\,mmol\,kg^{-1}$	1.7 ± 0.7	27 ± 9
24 h after TAO[†], $1\,mmol\,kg^{-1}$	1.2 ± 0.7	40 ± 18
TAO[†], $1\,mmol\,kg^{-1}$ daily, for 4 days	0.3 ± 0.1	168 ± 58

[†]abbreviation: TAO, triacetyloleandomycin
(From Pessayre, D. *et al.* (1981) *Biochem. Pharmacol.*, **30**, 559–64.)

On prolonged usage, this compound then inhibits drug oxidation and modulates the pharmacological activity of hexobarbitone (Table 3.18).

Accordingly, it has been postulated that the drug–drug reactions referred to above, can be rationalized by complexation and subsequent inhibition of cytochrome P-450. Interestingly, a related antibiotic oleandomycin (three free hydroxyl groups, not acetylated) shows similar properties to triacetyloleandomycin in that oleandomycin can also induce its own cytochrome P-450-dependent metabolism. However, compared to triacetyloleandomycin,

oleandomycin is both a weaker inducer of microsomal enzymes and also a much poorer substrate for the induced cytochrome *P*-450, resulting in diminished inactive cytochrome *P*-450 complex formation. This reduced activity of oleandomycin is consistent with the observation that no severe drug–drug interactions have been reported in Man, and it indicates that oleandomycin may be a safer substitute for triacetyloleandomycin in patients who receive other drugs metabolized by cytochrome *P*-450.

3.3.4 INHIBITION OF DRUG METABOLISM: MISCELLANEOUS DRUGS AND XENOBIOTICS

The inhibition of drug metabolism is by no means confined to the above groups of compounds, and, as shown in Table 3.19, many drugs and xenobiotics of diverse chemical structure can act through a variety of mechanisms to decrease the biotransformation of drugs.

Again, the liver appears to be the most important and susceptible target organ for inhibition of drug metabolism, and the data shown in Table 3.19 are only representative of the many reported instances of decreased drug metabolism.

3.4 Conclusions

The study of drug metabolism is both a complex and challenging one. This chapter has highlighted some of the *chemical* factors that are responsible for either the induction or inhibition of drug metabolism, and it is clear that these factors make a significant and complex contribution to modulating drug biotransformation. Awareness of the extent of induction and inhibition of drug metabolism is complicated by the observation that the body burden of potentially regulatory chemicals is unknown to any degree of accuracy, primarily because of the significant role played by environmental chemicals. Because of the variable exposure of man to pharmaceutical products and environmental chemicals, it is not absolutely certain that we can define 'basal levels' of drug metabolism in any given population or ethnic group. However with the refinement of epidemiological and animal studies in drug metabolism, we can confidently look forward to the future when at least we will have fully catalogued and largely understood the influence of pharmaceuticals and chemicals on drug metabolism. Whether or not this information will be acted upon, however, is a different matter.

Table 3.19 Miscellaneous drugs and xenobiotics that inhibit drug metabolism

Drug/xenobiotic	Use or occurrence	Nature of inhibitory action
Amantadine	Anti-viral drug	Specific mode of action unknown, may alter synthesis or degradation of cytochrome P-450
7,8-Benzoflavone		Complex action, relatively specific competitive inhibitor of cytochrome P-448
Carbon disulfide	Vulcanisation of rubber, intermediate in rayon manufacture, occupational exposure significant	Denaturation and loss of hepatic cytochrome P-450, sulfur binding to microsomal proteins, possibly induces lipid peroxidation
Carbon tetrachloride	Solvent	Loss of liver microsomal enzymes, lipid peroxidation, activated by cytochrome P-450 dependent metabolism (carbon–halogen bond cleavage)
Cimetidine	Anti-ulcer drug	Mechanism obscure, binds to cytochrome P-450 (competitive inhibitor?)
Chloramphenicol	Broad spectrum antibiotic	Competitive inhibitor of cytochrome P-450, also non-competitive inhibition due to covalent binding to apoenzyme of cytochrome P-450 (suicide substrate)
Cyclophosphamide	Anti-cancer and immunosuppressant drug	Denaturation of cytochrome P-450 by alkylation of sulfhydryl groups in active site
Disulfiram	Therapy of alcoholics	Blocks ethanol oxidation at stage of acetaldehyde by inhibiting aldehyde oxidase
Ellipticine	Anti-cancer drug	Potent competitive inhibitor of cytochrome P-448
Indomethacin	Anti-inflammatory drug	Depletes cytochrome P-450 by unknown mechanism
MAO inhibitors	Anti-depressant drugs	Inhibit monoamine oxidase (MAO) and enzymes of drug metabolism
Metyrapone	Diagnosis of pituitary function	Binds tightly to and inhibits cytochrome P-450
Parathion	Insecticide	Haem loss and binding of atomic sulfur to cytochrome P-450
Tilorone	Anti-viral agent (interferon-inducer)	Alters cytochrome P-450 turnover, probably by increasing its degradation

3.5 Further reading

TEXTBOOKS AND SYMPOSIA

Boobis, A. R. *et al.* (eds) (1985) *Microsomes and drug oxidations*, Taylor and Frances, London.

Bowman, W. C. and Rand, M. J. (1980) *Textbook of pharmacology*, 2nd edn, Blackwell Scientific Publications, Oxford.

Coon, M. J., Conney, A. H., Estabrook, R. W., Gelboin, H. V., Gillette, J. R. and O'Brien, P. J. (eds) (1980) *Microsomes, drug oxidations and chemical carcinogenesis*, Vols. 1 and 2, Academic Press, New York.

Hietanen, E., Laitinen, M. and Hanninen, O. (eds) (1982) *Cytochrome P-450, biochemistry, biophysics and environmental implications, developments in biochemistry*, Vol. 23, Elsevier Biomedical Press, Amsterdam.

Jenner, P. and Testa, B. (1981) *Concepts in drug metabolism*, Marcel Dekker, New York.

La Du, B. N., Mandel, H. G. and Way, E. L. (eds) (1971) *Fundamentals of drug metabolism and drug disposition*, Williams and Wilkins, Baltimore.

Parke, D. V. (ed.) (1975) *Enzyme induction*, Plenum Press, London.

Parke, D. V. and Smith, R. L. (eds) (1977) *Drug metabolism: from microbe to Man*, Taylor and Francis, London.

Rydström, J., Montelius, J. and Bengtsson, M. (eds) (1984) *Extrahepatic drug metabolism and chemical carcinogenesis*, Elsevier, Amsterdam.

Siest, G. (ed) (1985) *Drug metabolism: molecular approaches and pharmacological implications*, Pergamon Press, Oxford.

Vereczkey, L. and Magyar, K. (eds) (1985) *Cytochrome P-450, biochemistry, biophysics and induction*, Elsevier/Akademia kiado, Amsterdam and Budapest.

REVIEWS AND ORIGINAL ARTICLES

Adesnick, M., Bar-Nun, S., Maschio, F., Zunich, M., Lippmann, A. and Bard, E. (1981) Mechanism of induction of cytochrome *P-450* by phenobarbital. *J. Biol. Chem.*, **256**, 10340–5.

Bock, K. W., Josting, D., Lilienblum, W. and Pfeil, H. (1979) Purification of rat liver microsomal UDP–glucuronyltransferase. Separation of two enzyme forms inducible by 3-methylcholanthrene or phenobarbital. *Eur. J. Biochem.*, **98**, 19–26.

Boobis, A. R. and Davis, D. S. (1984) Human cytochrome *P-450*. *Xenobiotica*, **14**, 151–85.

Cinti, D. L. (1978) Agents activating the liver microsomal mixed-function oxidase system. *Pharmacol. Ther.*, **(A) 2**, 727–49.

Conney, A. H. (1967) Pharmacological implications of microsomal enzyme induction. *Pharmacol. Rev.*, **19**, 317–66.

De Matteis, F. (1978) Loss of liver cytochrome *P-450* by chemicals. In *Heme and hemoproteins* (eds F. De Matteis and W. N. Aldridge), Handbook of Experimental Pharmacology, Vol. 44, Springer-Verlag, New York, pp. 95–127.

Eckström, G., von Bahr, C., Glaumann, H. and Ingelman-Sundberg, M. (1982) Inter-individual variation in benzo[*a*]pyrene metabolism and composition of cytochrome

P-450 as revealed by SDS-gel electrophoresis of human liver microsomal fractions. *Acta Pharmacol. Toxicol.*, **50**, 251–60.

Franklin, M. R. (1977) Inhibition of mixed-function oxidations by substrates forming reduced cytochrome *P*-450 metabolic-intermediate complexes. *Pharmacol. Ther.*, (A)**2**, 227–45.

Gelboin, H. V. (1980) Benzo[*a*]pyrene metabolism, activation and carcinogenesis: role and regulation of mixed-function oxidases and related enzymes. *Physiol. Rev.*, **60**, 1107–66.

Gonzalez, F. J. and Kasper, C. B. (1982) Cloning of DNA complementary to rat liver NADPH–cytochrome c (*P*-450) oxidoreductase and cytochrome *P*-450 mRNAs. Evidence that phenobarbital augments transcription of specific genes. *J. Biol. Chem.*, **257**, 5962–8.

Guengerich, F. P. (1979) Isolation and purification of cytochrome *P*-450 and the existence of multiple forms. *Pharmacol. Ther.*, (A)**6**, 99–121.

Guengerich, F. P. (1982) Microsomal enzymes involved in toxicology – analysis and separation. In *Principles and methods of toxicology* (ed. A. W. Hayes), Raven Press, New York, pp. 609–34.

Guengerich, F. P., Wang, P., Mason, P. S. and Mitchell, M. B. (1981) Immunological comparison of rat, rabbit and human microsomal cytochromes *P*-450. *Biochem.*, **20**, 2370–8.

Halpert, J. and Neal, R. A. (1981) Inactivation of rat liver cytochrome *P*-450 by the suicide substrates parathion and chloramphenicol. *Drug Metab. Rev.*, **12**, 239–59.

Jakoby, W. B. (1978) *Adv. Enzymol.*, **46**, 383–414.

Johnson, E. F. (1979) Multiple forms of cytochrome *P*-450: criteria and significance. In *Reviews in Biochemical Toxicology* (eds E. Hodgson, J. R. Bend and R. M. Philpot), Vol. 1, Elsevier Biomedical Press, New York, pp. 1–26.

Lu, A. H. Y. and West, S. B. (1980) Multiplicity of mammalian cytochromes *P*-450. *Pharmacol. Rev.*, **31**, 277–95.

Nebert, D. W. (1979) Multiple forms of inducible drug-metabolizing enzymes: a reasonable mechanism by which any organism can cope with diversity. *Molec. Cell. Biochem.*, **27**, 27–46.

Nebert, D. W. and Gonzalez, F. J. (1985) Cytochrome *P*-450 gene expression and regulation. *TIPS*, **April**, 160–164.

Nebert, D. W. and Negishi, M. (1982) Multiple forms of cytochrome *P*-450 and the importance of molecular biology and evolution. *Biochem. Pharmacol.*, **31**, 2311–17.

Netter, K. J. (1980) Inhibition of oxidative drug metabolism in microsomes. *Pharmacol. Ther.*, **10**, 515–35.

Okey, A. B. and Vella, L. M. (1982) Binding of 3-methylcholanthrene and 2,3,7,8-tetrachlorodibenzo-*p*-dioxin to a common Ah receptor site in mouse and hepatic cytosols. *Eur. J. Biochem.*, **127**, 39–47.

Ortiz de Montellano, P. R., Mico, B. A., Yost, G. S. and Correia, M. A. (1978) Suicidal inactivation of cytochrome *P*-450: covalent binding of allylisopropylacetamide to the heme prosthetic group. In *Enzyme activated irreversible inhibitors* (eds N. Seiter, M. J. Jung and J. Koch-Wear), Elsevier Biomedical Press, Amsterdam, pp. 337–52.

Ortiz de Montellano, P. R. and Correia, M. A. (1983) Suicidal destruction of cyto-chrome *P*-450 during oxidative drug metabolism. *Ann. Rev. Pharmacol. Toxicol.*, **23**, 481–503.

Park, B. K. (1982) Assessment of the drug metabolism capacity of the liver. *Brit. J. Clin. Pharmacol.*, **14**, 631–51.

Pessayre, D., Descatoire, V., Tinel, M. and Larvey, D. (1982) Self-induction by oleando-mycin of its own transformation into a metabolite forming an inactive complex with reduced cytochrome *P*-450: comparison with trioleandomycin. *J. Pharmacol. Exp. Ther.*, **221**, 215–21.

Picket, C. B., Donohue, A. M. and Hales, B. F. (1982) Rat liver glutathione-*S*-trans-ferase B: the functional mRNAs specific for the YaYc subunits are induced differ-entially by phenobarbital. *Arch. Biochem. Biophys.*, **215**, 539–43.

Rees, D. E. (1979) The mechanism of induction of the microsomal drug hydroxylation system in rat liver by phenobarbitone. *Gen. Pharmacol.*, **10**, 341–50.

Snyder, R. and Remmer, H. (1979) Classes of hepatic microsomal mixed-function oxidase inducers. *Pharmac. Ther.*, **7**, 203–44.

Testa, B. and Jenner, P. (1981) Inhibitors of cytochrome *P*-450s and their mechanisms of action. *Drug Metab. Rev.*, **12**, 1–117.

Wang, P., Mason, P. S. and Guengerich, F. P. (1980) Purification of human liver cytochrome *P*-450 and comparison to the enzyme isolated from rat liver. *Arch. Biochem. Biophys.*, **199**, 206–19.

4

Factors affecting drug metabolism: internal factors

4.1 Introduction

Many factors affect the rate and pathway of metabolism of drugs, and the major influences can be sub-divided into internal (physiological and pathological) and external (exogenous) factors as indicated below:

Internal: species, genetic (strain), sex, age, hormones, pregnancy, disease.
External: diet, environment.

The internal factors will be discussed in this chapter, and diet and environment in the following chapter. Each of these factors will be examined in turn and their influences on drug metabolism highlighted by the use of examples. It should be remembered that this is not an exhaustive list and that examples of other factors affecting drug metabolism can be found in the literature. It can also be seen that certain categories overlap, such that species, strain, genetic and sex differences in drug metabolism have some common features as do hormonal influences on drug metabolism and sex differences; wherever this occurs the reader will be referred to the other section of possible interest. We begin with a look at the way in which the make-up of the animal in question affects the way in which it metabolizes drugs:

4.2 Species differences

Studies on the various differences in drug metabolism abound in the literature and are variously treated from the point of view of evolutionary development to the effects of these metabolic differences on the toxicity of the compound.

Species differences occur in both phase I and phase II metabolism and can be either quantitative (same metabolic route but differing rates) or qualitative (differing metabolic routes). A few examples of each of these cases are given in Table 4.1.

Table 4.1 The species variation in hexobarbitone metabolism, half-life and sleeping time

	Sleeping time (mins)	Hexobarbitone half-life (mins)	Hexobarbitone metabolism (units)
Mice	$12 \pm 8^{\dagger}$	19 ± 7	16.6
Rats	90 ± 15	140 ± 54	3.7
Dog	315 ± 105	260 ± 20	1
Man		~ 360	

†mean $\pm$ (standard deviation)
(Data from Quinn, G. P. *et al.* (1958) *Biochem. Pharmacol.*, **1**, 152–9. Reprinted with permission of Pergamon Press.)

In this example (Table 4.1) the oxidative metabolism of hexobarbitone is shown to vary widely between species and to be inversely related to the half-life and duration of action of the drug. It should be noted that there is not always a direct relationship between metabolism, half-life and action of a drug. These problems are more extensively discussed in Chapter 7. In this case however, this would seem to indicate that Man metabolizes hexobarbitone at a slower rate than the dog, and that the rate of elimination of the drug from the body is dependent on metabolism of the drug.

Phenol is metabolized by conjugation to glucuronic acid and/or sulfate, and the relative proportion of each metabolite depends on the species studied (Table 4.2).

As can be seen from Figure 4.1, oxyphenbutazone is rapidly metabolized in the dog ($t_{1/2} \sim 30$ mins) whilst in Man the rate of metabolism is rather slow ($t_{1/2} \sim 3$ days). This is an extreme example but clearly indicates the possible range of species differences.

The 7-hydroxylation of coumarin is catalysed by human, guinea pig, cat and rabbit liver but not in rat or mouse liver.

The anticoagulant, ethyl biscoumacetate, is rapidly metabolized by rabbit and Man but the resultant metabolites are different (Figure 4.2): the

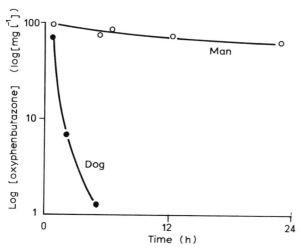

Figure 4.1 Plasma levels of oxyphenbutazone in Man and dog. (From Burns, J. J. (1962) In *Metabolic factors controlling duration of drug action* (eds B. B. Brodie and E. G. Erdös), Pergamon, Oxford, p. 278. Used with permission of Pergamon Press.)

Table 4.2 The species variation in the relative proportions of phenol conjugation to glucuronide and sulfate

	Phenol conjugation[†]	
	Glucuronide	Sulfate
Cat	0	87
Man	23	71
Rat	25	68
Rabbit	46	45
Pig	100	0

[†]Expressed as excretion of a particular conjugate as a percentage of total excretion of drug.
(Data from various sources; see Section 5.4.)

hydroxylated product in Man and the free acid in the rabbit (but both products are inactive). The two examples given above show qualitative differences in drug metabolism due to differences in phase I metabolism. Similar qualitative differences have been shown for phase II metabolism.

Sulfadimethoxine is converted to the glucuronide in Man but no glucuronide formation is evident in rat, guinea pig or rabbit.

All the above are simple examples of one or two enzymes acting on one compound. The situation can, howevere, become quite complex when a large

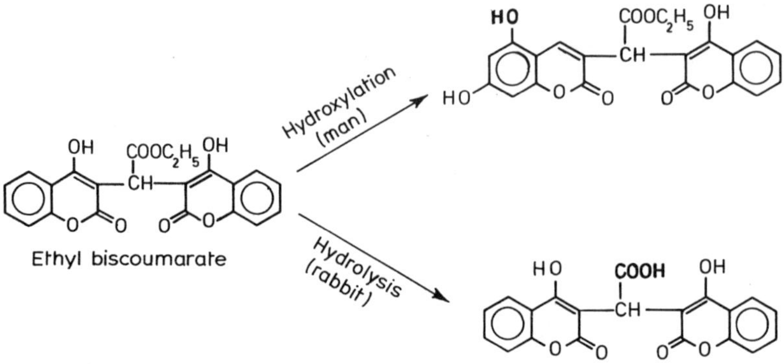

Figure 4.2 The metabolism of ethyl biscoumacetate in Man and rabbit.

number of reactions are involved in the metabolism of one compound. Such a compound is amphetamine, the overall metabolism of which is shown in Figure 4.3.

The rat mainly hydroxylates amphetamine leading to conjugated products on the phenol group whereas the rabbit, guinea pig (and Man) mainly de-aminate amphetamine. The guinea pig further oxidizes the ketone to benzoic acid, and excretes conjugates of benzoic acid. The rabbit has been shown to reduce the ketone and excrete the subsequent conjugates of the alcohol.

Thus it can be seen that different species may differ in their routes of metabolism as well as in the rates at which the metabolism occurs. Most of the data cited are for mammalian species but it should be remembered that lower animals (fishes, reptiles, birds, insects) and even micro-organisms can metabolize drugs. Little comparative work has been done on these species but

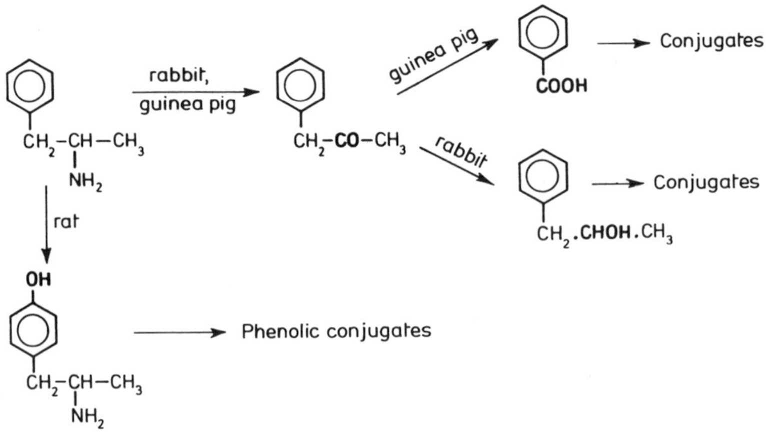

Figure 4.3 The metabolism of amphetamine in rabbit, guinea pig and rat.

in general it is seen that fish have a lower drug-metabolizing capacity than birds which are themselves less able to metabolize drugs than mammals. Species differences in drug metabolism are becoming increasingly important, as suitable models of human toxicity are sought by the pharmaceutical and other industries. For such purposes an animal model is required that as nearly as possible mimics the metabolism of the compound seen in Man. This animal model may be different for the different compounds under study.

4.3 Genetic differences

As has just been discussed major differences in drug metabolism can occur between different species. Such differences can also occur, however, within one species although generally not to such a marked extent. These differences are best noted in the various inbred strains of rats and mice, and are due to the different genetic make-up of the different strains of animals. These inbred strains act as models for other genetic variations in drug metabolism.

The classical example of strain differences in drug metabolism is that of hexobarbitone metabolism in the mouse (see Table 4.3). It is noted that there is a 2.5-fold difference in sleeping time and that the values for the animals in the inbred groups are close to each other whereas the outbred group show a wide variation in sleeping time, thus giving further evidence for a genetic control of drug metabolism.

Table 4.3 Hexobarbitone sleeping time in various strains of mouse

Strain	Sleeping time (mins)
A/NL	48 ± 4[†]
BALB/cAnN	41 ± 2
C57L/HeN	33 ± 3
C3HFB/HeN	22 ± 3
SWR/HeN	18 ± 4
Swiss (outbred)	43 ± 15

[†]mean $\pm$ (standard deviation)
All animals were age-matched males and were given a standard dose of hexobarbitone.
(Data from various sources; see Section 5.4.)

The marked strain differences in the mouse (noted above) have also been extended to include differences in the induction of drug metabolism (see Chapter 3). Using two strains of mouse it was shown that one (strain C57) responds to treatment with 3-methylcholanthrene (3-MC, a polycyclic hydrocarbon inducer of aryl hydrocarbon hydroxylase) whilst the other (strain DBA)

Table 4.4 Effect of cross-breeding on the inducibility by polycyclic hydrocarbons of aryl
hydrocarbon hydroxylase in mice

Strain	% Inducible
C57 $(Ah^dAh^d)^†$	100
DBA $(Ah^bAh^b)^†$	0
F1 (C57 × DBA) $(Ah^bAh^d)^†$	100
F1 × C57	100
F1 × DBA	50
F1 × F1	75

†Ah is the gene for inducibility for polycyclic hydrocarbons Ah^d – inducible, Ah^b – not inducible
(Data from various sources; see Section 5.4.)

does not. Cross breeding of the strains (see Table 4.4) has shown that the inheritance of inducibility is an autosomal dominant (Ah^d). The biochemical mechanism of this induction is discussed in Chapter 3.

In the rat, strain differences centre mainly around the genetically deficient Gunn rat which is unable to form many of the glucuronides produced by other strains of rats. Interbreeding of Gunn and normal rat strains leads to glucuronidation capacities intermediate between the two, indicating that neither trait is dominant.

It is obvious that such genetic control of drug metabolism can only be studied in genetically pure (i.e. inbred) animals; such experiments cannot be performed in Man. Some observations on possible genetic control of drug metabolism in outbred populations can, however, be done using breeding experiments (in animals) and family epidemiological data (in humans).

In rabbits, a genetically determined abnormality in the enzyme atropinase has been shown. Certain rabbits can rapidly metabolize atropine by means of a plasma esterase, the production of which is controlled by a gene that is autosomal and autonomous (i.e. a homozygote has 100% activity, a heterozygote 50% activity).

In Man the possibility of showing a pure genetic influence on drug metabolism is hampered by interfering influences from environmental sources (it is impossible to keep humans in controlled conditions of environment, diet, etc. during their life-span). It has, however, been possible to show probable genetic effects on drug metabolism.

It has been known for a long time that large variations in drug metabolism occur in Man (such as 14-fold variation in bishydroxycoumarin half-life) but only recently have discrete genetic sub-populations been uncovered. One such sub-population is the group of 'isoniazid slow acetylators'. The acetylation of

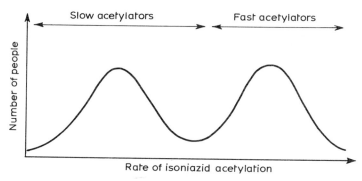

Figure 4.4 The distribution of isoniazid acetylation in the Caucasian population. Note the well-separated bimodal curve.

isoniazid in the human population exhibits a bimodal distribution (Figure 4.4) with about half the Caucasian population 'fast acetylators' and half 'slow acetylators'.

Family studies show that 'slow acetylation' is an autosomal recessive trait. The unusually high incidence of this recessive trait in the population indicates that 'slow acetylation' must confer some sort of advantage or be closely linked to a gene giving such an advantage.

In respect of phase I metabolism by cytochrome P-450, it has long been thought that some sort of genetic control was in operation, based on the 'twin' studies of Vessell and others. It was found that identical twins resembled each other very closely in terms of drug metabolism whereas fraternal twins (twins developed from two different eggs) showed variations similar to the general population. Also the rates of metabolism of desmethylimipramine, nortriptyline, phenylbutazone and dicoumarol show good mutual correlation, indicating a common mechanism of control of their metabolism. Recently a definite genetic polymorphism in cytochrome P-450-dependent drug oxidation has been seen using the marker substrate, debrisoquine. The 4-hydroxylation of this compound shows a bimodal distribution in the population (Figure 4.5).

Again twin, family and population studies have indicated that the 'poor metabolizer' (PM) trait is recessive. In this case, however, no advantage appears to be linked to the PM trait as these are in low frequency in the population. The metabolism of a number of other drugs has now been linked to debrisoquine 4-hydroxylation so that poor metabolizers of debrisoquine also show low metabolism of sparteine, phenytoin, phenformin and phenacetin. If these correlations hold true then it can be seen that a simple test (debrisoquine 4-hydroxylation) could be used to pinpoint patients at risk due to low metabolism of the drug to be administered. Other individual differences in oxidative

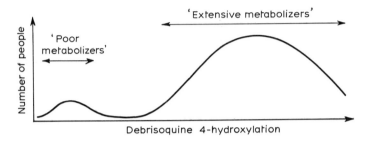

Figure 4.5 The distribution of the rate of metabolism of debrisoquine in the Caucasian population.

drug metabolism do not correlate to debrisoquine metabolism and may represent other genes controlling cytochrome *P*-450.

Thus it can be seen that genetic differences within a population most likely affect the rate at which drugs are metabolized; there is evidence to support direct genetic control of some oxidative and conjugative reactions. The importance of this genetic control is still under debate but may increase as more drug metabolism is found to be genetically controlled (see Chapter 7 for further discussion).

4.3.1 MECHANISM OF CONTROL OF SPECIES AND GENETIC DIFFERENCES

It has been seen that different species metabolize drugs differently and also that, within a species, strains or sub-populations can show marked changes in drug metabolism. What are the underlying mechanisms behind these differences? Various possibilities can be considered:

(1) Changes in amount or activity of the enzyme(s) involved.
(2) Changes in amount or nature of natural inhibitor(s) or activator(s).
(3) Changes in amount or accessibility of co-factor(s).
(4) Presence or absence of reversing enzyme(s).

Of these possibilities, changes in amount or activity of the enzyme(s) involved is by far the best-proven reason; for instance, if glucuronide conjugation is taken as an example. It was noted earlier in this chapter that the cat is noticeably devoid of phenol glucuronyltransferase activity but does have a normal bilirubin glucuronyltransferase. This has been shown to be due to the enzyme(s) in the cat not using phenols as substrate, i.e. a different enzyme in the cat as compared to other species. The Gunn rat, however, is deficient in many glucuronyltransferase activities and has been shown to be also deficient in the enzyme(s) responsible for this activity. Thus it appears that there can be different forms of the same enzyme in different species and even within one species. The possibility of multiple forms of drug-metabolizing enzymes has subsequently been proved by isolating, characterizing and comparing the various forms of glucuronyltransferase and cytochrome P-450 and showing that they do, indeed, show differing substrate specificity as was predicted.

It is now becoming clear, particularly from induction studies (see Chapter 3) that differences in cytochrome P-450 isoenzymes are related to the function of a number of genes (such as the Ah locus) and that genetic control of drug metabolism is, as expected, mediated via activation/repression of these genes.

In one instance at least, however, differences in the enzyme are not responsible for a species difference: this is the inability of dog liver to acetylate sulfonamides (Figure 4.6). It has been suggested that a reversing enzyme, a deacetylase, converts the acetyl derivative back to the original compound or that a natural inhibitor exists in the dog.

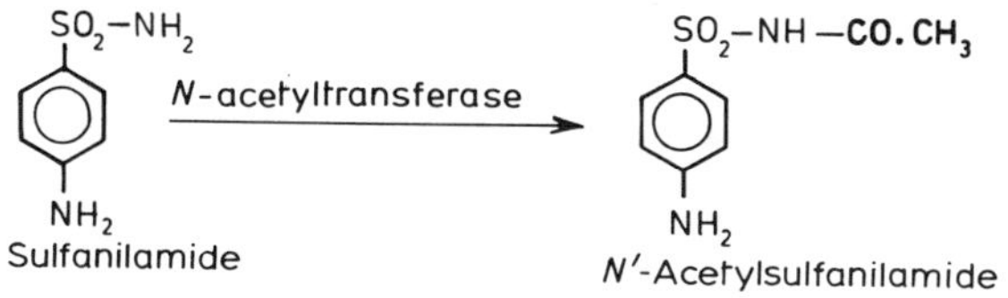

Figure 4.6 The acetylation of sulfanilamide.

Some progress is being made in the understanding of the genetic control of drug metabolism but much work still needs to be done particularly at the molecular level to fully elucidate the mechanisms involved in this control.

4.4 Sex differences

One aspect of 'genetic' control of drug metabolism has not yet been mentioned and that is sex. As will be seen, however, this is not a purely genetic control but more involves hormonal influences on drug metabolism (see later in this chapter).

Sex differences in drug actions were first noted by Nicholas and Barron in 1932 who saw that female rats required only half the dose of barbiturate needed by male rats to induce sleep. Later studies indicated that this was due to the reduced capacity of the female to metabolize the barbiturates. Such sex differences in drug metabolism have now been shown for a wide range of substrates including the endogenous sex steroids (for review see Gustafsson *et al.* (1980) – details in Section 5.4). Sex differences in drug metabolism have also been noted in the mouse for ethylmorphine and steroid metabolism, and in Man for antipyrine, diazepam and steroid metabolism although not to such a marked extent as in the rat. In general the sex differences seen in the mouse are the opposite of those seen in the rat whereas Man shows a similar sex-differentiated pattern to the rat.

Sex differences in the rat tend to follow a general pattern of the male metabolizing faster than the female particularly with regard to phase I metabolism but there are exceptions such as the 3-hydroxylation of lignocaine.

In phase II metabolism, the conjugation of 1-naphthol to form its glucuronide is greater in the male.

4.4.1 MECHANISM OF CONTROL OF SEX DIFFERENCES

In 1958 it was proposed that androgens were the regulators of the sex differences in drug metabolism in the rat when the androgen dependence of ethylmorphine, *p*-nitroanisole and hexobarbitone metabolism was noted (Figure 4.7).

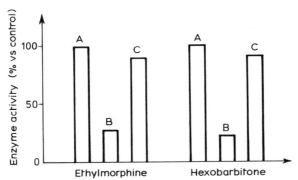

Figure 4.7 The effect of castration (B) and androgen-replacement therapy (C) on the hepatic microsomal metabolism of ethylmorphine and hexobarbitone in the rat; A is control. (From Brodie, B. B. *et al.* (1958) *Biochem. Pharmacol.*, **1**, 152. Used with permission of Pergamon Press.)

The androgen dependence of drug metabolism has recently been challenged and a dual control of drug metabolism involving androgens in the male (acting via the hypothalamo-pituitary hormonal axis) and a pituitary factor in the female has been proposed (for review see Gustafsson *et al.* – details in Section 5.4) as illustrated in Figure 4.8).

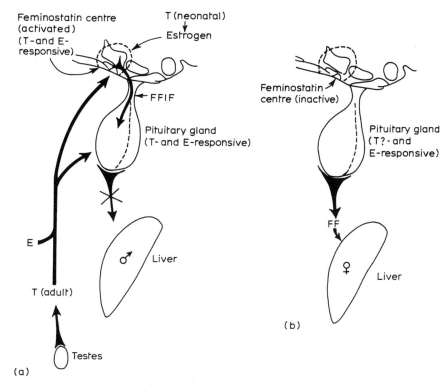

Figure 4.8 The control of sex differences in drug metabolism in the rat. (a) Male. (b) Female. Abbreviations: T, testosterone; E, estradiol; FFIF, feminostatin; FF, feminizing factor.

In the male, a hypothalmic centre releases a factor that inhibits the release of a hormone from the pituitary thus leaving the liver in its native state (i.e. male).

In the female, the hypothalamic centre is inactive, therefore allowing release of the pituitary factor ('feminizing factor') which changes the liver to a female state. The 'feminizing factor' is thought to be growth hormone.

Whether or not this hypothalamic inhibitory centre is active depends *not* on the genotypic sex of the animal (i.e. XX or XY) but on events which occur in the perinatal period. This is best illustrated by an example. The 15β-hydroxylase acting on steroid sulfates is hardly detectable in normal or castrated male animals (see Figure 4.9).

Neonatal castration of male animals, however, leads to a normal female level of enzyme. This can be reversed by treatment with testosterone perinatally but not by testosterone treatment in the adult period. Thus the presence or absence

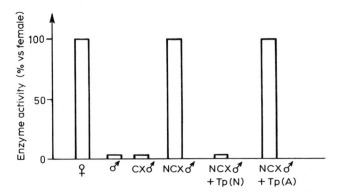

Figure 4.9 Effect of castration and androgen replacement therapy at various ages on
15β-hydroxylation of 5α-androstane-3α,17β-diol disulfate in the rat.
Abbreviations: CX, castrated; NCX, neonatal castration; Tp(N), testosterone
given in neonatal period; Tp(A), testosterone given in adult period. (Data
from J-Å. Gustafsson, personal communication.)

of androgen in the perinatal period determines whether an animal is male or
female with respect to drug metabolism – a process known as 'imprinting' (for
review see Skett and Gustafsson (1979) – details in Section 5.4).

The biochemical basis of the sex differences is not fully elucidated but seems
to be a complex interaction of differences in enzyme levels and activities and
changes in the lipid environment of the enzymes. Sex-related cytochrome
P-450 species have been isolated and seem to be involved in this control.

Sex differences in drug metabolism are of great importance when dealing
with rats and mice, but of less importance in a clinical context.

4.5 Age differences

The increased sensitivity of the young of many animals to drug action has long
been recognized such that neonatal animals show increased intensity and
duration of actions of drugs even when the dose is reduced to account for their
weight or surface area.

Studies on the development of drug-metabolizing capacity have indicated
that this increased sensitivity of neonates may be related to their very low
or, at times, unmeasurable drug-metabolizing capacity. Subsequent development of drug-metabolizing capacity depends on the substrate, species,
strain and, in some cases, sex of animal studied. To facilitate the understanding of this complex subject, phase I and II metabolism will be dealt with
separately, and the control of development discussed for each phase of
metabolism.

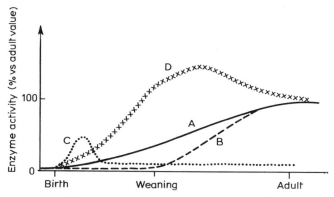

Figure 4.10 Developmental patterns for phase I metabolism.

4.5.1 DEVELOPMENT OF PHASE I METABOLISM

The various possibilities for development of phase I metabolism are indicated in Figure 4.10.

The activity can increase linearly between birth and adulthood (curve A), remain low until weaning and then increase to adult levels (curve B), increase rapidly early after birth and just as rapidly decline again to be very low in adult life (curve C) or increase rapidly from birth to reach levels above adult and subsequently fall to adult levels (curve D). Various combinations of, or variations on, this basic theme can also been seen.

In the rat, type A development is seen for many aromatic and aliphatic hydroxylation reactions, e.g. aniline 4-hydroxylation. Type B development is shown for some *N*-demethylation reactions but in the case of hydroxylation of methylbenzanthracene, type B development is followed for a time but then activity falls to a very low level. Type C development is seen for the hydroxylation of 4-methylcoumarin.

In the rat, the sex differences (see previous section) in drug metabolism exhibited by the adult confuse the developmental profile. Consider the 16α-hydroxylase acting on androst-4-ene-3,17-dione (Figure 4.11). The enzyme activity develops according to type B in both the male and the female but at 30 days of age (puberty in the female) the activity in female begins to disappear and by 40 days of age is undetectable, thus giving the sex differences seen in the adult period (♂ ≫ ♀).

In Man and primates a somewhat different developmental profile is seen with measurable levels of activity in mid-term foetuses, indicating an earlier start to the process of development in primates. It is, however, still quite clear that the foetus and neonate are less able to metabolize drugs than the adult

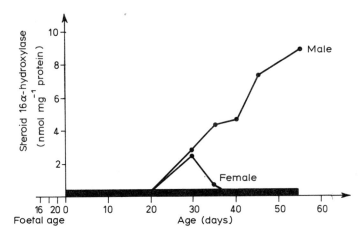

Figure 4.11 The development of the steroid 16α-hydroxylase in male and female rat liver. (From Sternberg, Å. (1976) *J. Endocr.*, **68**, 265–72. Used with permission of the author and publisher.)

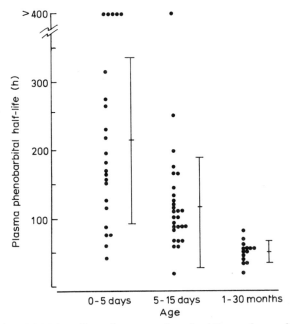

Figure 4.12 The effect of age on phenobarbitone plasma half-life in humans. (From Neims, A. H. *et al.* (1976) *Ann. Rev. Pharm. Tox.*, **16**, 427–45. Used with permission of Annual Reviews Inc. © 1976.)

as is evident from the diminishing half-life of phenobarbitone with increasing age (Figure 4.12).

(a) CONTROL OF DEVELOPMENT OF PHASE I METABOLISM

What are the biochemical changes associated with development of drug-metabolizing ability, and how are they controlled? These are two essential questions for our understanding of the ontogenesis of phase I metabolism.

Clues to the answer to the first question lie in the component of the mono-oxygenase system. The changes can be subdivided into cellular changes (morphological changes in the liver cell) and molecular changes (changes in the amount or type of the chemical components of the enzyme system).

Cellular changes are centred around two things: endoplasmic reticulum (ER) – the membranes where the enzyme system is found – and glycogen stores in the liver. In the prenatal rat there is no smooth ER and little glycogen; at birth a lot of glycogen appears but little smooth ER. Only at one week of age do we begin to see smooth ER appearing with attached glycogen granules (the significance of the glycogen is unclear), and this continues to develop until 6 weeks of age when a full adult pattern of cellular components is seen. This developmental pattern fits very well with the type A development of drug-metabolizing capacity seen earlier. In Man, smooth ER and glycogen begin to appear at 6 weeks of gestation exactly when drug-metabolizing capacity first becomes evident. It seems likely, therefore, that for some enzyme activities in some species, the development is related to appearance of smooth ER and glycogen deposits.

The molecular changes are those associated with the components of the enzyme system notably cytochrome P-450, NADPH–cytochrome P-450 reductase, cytochrome b_5, NADH–cytochrome b_5 reductase and phospholipid. The developmental pattern of cytochrome P-450 differs in various species. In the rat, the development of cytochrome P-450 levels follows that of the smooth ER and of type A development of drug-metabolizing capacity. In the ferret, cytochrome P-450 more follows type B development of metabolism. There is also evidence that the *type* (i.e. isoenzyme complement) of cytochrome P-450 changes during development, a fact that may also affect the enzyme activities measured.

The development of NADPH–cytochrome P-450 reductase follows that of cytochrome P-450 in most cases except that appreciable activity of this enzyme is found in newborn animals. In the rat and ferret NADPH–cytochrome c-reductase is found in the neonatal period, and the cytochrome P-450 reductase does not develop until later. This cytochrome c-reductase activity is thought to be associated with various azo reductase activities found in the neonatal period.

Cytochrome b_5 and its reductase has been little studied in development but

Table 4.5 The effect of reduced progesterone analogues on progesterone and coumarin metabolism in newborn rats

Progestagen added	Progesterone 16-hydroxylase	Coumarin 3-hydroxylase
None	$24.1 \pm 0.7^{\dagger}$	5.0 ± 0.3
5β-Pregnane-$3\alpha,20\alpha$-diol	$15.7 \pm 0.7^{*}$	$3.3 \pm 0.4^{*}$
5β-Pregnane-3α-ol-20-one	$15.5 \pm 1.0^{*}$	$2.3 \pm 0.3^{*}$
5β-Pregnane-3,20-dione	$16.8 \pm 0.6^{*}$	$3.1 \pm 0.3^{*}$

[†]activities expressed as nmoles metabolite formed per hour per mg protein; mean $\pm$ (standard deviation)
$* = p < 0.05$
(From Kordish, R. and Feuer, G. (1972) *Biol. Neonate*, **20**, 58–67, modified. Used with permission of S. Karger AG, Basel.)

are known to influence the activity of the monooxygenase system and thus may play a role.

Very little is known of the influence of phospholipid changes during development although in the rabbit liver a marked increase in linoleic acid content of phospholipids occurs after the first 10 days of life and this has been shown to be related to increases in drug metabolism.

Hormonal changes during development can also have a profound effect on drug metabolism. We have already seen the 'imprinting' of drug metabolism in the rat by androgens leading to sexual differentiation of enzyme activities in the adult period. It is, in fact, thought that the rapid but transient increase in activity seen for some enzymes in the first few days after birth is due to the androgen secreted at this time in order to 'imprint' the male.

The rise in enzyme activity seen after weaning (type B development) is also thought to be hormone-related – the hormone in this case being progesterone delivered to the infant in the mother's milk. Progestagens are, indeed, known to inhibit drug metabolism (see Table 4.5).

Growth hormone has also been shown to inhibit drug metabolism in the developing rat.

Even with all this wealth of information, the critical question: 'What is the rate-limiting step in the development of drug-metabolizing capacity?' remains unanswered. The answer is best summarized by Short who stated: '*It seems most likely that after birth the monooxygenase system develops largely as a unit*'. The rate-limiting factor to the development of this unit depends on the species, strain and sex of the animal and on the substrate under investigation.

4.5.2 DEVELOPMENT OF PHASE II METABOLISM

The development of phase II metabolism is of considerable importance as excretion of drugs and other xenobiotics is mainly in the form of conjugates

– the conjugation reactions being generally regarded as the true 'detoxification' reactions. Changes in the ability of the body to conjugate drugs therefore leads to large changes in toxicity of the drugs.

As with the phase I metabolism, phase II routes of metabolism are poorly represented in the foetal and neonatal animal, and mainly develop perinatally. For reasons of clarity this section will be split into glucuronidation reactions and other conjugation reactions.

(a) GLUCURONIDATION

The most thoroughly studied of the conjugation reactions is glucuronidation and here we are indebted to Professor G. Dutton for his group's excellent work on the development of glucuronidation. This group has found that there are two different developmental types (*not* corresponding to the types found for phase I metabolism), as shown in Figure 4.13.

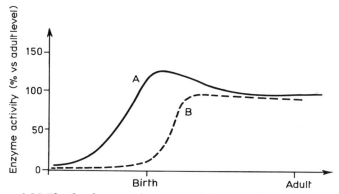

Figure 4.13 The developmental patterns of glucuronidation in the rat. Curve A is late foetal cluster (*p*-nitrophenol as substrate); B is neonatal cluster (bilirubin as substrate).

Type A development is characterized by a steadily increasing activity up until birth, reaching a peak around birth and then declining slightly to adult levels. Type B development is characterized by very low activity until birth, followed by a rapid rise to adult levels. Type A enzymes belong to the late foetal clusters of enzymes, and metabolize predominantly exogenous compounds (e.g. *p*-nitrophenol). Type B belongs to the neonatal cluster of Greengard, and metabolizes mainly endogenous compounds (e.g. bilirubin). In Man little glucuronidation activity is seen until after birth.

(b) CONTROL OF DEVELOPMENT OF GLUCURONIDATION

The study of the control of glucuronidation has led to the postulation of a number of reasons why enzyme activity appears to develop as it does. Some of these theories suggest that the differences are artefactual rather than real such as the suggestion that 'age-dependent activation' is the cause, i.e. variation in the conditions needed for optimal 'activation' of the enzyme with age. Also differing sedimentation properties of foetal, neonatal and adult microsomes can lead to artefactual results as can the differing sensitivity of the perinatal enzyme to destruction during preparation.

All of these possibilities have, however, been thoroughly tested as has the possibility of a natural inhibitor of the enzyme in the perinatal period, and none have stood up to the tests applied. The most likely explanation remains the most obvious, i.e. the animals lacking enzyme activity lack the enzyme.

The physiological control of development has also been studied in some detail. One series of studies involved the use of chick embryos which can readily be cultured to facilitate the investigation. In this case, glucuronyl-transferase activity is negligible until hatching and then undergoes a rapid increase, reaching adult levels in 1–3 days. If embryonic liver is cultured, its glucuronyltransferase activity increases to adult levels spontaneously and precociously. The process of maturation involves a morphological change in the cells and protein synthesis. This precocious increase in activity in culture does not occur if the liver is cultured in the presence of the chorioallantoic membrane, indicating that induction of enzyme activity can only take place after removal of the repressive influence of the embryonic environment. The nature of this repressive influence is unclear. Certain hormones were, however, shown to overcome this repressive influence such as corticosteroids (with thyroxine acting synergistically). In the chick, therefore, postnatal development is probably stimulated by corticosteroid production (and thyroxine).

In mammalian foetuses a similar mechanism of control was shown to be in operation. Embryonic liver cultured on chorioallantoic membrane, as before, maintained its embryonic character. A pituitary graft onto the membrane stimulated glucuronyltransferase activity to the adult level. Again cortico-steroids were shown to be the natural inducers by injection of the mother with hormones, and subsequent examination of the foetal liver.

This means of control applies to the late foetal cluster, i.e. glucuronyl-transferase activity towards *p*-nitrophenol and not the neonatal cluster. No evidence exists for hormones which control phase I metabolism (e.g. pro-gesterone and growth hormone) having any effect on phase II metabolism.

(c) OTHER PHASE II REACTIONS

Compared to glucuronidation very few data are available on the developmental patterns of other phase II reactions (i.e. sulfation, acetylation, amino acid conjugation, methylation and glutathione conjugation). The sulfo-conjugating enzymes (sulfotransferases) are thought to be high in foetal tissue (about adult levels) and, particularly in the case of steroid sulfotransferases, develop early in gestation. This is probably a function of their role in biosynthetic and transport pathways of metabolism rather than an excretory role. Hypothalamo-pituitary factors have been implicated in the control of development of steroid sulfo-transferases. An inhibitor of phenol sulfotransferases has also been found to be present at birth accounting for the apparent fall in activity of the enzyme seen around this period.

For acetylation it was found that premature infants acetylate sulfonamides less well than full-term infants, but this latter group are still below the activity of adults. In the rabbit, acetylation of isoniazid is low at 6 days, rising steadily to 14 days and then surges to adult levels between 21 and 28 days. It is suggested from kinetic data that different forms of the enzyme exist at different ages.

Amino acid conjugation and methylation are similar to acetylation, being low in foetal and neonatal tissues and developing steadily to adult levels.

Glutathione conjugation is of particular importance in being one of the major defence mechanisms in the body against xenobiotic electrophiles (many of which are mutagens and/or carcinogens). Early studies on the development of the enzyme responsible for glutathione conjugation (glutathione-*S*-transferase) showed a steady rise in activity from 3 days prenatally to 20 days postnatally in the rat, by which time adult levels had been reached. In Man an even earlier development of enzyme activity is thought to occur. Later studies have shown multiple forms of glutathione-*S*-transferase, one of these, glutathione-*S*-transferase B (ligandin), having been particularly well studied. Ligandin is absent in foetal animals and Man but subsequently appears in the perinatal period, and increases to reach adult levels in the first few weeks of life. Induction, by exogenous or endogenous compounds, of ligandin can also occur *in utero* particularly if other drug-metabolizing enzymes are lacking (e.g. Gunn rats; see Section 4.3, on genetic differences).

In summary, phase II metabolism is generally low or absent in foetal animals, and develops perinatally, reaching adult levels early in life. The multiplicity of the various enzymes involved should be remembered when studying these reactions in terms of development, as the different forms of the enzyme may develop at different times and different rates.

Age-related changes are seen by the clinician to be of major importance as special dosage schedules for infants are used which are unrelated to the dose for an adult on a weight basis. The reduced metabolic activity of the older patients has also been shown to be important but little account is taken of this in prescribing of drugs.

4.6 Hormonal control of drug metabolism

The two preceding sections of this chapter (on sex and age differences in drug metabolism) have indicated the central role that hormones can play in the control of drug metabolism, particularly the hormones of the pituitary and adrenal gland, and of the sex organs. In this section it is intended to expand this idea to include all the endocrine organs, to further examine the role of the pituitary, adrenal and sex glands and consider the thyroid and pancreas in terms of their effects on drug metabolism. The effects of pregnancy (as a major disturbance in the hormonal balance of the female body) on drug metabolism will also be discussed.

4.6.1 PITUITARY GLAND

The pituitary gland controls the release of hormones from the other endocrine organs (except in the case of the pancreas where other influences are more important), and thus any effects exerted by the endocrine organs will be mimicked by the pituitary gland. As has been stated previously, the pituitary gland also seems to have direct effects on drug metabolism by means of growth hormone (see Sections 4.4 and 4.5). Direct effects of other pituitary hormones have also been seen. Adrenocorticotrophic hormone (ACTH), luteinizing hormone (LH), follicle-stimulating hormone (FSH) and prolactin have been shown to affect hepatic steroid and drug metabolism. The pituitary gland, therefore, occupies a central role in the hormonal control of drug metabolism, and the individual effects of this organ will be discussed under the various endocrine glands that it controls.

4.6.2 SEX GLANDS

Sex glands in this context refer to the endocrine glands, the testes (in the male) and the ovaries (in the female). The effect of these organs on drug metabolism has already been covered in this chapter (see Section 4.4).

4.6.3 ADRENAL GLANDS

The adrenal glands have already been discussed in terms of glucocorticoid control of development of drug metabolism (see Section 4.5). The adrenal

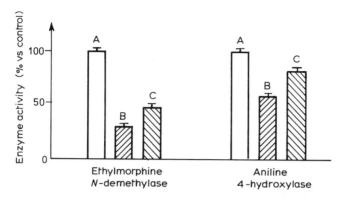

Figure 4.14 The effect of adrenalectomy and corticosteroid replacement therapy on the hepatic metabolism of ethylmorphine and aniline. A is control; B, results from adrenalectomy; C, adrenalectomy followed by corticosterone treatment. (From Furner, R. L. and Stitzel, R. E. (1968) *Biochem. Pharm.*, **17**, 121–7. Used with permission of Pergamon Press.)

glands are, however, also thought to be involved in the regulation of drug metabolism in the adult period.

Adrenalectomy has been shown to reduce the microsomal metabolism of a number of xenobiotics, whereas glucocorticoid replacement therapy can reverse the effect of adrenalectomy (see Figure 4.14).

Glucocorticoids have, however, been shown to mimic or potentiate the action of adrenalectomy in a number of instances. This apparent paradox in glucocorticoid action was resolved by Tredger who showed that the natural, short-acting glucocorticoids are inhibitory to drug metabolism, whereas the synthetic potent analogues (which are not so readily metabolized) are stimulatory (act as enzyme inducers).

It was argued that the effect of adrenalectomy is due to the removal of adrenal androgens (similar effect to castration) but the effect of the adrenal gland on drug metabolism would appear to be more complex than this. It is probable that the effects of adrenalectomy on drug metabolism are a result of changes in adrenal production of hormones (glucocorticoids, mineralocorticoids and adrenaline), the subsequent changes in pituitary outflow of hormones (ACTH) and other physiological changes induced by hypoadrenalism.

4.6.4 THYROID GLANDS

The thyroid glands, controlled by release of thyrotropin-releasing hormone (TRH), from the hypothalamus and subsequent release of thyroid-stimulating hormone (TSH) from the pituitary gland, are known to have some influence on

Table 4.6 Sex-dependency of the effect of thyroidectomy on hepatic drug metabolism

Enzyme activity	Effect of thyroidectomy	
	Male animals	Female animals
Alcohol oxidation	(Not determined)	Increase
Cytochrome P-450	Increase	Increase
Ethylmorphine N-demethylase	Decrease	Decrease
Benzo[a]pyrene hydroxylase	Decrease	Decrease
Aniline 4-hydroxylase	Decrease	Decrease
5β-Reductase	(No change)	Increase
11β-Hydroxysteroid dehydrogenase	Decrease	Increase

(Data from various sources; see Section 5.4.)

drug metabolism. The effect of thyroidectomy in the rat depends on the substrate being studied and on the sex of the animal used (see Table 4.6).

In a recent study lignocaine metabolism was shown to be increased by thyroidectomy in both male and female species, whereas imipramine and diazepam metabolism were unaffected in the male. Imipramine metabolism was enhanced in the female. The effects noted in the earlier studies could be reversed by L-thyroxine treatment but it was noted that high doses of hormone were *less* effective than low doses indicating that excess hormone (a thyrotoxic state) may be as inhibitory to drug metabolism as the hypothyroid state. Later evidence has tended to discount this possibility as no effects of excess L-thyroxine in normal animals was seen.

In the human, the thyroid gland has also been implicated in the control of drug metabolism. For the limited number of substrates used (antipyrine, paracetamol and aspirin), thyroidectomy always decreases their apparent metabolism. Further work may reveal a substrate dependence in effect, as seen in the rat.

The mechanism of thyroid control of drug metabolism is unclear but does not appear to involve cytochrome P-450 in changes in phase I metabolism as enzyme activity changes do not correlate with changes in cytochrome P-450. The multiplicity of cytochrome P-450 should be remembered here as the thyroid hormones may change the proportion of different isoenzymes without necessarily changing the overall amount.

Phase II metabolism can also be affected by thyroidectomy. Recent data have indicated that the glucuronidation of 1-naphthol is significantly lower in thyroidectomized rats of both sexes (Table 4.7). No data are available on the reversal of this effect by thyroid hormones and, thus, no definite conclusion can be drawn concerning the thyroid control of phase II metabolism.

Table 4.7 The effect of thyroidectomy (TX) on glucuronidation of 1-naphthol in liver cubes

Animal	1-Naphthol glucuronide formed $(min^{-1} g^{-1} liver)^{\dagger}$
Control male	1.70 ± 0.17
TX male	$1.27 \pm 0.12^*$
Control female	0.59 ± 0.08
TX female	$0.34 \pm 0.03^*$

†Results expressed as mean $\pm$ (standard deviation)
$^* = p < 0.05$

Thus the thyroid glands may play a role in the hormonal control of drug metabolism and, in the rat, may be involved in the sexual differentiation of drug metabolism (see Section 4.4).

4.6.5 PANCREAS

The pancreas produces and secretes one hormone of particular relevance to the control of drug metabolism, i.e. insulin. This is produced by the β-cells within the endocrine pancreas and is responsible for the maintenance of a suitable blood sugar level.

In the rat, treatment with streptozotocin (STZ) (see Figure 4.15 – a glucosyl-nitrosourea derivative), which destroys the β-cells of the pancreas causes marked changes in hepatic phase I and II metabolism (see Table 4.8).

Phase I metabolism, exemplified by diazepam and lignocaine hydroxylation and N-dealkylation, shows a marked decrease in activity (except lignocaine 3-hydroxylation) whereas phase II metabolism of 1-naphthol shows no change in activity. Other reports indicate that, with other substrates, phase II metabolism may also decline after STZ-treatment. As usual in the rat, the sex of the animal must be taken into consideration – all of the effects noted are only seen in the male.

Recent reports of a diabetes-specific form of cytochrome P-450 causing the changes noted in phase I metabolism following STZ-treatment indicate that

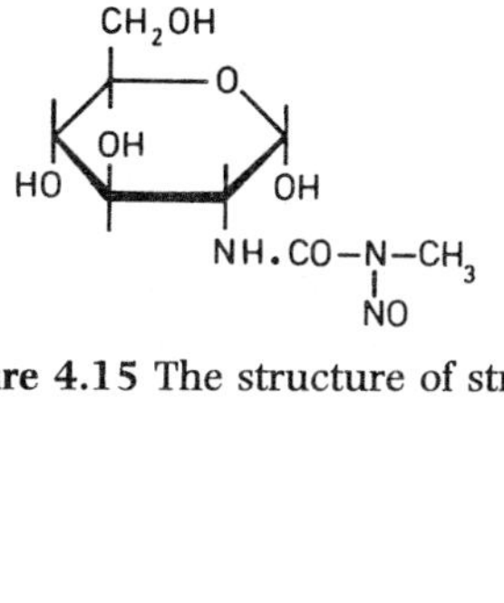

Figure 4.15 The structure of streptozotocin (STZ).

Table 4.8 The effect of streptozotocin (STZ)-induced diabetes on liver weight, blood glucose and drug metabolism in the male rat

	Control	STZ-treated	
Liver (% body weight)	$3.58 \pm 0.28^{\dagger}$	4.32 ± 0.47	**
Blood glucose (mM)	8.67 ± 0.68	32.13 ± 2.54	***
Cytochrome P-450 (nmoles mg^{-1})	0.56 ± 0.06	0.54 ± 0.08	n.s.
Diazepam 3-hydroxylase (pmoles min^{-1} g^{-1} protein)	60.3 ± 21.4	35.6 ± 4.8	*
Diazepam N-demethylase (pmoles min^{-1} g^{-1} protein)	32.4 ± 7.6	19.4 ± 5.1	*
Lignocaine 3-hydroxylase (pmoles min^{-1} g^{-1} protein)	35 ± 6	31 ± 16	n.s.
Lignocaine N-de-ethylase (pmoles min^{-1} g^{-1} protein)	317 ± 118	182 ± 65	*
1-Naphthol glucuronidation (nmoles product min^{-1} g^{-1} liver)	1.42 ± 0.22	1.57 ± 0.15	n.s.

†mean $\pm$ S.D. (of at least 4 values)
* $= p < 0.05$; ** $= p < 0.01$; *** $= p < 0.001$; n.s. $=$ not significant, $p > 0.05$

the unchanged cytochrome P-450 level after treatment may hide a change in isoenzyme proportions. The diabetes-dependent isoenzyme has been purified and characterized, and has been shown to be different to those already purified from normal animals.

Replacement therapy with insulin can reverse the effects of diabetes caused by streptozotocin (see Figure 4.16).

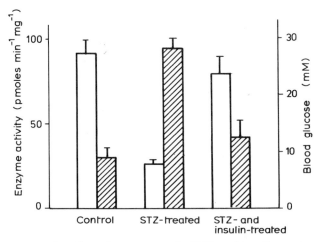

Figure 4.16 The effect of streptozotocin (STZ) and insulin treatment on blood glucose levels and the N-de-ethylation of lignocaine in the rat liver. Plain block-diagrams represent enzyme activity; hatched blocks, blood glucose.

There appears to be a good inverse relationship between blood glucose levels and phase I metabolism and thus it can be inferred that a good direct relationship exists between insulin levels and phase I metabolism.

Little has been reported on the effects of diabetes on drug metabolism in Man: what has been published shows a very confused picture – perhaps due to the complex nature of the disease state in Man.

4.6.6 SUMMARY OF EFFECTS OF HORMONES

A summary of the possible hormonal control of drug metabolism is shown in Figure 4.17. It would appear that thyroid, pituitary and adrenal hormones (except adrenal androgens) and insulin act directly on the liver, whereas androgens and oestrogens exert their effects on the liver by interaction with the hypothalamo-hypophyseal axis, modifying the release of the pituitary hormones.

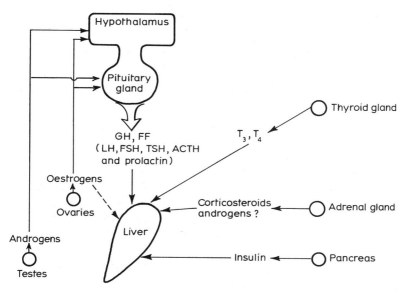

Figure 4.17 Hormonal control of drug metabolism. Abbreviations: GH, growth hormone; FF, feminizing factor; T_3, tri-iodothyronine; T_4, thyroxine.

The hormonal control of drug metabolism is, as can be seen from the above summary, quite complex and is made more so by the numerous interactions of the hormones involved (e.g. GH and insulin have been shown to be mutually antagonistic). The above description should, therefore, be regarded as an approximation to the actual situation and not as a fixed set of facts. The importance of hormonal control of drug metabolism is well established in rats and mice but has been little regarded in clinical practice, perhaps due to lack of research in this field in the human.

4.6.7 PREGNANCY

Pregnancy is a natural condition when the hormonal balance of the female body is grossly upset. The oestrous (menstrual) cycle ceases and there are large changes in blood levels of peptide and steroid hormones. It, therefore, seems fitting to discuss the effects of pregnancy on drug metabolism under the heading: hormonal control.

The study of drug metabolism during pregnancy in the human is rather difficult due to the obvious ethical considerations of administering drugs to a pregnant woman. Most of the work, therefore, has been done in animal models.

Table 4.9 The effect of pregnancy on the metabolism of coumarin and progesterone in the rat

	Non-pregnant	Pregnant
Coumarin 3-hydroxylase	18.61 ± 1.92	10.28 ± 1.05*
Progesterone 16α-hydroxylase	6.68 ± 0.15	4.63 ± 0.33*
Progesterone 5α-reductase	15.38 ± 0.26	21.86 ± 0.47*

Results expressed as nmoles product $h^{-1} g^{-1}$ protein; mean $\pm$ (standard deviation)
* $= p < 0.05$
(From Kordish, R. and Feuer, G. (1972) *Biol. Neonate*, **20**, 58–67, modified. Used with permission of S. Karger AG, Basel.)

In the rat, pregnancy causes a general decrease in drug metabolism, e.g. 3-hydroxylation of coumarin, but a more complex change in the metabolism of the endogenous progestagen, progesterone (Table 4.9). These changes were shown to be due to progesterone or its metabolites that are found in blood in high concentrations during pregnancy. This is the same phenomenon seen in suckling infants (see Section 4.5, on age differences in drug metabolism) where progestagens in the mother's milk are thought to inhibit drug metabolism in the young animal in certain cases.

4.6.8 TEMPERATURE AND pH

Before moving on from physiological factors to pathological factors affecting drug metabolism, two other items should be briefly mentioned; these are the effects of temperature and pH on drug metabolism.

Temperature and pH are physical factors that affect the action of all enzymes, and thus it can be assumed that they exert an effect on drug metabolism. Indeed if the temperature and pH optima of various drug-metabolizing enzymes

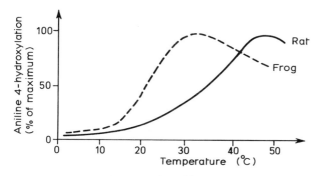

Figure 4.18 The temperature dependence of aniline 4-hydroxylation in the rat (warm-blooded) and the frog (cold-blooded).

are investigated, some interesting correlations with the environment of the enzymes are seen. For instance, cytochrome P-450-dependent metabolism in the rat exhibits a temperature optimum around 40–45 °C (the rat's normal body temperature) whereas the frog has a much lower temperature optimum (about 30 °C; see Figure 4.18) perhaps owing to the fact that the frog is a cold-blooded animal.

This is taken to extremes by a fish inhabiting Arctic waters, which has a steroid-metabolizing enzyme with temperature optimum at 0 °C and denaturation temperature of 20 °C, and the pseudomonad (bacterium) that lives in hot springs, with a cytochrome P-450-like enzyme with temperature optimum at 80 °C.

The same can be said to be true of pH, such that liver enzymes tend to have a pH optimum around 7.4 (the normal pH in the liver), whereas the gut enzymes (e.g. pepsin) have a pH optimum around 2.

One interesting example is the bladder β-glucuronidase which hydrolyses glucuronides in the urine and slows down excretion of a number of drugs (e.g. salicylates). (See Figure 4.19.) This β-glucuronidase has a low optimum pH; acidification of the urine causes increased activity of the enzyme, and thus less drug is excreted.

4.7 Effects of disease on drug metabolism

The liver is the major site of drug metabolism in the body and it is, therefore, safe to say that diseases affecting the liver are those most likely to affect drug metabolism. A list of liver diseases that have been indicated to affect the metabolism of drugs is shown in Table 4.10.

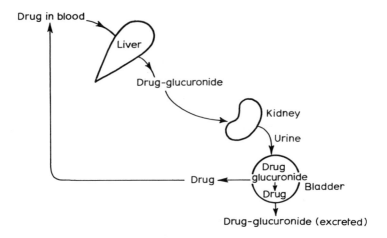

Figure 4.19 The urino-hepatic circulation of drugs.

Table 4.10 Diseases of the liver that affect drug metabolism

Cirrhosis
Alcoholic liver disease
Viral hepatitis
Porphyria
Hepatoma

The problems of alcoholic liver disease are complex and overlap in the later stages with cirrhosis, but the earlier stages are very different and, thus, this is treated as a separate disease.

In this section each disease will be looked at in turn, and then a general summary included to draw together the various aspects of disease influences on drug metabolism. It will be appreciated that the majority of the data are clinical as diseases of Man are the most widely studied.

4.7.1 CIRRHOSIS

In cirrhosis, parts of the liver are replaced by fibrous tissue, and the number of functional hepatocytes is reduced. It is therefore not unreasonable that drug metabolism is impaired in this condition and, indeed, the conversion of chlordiazepoxide to its primary metabolite, desmethylchlordiazepoxide, is slower in cirrhotic patients.

This appears to be true also for the conversion of diazepam to desmethyl-diazepam. Oxazepam and lorazepam metabolism – which is purely glucuronidation – is, however, not affected by cirrhosis.

The N-dealkylation of lignocaine is grossly affected by cirrhosis, as is the oxidation of propranolol with a much longer half-life for each drug. The same increase in elimination half-life is seen for theophylline and tolbutamide (an oral hypoglycemic). The problem of equating plasma half-life with metabolism is evident here as both lignocaine and propranolol are highly extracted drugs and, thus, the blood flow through the liver is important (see Chapter 7).

Various drugs which are normally metabolized by the liver are not affected with respect to their metabolism by cirrhosis. Morphine, for example, is converted to its glucuronide by the liver; this conversion is unaffected by cirrhosis. In one instance the activation of a prodrug is impaired by cirrhosis: the conversion of prednisone (the prodrug) to prednisolone (the active drug) is slower in cirrhotic patients.

One other aspect of cirrhosis should also be considered and that is enzyme induction by drugs and other xenobiotics. It is well known that many drugs can increase the rate at which they and other drugs are metabolized (see Chapter 3). The cirrhotic condition can greatly diminish the degree of increase in drug metabolism. For example, phenobarbitone pretreatment of normal subjects markedly increases the metabolism of antipyrine whereas similar pretreatment of cirrhotic patients has little effect. Glutethimide can, however, induce antipyrine metabolism in cirrhotic patients. This apparent paradox can be explained in terms of the multiplicity of drug-metabolizing enzymes, the differing degrees of cirrhosis and the different inducing agents used. The effect of cirrhosis on enzyme induction, therefore, remains unclear.

Table 4.11 summarizes the effect of cirrhosis on drug metabolism. It is noted that cirrhosis appears to depress phase I but have no effect on glucuronidation.

Table 4.11 The effect of liver cirrhosis on drug metabolism

Drugs affected	(Metabolic route)	Drugs not affected	(Metabolic route)
Chlordiazepoxide	(N-Demethylation)	Oxazepam	(Glucuronidation)
Diazepam	(N-Demethylation)	Lorazepam	(Glucuronidation)
Barbiturates	(Oxidation)	Morphine	(Glucuronidation)
Antipyrine	(Oxidation)	Paracetamol	(Glucuronidation)
Glutethimide	(Oxidation)		
Methadone	(Oxidation)		
Salicylates	(Glycine conjugation)		

(Data from various sources; see Section 5.4.)

4.7.2 ALCOHOLIC LIVER DISEASE

Chronic alcohol administration can lead to a condition similar to that of cirrhosis with large portions of the liver replaced by fibrous masses following the death of the parenchymal cells. Before this stage is reached, however, alcohol administration can markedly affect drug metabolism.

The stages of alcohol's effect on drug metabolism are summarized in Figure 4.20.

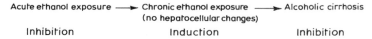

Acute ethanol exposure ⟶ Chronic ethanol exposure ⟶ Alcoholic cirrhosis
(no hepatocellular changes)

Inhibition   Induction   Inhibition

Figure 4.20 The stages in the development of the effect of ethanol on hepatic drug metabolism.

Acute ethanol exposure, in general, decreases drug metabolism such that drugs metabolized primarily by phase I routes (e.g. chlordiazepoxide, diazepam, aminopyrine, pentobarbitone and chlorpromazine) or phase II routes (e.g. lorazepam, p-nitrophenol, harmol and paracetamol) exhibit longer half-lives if administered with ethanol.

The inhibition of phase I metabolism is thought to be due to ethanol binding to cytochrome P-450 (the liver actually has a cytochrome P-450-dependent ethanol oxidizing system (MEOS)) in a competitive manner. Inhibition of electron flow from the reductase to cytochrome P-450 has also been seen. Ethanol seems to inhibit the metabolism of type II binding substrates more than type I binding substrates. The alteration of the NADP/NADPH ratio, and the disturbance of the lipid environment, have also been put forward as possible explanations of the effect of ethanol on phase I metabolism. A number of workers have suggested a mediating role of the adrenal gland in the effects of ethanol.

The inhibition of phase II metabolism is not due to inhibition of the enzymes involved. In the case of glucuronidation, ethanol is thought to increase the NADH/NAD ratio (via oxidation of ethanol by alcohol dehydrogenase). This in turn inhibits the production of the co-factor for glucuronidation, UDP–glucuronic acid (which requires NAD). (See Figure 4.21.)

In one reaction, acute ethanol administration has been shown to increase

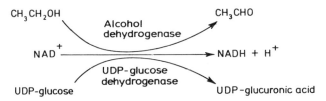

Figure 4.21 The interaction of ethanol with UDPGA production.

Table 4.12 The effect of chronic ethanol treatment on the plasma half-life of drugs

Drug	Decrease in $t_{1/2}$ following chronic ethanol exposure (%)
Meprobamate	40
Pentobarbitone	25
Phenytoin	30
Warfarin	35
Antipyrine	25

(Data from various sources; see Section 5.4.)

activity; that is, in the acetylation of sulfadimidine. No explanation for this effect was given.

Chronic ethanol exposure in the absence of pathological changes in the liver is usually associated with enhanced drug metabolism. Ethanol is classed as a microsomal enzyme inducer of a type different to both phenobarbitone and the polycyclic hydrocarbons (see Chapter 3). It has been shown to induce phase I and II metabolism.

The metabolism of meprobamate, phenytoin, warfarin, antipyrine and pentobarbital was increased following one month's pretreatment with ethanol (Table 4.12).

The marked increase in cytochrome *P*-450 after chronic ethanol exposure indicates that induction of the terminal oxidase may be responsible for the increased drug metabolism that is seen.

Once the extent of alcoholic liver disease has become extensive, a pattern of effects similar to cirrhosis is seen such that the metabolism of diazepam, paracetamol and lignocaine is reduced.

4.7.3 VIRAL HEPATITIS

Little is known of the effects of viral hepatitis, but what information is available suggests that this condition causes a decrease in hepatic drug metabolism. Chlordiazepoxide clearance is decreased in viral hepatitis as is the clearance of meperidine (pethidine). Clearance of lignocaine is unaffected by viral hepatitis whereas tolbutamide exhibits an enhanced clearance in this condition (see discussion of drug clearance in Chapter 7).

4.7.4 HEPATOMA

A hepatoma is a cancerous growth derived from the liver parenchymal cells. The drug-metabolizing capacity of the tumour cells, however, is very much less than the corresponding normal cells. This is a typical loss of differentiated function in de-differentiated cells.

Table 4.13 The steroid 5α-reductase activity of various rat hepatomas

Hepatoma (code no.)		5α-Reductase activity (% vs control liver)
44		3.6
38B	Growth rate increasing	2.6
7795		2.0
5123A		1.5
7288C		1.0
7777		0.6
42A		0.2

(From Houglum, J. E. *et al.* (1974) *Cancer Res.*, **34**, 938–41. Used with permission of the authors and Cancer Research Inc.)

The loss of differentiated function is noted for the metabolism of aniline to 4-aminophenol. The level of aniline metabolism in the tumours was similar to that in foetal and regenerating liver.

The faster growing (i.e. less differentiated) the tumour the less drug metabolism was evident. This was shown particularly well with the 5α-reduction of testosterone (Table 4.13).

Metabolism of oestrogens, methadone, benzphetamine and 4-nitroanisole are also found at much reduced levels in hepatoma tissue.

One interesting point emerged from these studies and that was that the unaffected liver tissue of the animal with the hepatoma also showed a reduced capacity to metabolize drugs. The decreases were not as dramatic as those of the hepatoma itself but the presence of a de-differentiated hepatoma could reduce hepatic drug metabolism by 20%. This has recently been challenged by Sultatos and Vessell who showed enhanced drug metabolism in liver tissue surrounding a hepatoma.

The answer to this paradox lies (say the authors) in the fact that previous studies have used intramuscularly implanted hepatomas whereas they used intrahepatic hepatomas. This enhancement of drug metabolism in tumour-adjacent tissue would seem to extend to Man (Table 4.14).

Table 4.14 Drug metabolism in hepatoma tissue and surrounding normal liver tissue

Tissue studied	Ethylmorphine N-demethylase (% vs control tissue)	Aniline hydroxylase (% vs control tissue)
Normal liver	100	100
Tumour	70	27
Tumour-adjacent liver	250	290
Far-removed liver	100	100

(From Sultatos, L. G. and Vessell, E. S. (1980) *P.N.A.S.*, **77**, 600–3. Used with the permission of the authors.)

The changes in drug-metabolizing capacity – seen in hepatoma lines and liver adjacent to hepatomas – are related to changes in cytochrome *P*-450 levels: markedly decreased in hepatoma tissue but elevated in histologically normal liver tissue close to a tumour. Little difference appears to exist between the drug-metabolizing system of the tumour and normal tissue, each can be induced and inhibited similarly and, thus, the only difference lies in the amount of enzyme present.

4.7.5 PORPHYRIA

Porphyria is a set of disorders of porphyrin metabolism (precursors of the haem in haemoproteins) whereby porphyrins or precursors build up in the tissues and are excreted in increased amounts. The types of porphyria of interest here are the hepatic porphyrias. The main defect lies in a deficiency of haem production or failure of the feedback mechanism on the rate-limiting step, ALA-synthetase.

As haem is required for the production of cytochrome *P*-450 (the main enzyme involved in phase I metabolism) it is safe to assume that porphyria brings with it the possibilities of disturbances in drug metabolism. Little work has, however, been done in this field.

4.7.6 SUMMARY OF EFFECTS OF LIVER DISEASES ON DRUG METABOLISM

As has been seen, diseases of various types generally decrease the liver's ability to metabolize drugs (with the notable exception of chronic ethanol exposure). The possible reasons for this decreased capacity are listed below:

(1) Decreased enzyme activity in liver.
(2) Altered hepatic blood-flow (intra/extrahepatic shunting).
(3) Hypoalbuminaemia (leading to lower plasma binding of drugs).

Of these reasons only (1) is really to be classed as a change in metabolism of the drug but the other two can lead to changes in metabolism and, thus, must be considered.

Two theories have been put forward to explain the poor metabolism in cirrhotic patients: one – the 'sick cell' theory – maintains that blood flow through the liver is normal but the cells are deficient in drug-metabolizing enzymes, whereas the other – the 'intact hepatocyte' theory – says that the cells are normal but do not receive the normal blood flow due to shunting of blood past some parts of the liver (to get round the fibrous masses). Both theories have some evidence in favour of them, such as reduced cytochrome *P*-450 levels and drug-metabolizing enzyme activity in cirrhotic rats ('sick cell' theory) and increased (9 times normal) intrahepatic shunting in cirrhotic animals ('intact hepatocyte' theory). It is probable that both theories are correct and vary in importance depending on the stage of cirrhosis and on the substrate, animal, etc. being studied.

Other non-hepatic diseases should also be considered in terms of influence on drug metabolism; these particularly include the hormonal diseases such as hyperthyroidism, pituitary insufficiency (dwarfism), adrenal insufficiency, pituitary, thyroid or adrenal tumours, diabetes and the genetic abnormalities of sexual development. All of the above mentioned disease states have been shown to influence drug metabolism (most of which have been discussed to a greater or lesser extent in Section 4.6).

The health of the patient/animal can thus play a major role in the drug-metabolizing capacity of the liver of that patient/animal and, together with age, probably represents the major consideration when deciding the dose of drug to be given to a patient or, indeed, whether a drug should be given at all.

It has now been shown how the physiological and pathological make-up of the animal can influence the way in which it metabolizes drugs. In the next chapter it is intended to discuss the other major controlling influences on drug metabolism: the external factors.

Further reading for this chapter will be found after Chapter 5.

5

Factors affecting drug metabolism: external factors

In the previous chapter, it has been shown how physiological and pathological factors can affect drug metabolism and how these factors vary in importance. There are, however, factors outside the body that can also have a profound influence on drug metabolism. The body can be exposed to these factors by design (e.g. substances taken as food, alcohol and tobacco smoke) or by accident (air, water and food contaminants or pollutants). The first group will be referred to as dietary factors and the second group as environmental factors. The substances to be examined under each heading are listed in Table 5.1.

Table 5.1

Dietary factors	Environmental factors
Protein	Petroleum products
Fat	Pyrolysis products
Carbohydrate	Heavy metals
Vitamins	Insecticides, herbicides
Trace elements	Industrial pollutants
Essential elements	
Pyrolysis products	
Tobacco smoke	
Alcohol	

5.1 Dietary factors

In discussing dietary factors, the influence of the staple diet on drug metabolism will first be discussed: that is, the effects of changes in the major dietary components (protein, fat and carbohydrates).

5.1.1 PROTEIN

The normal proportion of protein in an animal's diet is about 20%; animals kept on a diet containing this amount of protein show normal development of drug-metabolizing enzymes. If, however, rats are fed on a 5% protein (casein) diet then oxidative drug-metabolizing capacity decreases (Table 5.2). The decrease in drug metabolism is partially due to decreases in overall microsomal protein and partially to specific effects on the enzymes still remaining. Elegant work by Campbell *et al.*, using isolated mixed-function oxidase component (cytochrome *P*-450, reductase and phospholipid) in cross-over experiments, has indicated that it is a fault in the protein components and not the lipid component that is responsible for the decrease in drug metabolism.

Table **5.2** The effect of feeding a 5% and 20% casein diet on the hepatic ethylmorphine *N*-demethylase activity in the rat

	Enzyme activity (nmoles HCHO per 100 g bw per 10 mins)
Control (20% casein)	10.5
5% Casein (4 days)	6.0
5% Casein (8 days)	< 1.0

The interaction between the cytochrome *P*-450 and the reductase appears to be the key to this effect. Re-feeding a 20% protein diet reverses the effects of the 5% protein diet, indicating that this is not an irreversible effect.

A correlation with this *in vitro* effect has been found *in vivo*, where a low protein diet delayed the clearance of phenobarbitone from rats. In many other cases, however, little correlation has been seen between the effects of protein on microsomal metabolism of a drug and the effect of the drug *in vivo*. One example of this is the hepatotoxicity of aflatoxin, the toxicity of which depends on phase I metabolism forming an epoxide. Both phenobarbitone treatment (an inducer of phase I metabolism) and low protein diet (an inhibitor of phase I metabolism) decrease production of the epoxide and thus reduce the hepato-toxicity of aflatoxin. A number of possible explanations for this have been put forward such that the metabolism measured *in vitro* at saturating sub-strate concentrations does not necessarily reflect the *in vivo* metabolism at lower concentrations, or that the rate-limiting step for epoxide appearance/ hepatotoxicity may not be epoxide formation – it may be epoxide disappearance, for instance. These possibilities must be taken into account when dealing with correlations of *in vitro* and *in vivo* data (for further discussion of this point see Chapter 7).

Contrary to the effect of protein deficiency on oxidative drug metabolism, the same treatment causes an increase in glucuronide conjugation of some substrates, notably 4-nitrophenol and 2-aminophenol.

5.1.2 FAT

Lipids are required by the drug-metabolizing enzymes as membrane components and, possibly, for specific interactions. It is thought that phosphatidylcholine (an acidic lipid component of endoplasmic reticulum) is needed for metabolism of ethylmorphine and hexobarbitone. Phenobarbitone induction of hepatic drug metabolism is also associated with marked increases in microsomal phospholipids – a causal relationship? Lipids can also act as inhibitors of drug metabolism; steroids and fatty acids may bind to cytochrome *P*-450 and act as competitive inhibitors.

What effect does dietary lipid have on these phenomena? It was found that diets deficient in the essential fatty acids, notably linoleic acid, caused a reduction in the metabolism of ethylmorphine and hexobarbitone, and that subsequent addition of corn oil (containing linoleic acid) to the diet could reverse this effect. It is linoleic acid and arachidonic acid that seem to be particularly important in the control of drug metabolism. Treatment with corn oil or polyunsaturated fatty acids, for instance, increases microsomal content of these fatty acids and also increases drug-metabolizing capacity.

Various explanations of these effects have been put forward such as the theory that essential fatty acids are needed for the interaction of substrate with the active site of cytochrome *P*-450, the essential fatty acids in this case being incorporated into phospholipids. No consistent effects of deprivation of, or supplementation with, essential fatty acids on substrate binding to cytochrome *P*-450 (either for type I or II substrates) has been seen. An effect mediated via a direct effect on the amount of cytochrome *P*-450 has also been postulated, as deficiencies in essential fatty acids lead to decreased concentrations of cytochrome *P*-450 in some instances (see Figure 5.1).

One dietary aspect of lipids not yet discussed is the influence of co-factors needed for methylation of phospholipids – the lipotropes. The major phospholipid in liver microsomes is phosphatidylcholine; this is biosynthesized from phosphatidylethanolamine using the enzyme, phosphatidylethanolamine-*N*-methyltransferase and the co-factor, *S*-adenosylmethionine (SAM) (Figure 5.2).

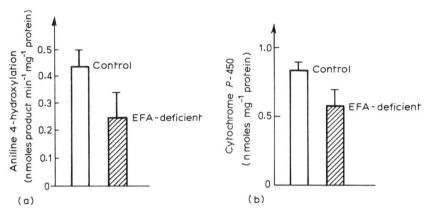

Figure 5.1 The effect of essential fatty acid (EFA) deficiency on (a) aniline 4-hydroxy-
lation and (b) cytochrome P-450 levels in liver. (From Kaschnitz, R. (1970)
Hoppe-Seyler's Z. Physiol. Chem., **351**, 771–4. Used with permission of the
author and Walter de Gruyter and Co.)

SAM is synthesized from L-methionine and ATP. Inhibition of this system leads
to deficiencies in transport of liver triglycerides and thus triglycerides build up
in the liver (a condition referred to as 'fatty liver'). Lack of L-methionine in the
diet, therefore, leads to 'fatty liver'. A markedly reduced capacity of the liver to
metabolize aflatoxin B_1 (a hepatocarcinogen) has been shown to be associated with 'fatty liver' induced in this way as has the reduced metabolism of
monocrotaline (a hepatotoxin).

In this context, choline deficiency has also been shown to decrease drug
metabolism: this decrease is paralleled by decreases of phosphatidylcholine in
liver microsomes. The overall impression of the influence of dietary fat on drug
metabolism is that anything that can affect the amount or fatty acid composition of hepatic microsomal phosphatidylcholine can affect the capacity
of the liver to metabolize drugs. Increases in phosphatidylcholine or unsaturated fatty acid content of phosphatidylcholine tend to increase drug
metabolism.

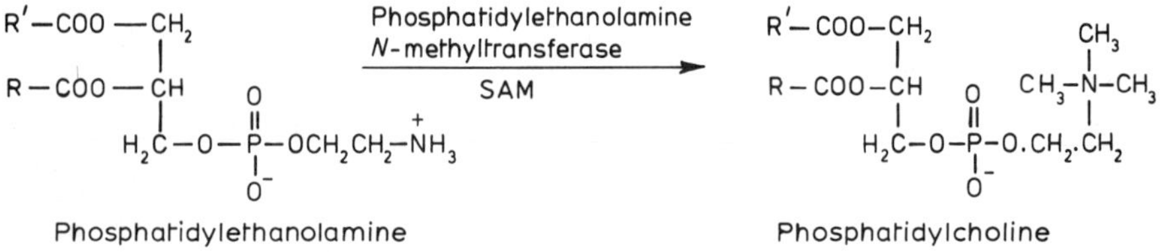

Figure 5.2 The final steps in the biosynthesis of phosphatidylcholine.

5.1.3 CARBOHYDRATE

Carbohydrates seem to have few effects on drug metabolism although high intake of glucose, particularly, can inhibit barbiturate metabolism and, thus, lengthen sleeping time. Glucose excess has also been shown to decrease hepatic cytochrome *P*-450 content and to lower biphenyl-4-hydroxylase activity.

It has been suggested that carbohydrate manipulations are effective by more diverse effects on intermediary metabolism and hormone balance, and not by a direct effect on the liver.

Although examples have been given of the effects of protein, fat and carbohydrate on drug metabolism, it is clear from the literature that the individual influence of these macronutrients is difficult to assess as each influences the use of the other and, thus, an effect of one component may be due to changes it caused in another. This may be illustrated by looking at one particular aspect of diet, starvation. Starvation of female rats caused marked rises in some enzyme activities (contrast this with the effect of isocaloric protein deficiency) while having little effect on other activities (Table 5.3).

Table 5.3 The effects of starvation on drug metabolism in rats

Enzyme	Change (%) after starvation
Aminopyrine *N*-demethylase	+114
4-Nitroanisole *O*-demethylase	+90
Aniline 4-hydroxylation	+94
Zoxazolamine hydroxylation	+15
Dichlorophenolindophenol reductase	+7

(Data from various sources: see Section 5.4.)

It would appear that starvation can actually induce the synthesis of microsomal proteins in contrast to the marked loss of protein from the liver as a whole. This effect may be specific for the rat as starvation of both mice and guinea pigs causes a marked decrease in drug-metabolizing capacity. In the latter cases it was oxidative metabolism that was affected most and the effects were said to be due to reduction of the NADPH/NADP ratio, so reducing the availability of the co-factor for oxidative metabolism. Thus changes in macronutrients can markedly effect the drug-metabolizing capacity of the liver.

Apart from the above mentioned macronutrients there are many other components of the diet that can affect drug metabolism. The most noticeable of these are the so-called micronutrients: vitamins and minerals. These will be considered separately. Of the many vitamins, those of the A, B, C and E groups will be mentioned; and, of the minerals, calcium, magnesium, iron and various trace elements will be particularly covered. All these have been shown to have some effects on drug metabolsim.

5.1.4 VITAMINS

Vitamins are an essential part of the diet and are needed for the synthesis of proteins and lipids, both of which are vital components of the drug-metabolizing enzyme system. It is, therefore, not surprising that changes in vitamin levels, particularly deficiencies, cause changes in drug-metabolizing capacity. The vitamins indicated to be involved in drug metabolism are listed in Table 5.4.

Table 5.4 Vitamins affecting drug metabolism

Vitamin A
Vitamin B group
niacin
riboflavin
thiamine
Vitamin C
Vitamin E

(a) VITAMIN A

Vitamin A deficiency was found to decrease drug metabolism. For example, it was seen that rats fed a vitamin A-free diet had lower levels than the control of aniline 4-hydroxylase and aminopyrine N-demethylase. This was shown to be related to reduced cytochrome P-450 levels. It was suggested that vitamin A deficiency affects the structure of the membrane and not protein synthesis. How this fits with the decrease in the protein, cytochrome P-450, is not explained.

(b) NIACIN (NICOTINIC ACID)

Niacin is a precursor of the co-factors, nicotinamide adenine dinucleotide phosphate (NADPH), which is the electron donor for oxidative drug metabolism, and NAD, which is required for the oxidation of UDP–glucose to UDP–glucuronic acid (for use in glucuronidation). Thus, it should not be surprising that deficiencies in this vitamin can cause alterations in drug-metabolizing capacity. Little work has, however, been done on this subject and no relationship to drug metabolism has been seen.

(c) RIBOFLAVIN (VITAMIN B_2)

Riboflavin is an essential component in the flavoprotein NADPH–cytochrome P-450-reductase, which is itself a component of the mixed-function oxidase

Table 5.5 The effect of riboflavin deficiency on hepatic drug
metabolism

Activity	% vs control
Aminopyrine N-demethylase	$124 \pm 15^{\dagger}$
Aniline 4-hydroxylase	152 ± 15
4-Nitrophenol glucuronyltransferase	74 ± 11
2-Aminophenol glucuronyltransferase	159 ± 80

[†]mean $\pm$ (standard deviation)

system. A deficiency of riboflavin, therefore, would be expected to reduce
NADPH–cytochrome P-450 reductase content and thus decrease drug-
metabolizing capacity. This expectation was justified by the reduced azo-
reduction of 4-dimethylaminoazobenzene in vitamin-B_2-deficient rats.

In fact, hepatic azo-reductase activity dropped 85–90% when rats were
maintained on a low riboflavin diet – a dramatic effect. The hepatic azo-
reductase is a flavoprotein enzyme.

In contrast to this study, however, other reports indicate that riboflavin
deficiency can enhance drug-metabolizing capacity. Oxidation of aminopyrine and aniline increases in riboflavin deficiency whereas the effects
on glucuronidation were variable (Table 5.5). It was suggested that disappearance of a flavin-like inhibitor caused the increase in oxidative
activity.

Thus it seems that riboflavin deficiency reduces drug metabolism related to
flavoproteins but increases that related to cytochrome P-450 oxidative
metabolism.

(d) THIAMINE (VITAMIN B_1)

Thiamine is not directly involved in drug metabolism but is essential for
carbohydrate metabolism. Despite the apparent lack of connection to drug
metabolism, thiamine does affect the capacity of the liver to metabolize drugs.

Thiamine deficiency has been shown to increase the metabolism of aniline
and reduce hexobarbitone metabolism. Excess thiamine inhibits aniline and
ethylmorphine metabolism.

The effect of thiamine is related to changes in the microsomal cytochromes
(P-450 and b_5) and NADPH–cytochrome P-450 reductase levels. The effects
were not similar to starvation although it was suggested that the effects of
thiamine were mediated via a reduction in blood glucose. More recently
thiamine has been found to change the type of cytochrome P-450 present and
this could account for the effects seen.

(e) VITAMIN C

Of the animal species studied in terms of drug metabolism, only Man, monkey and guinea pig show a nutritional requirement for vitamin C and, thus, only these animals have been used in the study of vitamin C's effects on drug metabolism.

Vitamin C deficiency has been well studied following the early observation that guinea pigs deficient in the vitamin were more sensitive to the effects of pentobarbitone and procaine. As would be expected from this increased sensitivity, vitamin C deficiency causes marked reductions in drug-metabolizing capacity (see Table 5.6).

Table 5.6 The effect of vitamin C deficiency on hepatic drug metabolism in the guinea pig

	Control	Vitamin C deficient	
Aniline 4-hydroxylase[†]	1.6 ± 0.2	0.8 ± 0.2	***
Aminopyrine N-demethylase	3.9 ± 0.1	1.7 ± 0.3	***
4-Nitroanisole O-demethylase	3.2 ± 0.4	1.1 ± 0.2	***
Cytochrome P-450[‡]	0.5 ± 0.1	0.3 ± 0.03	**
Cytochrome b_5	0.03 ± 0.004	0.02 ± 0.006	*

[†]results expressed as μmoles product per hour per 100 mg protein
[‡]expressed as nmoles mg^{-1} protein
All results: mean ± (standard error); * = $p < 0.05$; ** = $p < 0.01$; *** = $p < 0.001$.
(From V. G. Zannoni, 1978; used with permission.)

Addition of vitamin C to *in vitro* incubations did not reverse the effects of the deficiency, indicating that vitamin C is not directly involved in drug metabolism. Reduced levels of cytochrome P-450 have been detected in vitamin C-deficient animals and abnormal binding spectra have been seen, the binding spectra could be returned to normal using ascorbyl palmitate (the fatty acid derivative of vitamin C). It may, thus, be that vitamin C is involved in the maintenance of the membrane structure of the endoplasmic reticulum.

There is also evidence to suggest that vitamin C is involved in the biosynthesis of haem and thus directly in the synthesis of the microsomal cytochromes. This gives another possible reason for vitamin C's requirement in drug metabolism. Neither of these proposed mechanisms of action of vitamin C have been proved as yet but it is certain that the vitamin is an essential dietary component for the maintenance of drug metabolism.

(f) VITAMIN E

Deficiencies of vitamin E reduce drug-metabolizing capacity when assayed with a variety of substrates but, again, as with the other vitamin deficiencies no definite biochemical reasons can be put forward. Two interesting theories have been advanced. The first states that vitamin E is required for haem biosynthesis notably for the function of the enzyme δ-aminolaevulinic acid dehydratase, and, indeed, microsomal cytochrome P-450 does fall during vitamin E deficiency. The second theory is based on the proposed role of vitamin E in the body as an inhibitor of the oxidation of selenium-containing proteins (selenium can act instead of sulfur in some instances, a selenide group replacing the sulfhydryl group). It was speculated that a non-haem iron protein (similar to ferredoxin but containing selenium instead of sulfur) may be involved in microsomal drug oxidation although no such requirement for a non-haem iron protein has been seen. Evidence for this theory comes from the observation that phenobarbitone-induction of drug metabolism is accompanied by a large increase in selenium incorporation, an effect which is inhibited by vitamin E deficiency. Phenobarbitone, however, affects many more enzymes than those involved in drug metabolism, and the effect noted above may be related to one of those.

Vitamins of the A, B, C and E class are, therefore, not only dietary requirements for good health but also for the maintenance of normal levels of drug metabolism. Both excesses and deficiencies of these vitamins can cause marked alterations in the way in which the body handles drugs. The significance of this to clinical practice in the malnourished, for example, is obvious.

5.1.5 MINERALS

Minerals are the metallic and non-metallic elements needed in the diet to maintain good health. Those which have been shown to affect drug metabolism are: iron, calcium, potassium, magnesium, zinc, copper, selenium and iodine.

The effects of mineral deficiency are shown in Table 5.7.

The effects of calcium deficiency take a long time to develop (40 days) but little information is available as to why these effects are seen.

Magnesium deficiency, often found in conjunction with calcium deficiency, gives a specific effect and is not related to decreased food intake or starvation effects. Various explanations for the effect of magnesium deficiency have been put forward. Decreases in NADPH–cytochrome P-450 reductase have been correlated to a reduced ability to metabolize drugs and decreased liver magnesium levels. In many studies, however, no decrease in liver magnesium levels is evident and alternative explanations are needed. One such explanation is found in the interaction of magnesium, thyroid hormones and phospholipids. Thyroid hormone levels are depressed in magnesium-depleted animals, a change that can lead to decreased drug metabolism (see Chapter 4).

Table 5.7 The effects of mineral deficiencies on hepatic drug metabolism

Mineral	Effect of deficiency on drug metabolism	Enzymes affected
Calcium	Decrease	Aminopyrine N-demethylase
	Decrease	Nitroreductase
	Decrease	Hexobarbitone oxidation
Magnesium	Decrease	Aniline 4-hydroxylation
	Decrease	Aminopyrine N-demethylase
	No change	Nitroreductase
	No change	Pentobarbitone oxidation
	Decrease	Cytochrome P-450
Iron	Increase	Hexobarbitone oxidation
	Increase	Aminopyrine N-demethylation
	Increase	Cytochrome b₅
	No change	Cytochrome P-450
	Increase/no change	Aniline 4-hydroxylation
	No change	Nitroreductase
	No change	Glucuronyltransferase
Potassium	No change	Aniline 4-hydroxylation
	No change	Aminopyrine N-demethylation
	No change	Nitroreductase
Copper	Decrease	Aniline 4-hydroxylation
	Increase	Benzo[a]pyrene hydroxylation
	Decrease	Hexobarbitone oxidation
	Decrease	Zoxazolamine 6-hydroxylation
Zinc	Decrease	Aminopyrine N-demethylase
	Decrease	Pentobarbitone oxidation
	Decrease	Cytochrome P-450
Selenium	No change	Ethylmorphine N-demethylase
	No change	Biphenyl 4-hydroxylase
	No change	Pentobarbitone oxidation
Iodine	Increase	Aminopyrine N-demethylase
	Increase	Hexobarbitone oxidation
	Increase	Benzo[a]pyrene hydroxylation
	Increase	Aniline 4-hydroxylation
	No change	Glucuronyltransferase

(Data from various sources; see Section 5.4.)

Magnesium-depleted diets also markedly reduce microsomal content of lyso-phosphatidylcholine and, to a lesser extent, phosphatidylcholine – an affect also associated with decreased drug-metabolizing capacity. The possibility that magnesium affects drug metabolism via thyroid hormones which act through an effect on phospholipid metabolism must be considered.

Potassium deficiency gives changes in the effect or half-life of a number of drugs (see Table 5.8). This has been found to be due to changes in renal clearance and not changes in drug metabolism (see Table 5.7).

Table 5.8 The effect of potassium deficiency on pentobarbitone sleeping time and antipyrine half-life in the rat

Diet	Pentobarbitone sleeping time (mins)	Antipyrine half-life (mins)
Control	90 ± 8	80 ± 4
K^+-deficient	142 ± 11*	122 ± 6*
K^+-deficient $+ K^+$	101 ± 12	90 ± 7

*$= p < 0.05$; mean $\pm$ (standard deviation)
(From Becking, G. C. (1978) Dietary minerals and drug metabolism. In *Nutrition and drug interrelationships* (eds J. M. Hathcock and J. Coon), Academic Press, New York. Used with permission.)

Iron deficiency is unusual in that it causes an increase in drug-metabolizing capacity (see Table 5.7); excess iron in the diet can also inhibit drug metabolism. Iron levels in liver are inversely correlated to NADPH-dependent lipid peroxidation. As increased lipid peroxidation has been associated with decreased drug metabolism, this may offer an explanation of the effects of iron. Iron deficiency limits the degree of lipid peroxidation and thus allows more expression of the drug-metabolizing enzymes. The active form of iron may be ferritin as ferritin added directly to microsomal incubations can inhibit aminopyrine and aniline metabolism. Iron-deficient diets markedly decrease intestinal drug metabolism, and this may be of greater pharmacological and toxicological importance considering the protective role of the intestinal enzymes, particularly against the procarcinogenic polycyclic hydrocarbons.

The effects of copper deficiency on drug metabolism are variable (see Table 5.7) and no concensus is evident on the mechanism of these effects. Alterations in NADPH–cytochrome *P*-450 reductase or binding of substrate to cytochrome *P*-450 have been put forward as possible mechanisms, but these do not explain all of the effects seen. One interesting effect of copper deficiency on drug metabolism is the toxicity of parathion. Parathion is normally metabolized to the toxic compound, paraoxon, or to the relatively non-toxic 4-nitrophenol. In copper-deficient mice, parathion is found to be more toxic than in normal mice due to a reduced ability to produce the non-toxic 4-nitrophenol, thus allowing more of the substance to be converted to paraoxon.

It is interesting to note that excess copper has the same effect as copper deficiency, i.e. a reduced ability to metabolize drugs in some cases. Thus an optimum level of dietary copper exists for the maintenance of drug metabolism in the body.

Zinc deficiency leads to reduced drug metabolism for some substrates but no effects on others (e.g. aniline and zoxazolamine hydroxylation). The effects were related to reduced cytochrome *P*-450 levels. The liver content of zinc and copper are intimately linked and it may be that the effects of changes in dietary zinc on drug metabolism are due to subsequent changes in hepatic copper content (as previously described). Zinc-deficient diets also lead to extreme poor health in the animals: the effects seen may be a function of this malnutrition.

Selenium, as an essential trace element, is linked to vitamin E; the effects of both on drug metabolism are closely linked (see Section 5.1.4). No direct effects of selenium deficiency on drug metabolism have been seen but a role for dietary selenium in the biosynthesis of microsomal components has been suggested. Selenium deficiency impairs the ability of the liver to respond to pheno-barbitone treatment. In the presence of selenium a 3.65-fold induction is seen but this falls to 2.64-fold in selenium-deficient animals. As with copper, an optimal level of selenium in the diet exists, with excessive selenium intake also being inhibitory in drug metabolism. The biochemical reasons behind the effects of selenium are unclear with some, but not all, of the effects being related to vitamin E.

Little work has been done on the effects of iodine deficiency other than to note that certain drug-metabolizing enzyme activities are affected. An effect mediated via thyroid hormones, which require iodine for their synthesis, was suggested but rejected due to the opposing effects seen (see Chapter 4).

It can thus be seen that many micronutrients in deficiency or in excess can have noticeable effects on drug metabolism. The whole subject of the inter-action of dietary components and drug metabolism can become extremely complex even if one only examines the nutritional elements in the diet. A summary of the effects of macro- and micro-nutrients is given in Figure 5.3.

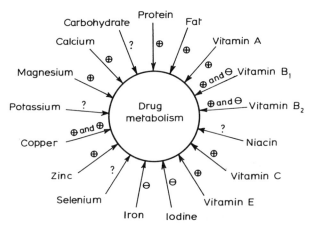

Figure 5.3 The effects of dietary nutrients on drug metabolism: a summary. Key: $\oplus$ = an increase in drug metabolism; $\ominus$ = a decrease in drug metabolism.

The importance of the effects of the factors discussed above on drug metabolism is greatest in conditions of deficiency and, thus, in cases of malnutrition. As this is particularly prevalent in Third World societies, it is here that these effects are mainly encountered.

5.1.6 NON-NUTRIENTS

When dealing with the effects of diet on drug metabolism, it must be remembered that food contains not only nutritional factors but also other chemical substances, and any examination of diet-related effects on drug metabolism should include studies on these substances. The most notable group of these substances naturally occurring in food are the pyrolysis products – chemicals formed by the cooking (literally burning) of the food.

The pyrolysis products that are formed in meat and fish, particularly when fried or charcoal-broiled, have recently been isolated as breakdown products of amino acids, mainly tryptophan. The structures of some of them are shown in Figure 5.4. All these compounds are known inducers of cytochrome *P*-448 (aryl hydrocarbon hydroxylase) and are also potential mutagens/carcinogens.

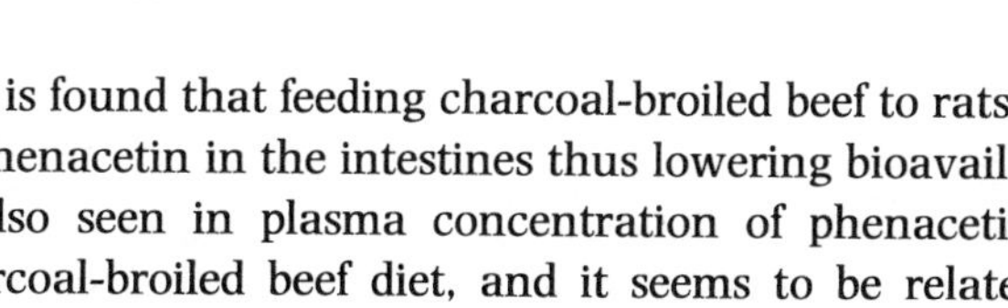

Figure 5.4 Tryptophan pyrolysis products found in fried or charcoal-broiled meat and fish.

It is found that feeding charcoal-broiled beef to rats induced the metabolism of phenacetin in the intestines thus lowering bioavailability of the drug. A fall is also seen in plasma concentration of phenacetin in humans fed on a charcoal-broiled beef diet, and it seems to be related to metabolism of the phenacetin. Further work has indicated that it is benzo[*a*]pyrene (a polycyclic hydrocarbon inducer of cytochrome *P*-450; see Chapter 3) in the charcoal-broiled beef that causes the effects seen. Recently these results have been extended to include the induction of antipyrine and theophylline metabolism in Man.

One other group of compounds which could also be considered in this category are the substances found in cabbages and brussels sprouts. These compounds are of the indole type (Figure 5.5) and are also enzyme inducers. The similarity to the tryptophan pyrolysis products is noticeable.

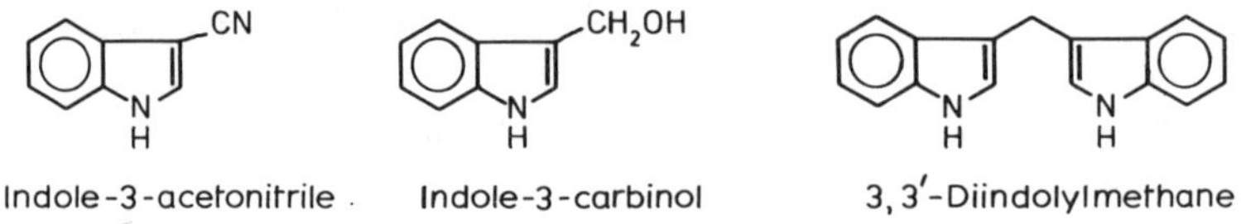

Figure 5.5 Indoles found in cabbage and brussels sprouts.

Dietary brussels sprouts and cabbage induce the hydroxylation of benzo[a]pyrene and hexobarbitone, the O-dealkylation of phenacetin (see above) and 7-ethoxycoumarin in the rat. Other vegetables not containing indoles did not induce drug metabolism. Studies in humans have shown a similar induction of phenacetin metabolism but also revealed apparent induction of antipyrine metabolism and paracetamol glucuronidation.

Thus, even non-nutrient components of food can have marked effects on drug metabolism. It is likely that more examples of the type illustrated above will be found and that induction and inhibition of drug metabolism by non-nutrient components of food is a common phenomenon.

5.1.7 TOBACCO SMOKING

Two other 'dietary' components can be considered: tobacco smoke and alcohol. The effects of alcohol have been discussed previously (see Chapter 4).

Tobacco smoking can be thought of as a different way of ingesting pyrolysis products (from the burning of the plant materials in tobacco) with the lungs the first site of interaction rather than the intestine as in the case of charcoal-broiled meat. The most common effect of tobacco smoking is an increase in biotransformation of drugs – an effect very similar to that seen for ingestion of charcoal-broiled meat. Indeed, there is a common factor: the polycyclic hydrocarbon, benzo[a]pyrene: this substance is found in both charcoal-broiled meat and tobacco smoke.

A marked effect on the plasma phenacetin level can be seen following tobacco smoking (cf. effect of charcoal-broiled meat on phenacetin plasma levels) (Table 5.9). The lower plasma level of phenacetin was due to increased metabolism either by the intestinal mucosa or 'first-pass' through the liver.

Another well-studied drug marker is antipyrine, the metabolism of which is directly related to its rate of excretion. Using antipyrine as a substrate, smoking was found to increase drug clearance and thus, by inference, the rate of metabolism of antipyrine. Stopping smoking returns the rate of metabolism of antipyrine to the pre-smoking level. The metabolism of a number of other drugs is affected by smoking whereas some have shown no change in metabolism following smoking; a summary of these is shown in Table 5.10. Thus tobacco smoking selectively induces the metabolism of some drugs.

Table 5.9 Mean plasma concentrations of phenacetin as a function of time in smokers and non-smokers

Time (h)	Phenacetin plasma concentration ($\mu g\,l^{-1}$)	
	Smokers	Non-smokers
1	0.35	0.8
2	0.45	2.25
3.5	0.1	0.4
5	0.05	0.15

(From Pantuck, E. J. *et al.* (1972) *Science*, **175**, 1248–50. Used with permission of the author and the American Association for the Advancement of Science. © 1972 AAAS.)

Table 5.10 The effect of tobacco smoking on the metabolism of drugs

Affected (increased)	Not affected
Nicotine	Diazepam
Theophylline	Phenytoin
Imipramine	Warfarin
Pentazocine	Nortriptyline

Tobacco smoke contains at least 3000 different chemicals, some of which are known enzyme inducers (such as the polycyclic hydrocarbons discussed above) and some known enzyme inhibitors (e.g. carbon monoxide, hydrogen cyanide). From the results obtained it is the induction effects of tobacco smoke that are prevalent. Animal experiments have indicated that the great majority, if not all, of the effects of tobacco smoking can be mimicked by treatment with benzo[*a*]pyeine (see Chapter 3). It, thus, seems likely that the major effects of tobacco smoking are due to induction of drug metabolism by benzo[*a*]pyrene and other such compounds.

Marihuana smoking produces identical effects to tobacco smoking and cannot be looked upon as a 'safer' habit in this respect.

A summary of the effects of the non-nutrient components of the diet on drug metabolism is given in Figure 5.6. It should be remembered that there are many more dietary non-nutrients such as colorants, anti-oxidants, flavourings which could also influence drug metabolism. Space limitations, however, restrict our coverage of this extensive subject.

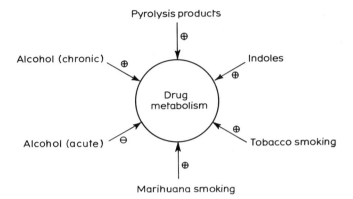

Figure 5.6 The influence of dietary non-nutrients on drug metabolism: a summary. Key: $\oplus$ = an increase in drug metabolism; $\ominus$ = a decrease in drug metabolism.

5.2 Environmental factors

Environmental factors are those influences in our surroundings that can affect drug metabolism; no conscious act is required to be influenced by them (cf. dietary factors). The environment is replete with substances which can affect drug metabolism, and those to be considered in this section are:

Heavy metals: lead, mercury, cadmium.
Industrial pollutants: tetrachlorodibenzodioxin (TCDD), solvents, polychlorinated biphenyls (PCBs).
Insecticides, herbicides: DDT, parathion, mirex.

Reviewers have different views concerning what constitutes an environmental factor and many include dietary factors in this category. One should not be confused by these differences in nomenclature. It should also be realized that there are a large number of environmental chemicals that could potentially affect drug metabolism; the representative examples of a number of groups of compounds discussed here are only a small part of this.

5.2.1 HEAVY METALS

Exposure of the human population to heavy metals can be related to occupation, diet (such as cadmium in vegetables) or other phenomena (e.g. lead in exhaust from petrol-driven vehicles). Most exposure is low level and long term and so cumulative exposure becomes important. These facts are rarely taken into account when examining heavy metal effects on drug metabolism in experimental animals.

Chronic exposure of rats to lead in the diet has little effect on drug-metabolizing capacity but does induce cytochrome *P*-450 levels. The increased level of cytochrome *P*-450 indicates that lead induces a form of enzyme that does not metabolize any of the substrates used; different substrates may show induction of drug-metabolizing capacity. Acute lead toxicity in rats is associated with reduced drug-metabolizing capacity. The situation found in human subjects was similar but only young children exhibited the inhibition of drug metabolism during acute lead toxicity. No measurement of cytochrome *P*-450 in humans was performed; thus, the possible induction of this enzyme by chronic lead exposure is still open to investigation.

Two possible explanations for the effect of acute lead exposure on drug metabolism have been put forward. If lead is added to incubations of microsomes the activity of NADPH–cytochrome *P*-450 reductase is inhibited and this could lead to inhibition of drug metabolism with certain substrates. Lead has also been shown to inhibit one of the enzymes involved in the synthesis of haem, δ-aminolaevulinic acid dehydratase, and thus could inhibit the production of the haem moiety in cytochrome *P*-450.

Little work has been done on mercury's effects on drug metabolism; what has been done has used excessively high doses of this toxic metal. Inorganic forms of mercury (Hg^{2+}) seem to induce drug metabolism (although the compound administered was mercuric acetate and the effect of the acetate ion was not investigated) whereas organic mercury (methylmercury) inhibits drug metabolism after chronic administration. No explanations for the effects of mercury were found.

The great majority of the work published on the interaction of heavy metals with drug metabolism has been done with cadmium. This is an industrial pollutant in the manufacture of a number of metals including zinc, and is a dietary pollutant in vegetables grown in cadmium-rich soil.

High intake of cadmium has been shown to be associated with inhibitions of drug-metabolizing enzymes. In the rat, however, an interesting sexual dimorphism of the effect has been seen (Table 5.11). The male rat responds to cadmium treatment with marked inhibition of all enzyme activities studied and a concomitant decrease in cytochrome *P*-450 levels. The female rat, on the other hand, shows no reduction in cytochrome *P*-450 levels and, indeed, marked induction of diazepam metabolism.

A hormonal control of cadmium sensitivity similar to that of drug metabolism in general (see Section 4.6) was found to operate: i.e. removal of androgens from the male by castration removed their sensitivity to cadmium.

Cadmium was shown to have many effects on the various components of the drug-metabolizing enzyme system. Cytochrome *P*-450 and cytochrome b_5 levels were reduced, and cytochrome *P*-450 could be converted to the inactive

Table 5.11 The effect of cadmium on hepatic drug metabolism in male and female rats

Enzyme	Change (%) in enzyme activities caused by cadmium	
	Male	Female
Diazepam 3-hydroxylase	− 58	+ 65
Diazepam N-demethylase	− 55	+ 66
Imipramine 2-hydroxylase	− 33	+ 9
Imipramine N-demethylase	− 55	− 4
Imipramine N-oxidase	− 60	+ 7
Cytochrome P-450	− 25	+ 3

cytochrome P-420 *in vitro*. The former effect seems to be due to cadmium's ability to induce haem oxygenase activity (the enzyme that breaks down the cytochromes P-450 and b_5). The fact that only males respond to cadmium with marked inhibition of drug metabolism suggests that the cadmium-sensitive cytochrome P-450 (or b_5) is sex-related. The alternative explanation that cadmium exerts its effects by reducing androgen levels does not hold, as androgen-replacement therapy cannot reverse the effects of cadmium although it is known that cadmium causes massive testicular damage and does drastically reduce plasma testosterone levels (Table 5.12).

So cadmium not only reduces plasma testosterone levels but also makes the liver non-responsive to androgens. Little work has been done on the inducing ability of cadmium in the female rat although it has been suggested that the female is less sensitive to the toxic effects of cadmium by virtue of having a cadmium-binding protein which takes up the metal and prevents it being toxic.

Heavy metals can, therefore, induce and/or inhibit drug metabolism depending on the species and sex of animal and substrate studied. The relevance of this animal data to the environmentally encountered low-level, long-term exposure

Table 5.12 The effect of cadmium and testosterone treatment on hepatic drug metabolism in the male rat

Parameter	+ Cd (% vs control)	+ Cd + testosterone (% vs control)
Cytochrome P-450	82	71
Diazepam 3-hydroxylase	75	72
Diazepam N-demethylase	64	66
Lignocaine 3-hydroxylase	292	229
Lignocaine N-de-ethylase	69	53
Plasma testosterone	17	78

is debatable and much more work is needed to be done to ascertain the effects of environmental exposure to these metals.

5.2.2 INDUSTRIAL POLLUTANTS

There are literally thousands of industrial pollutants that, in experimental animals, have been shown to affect drug metabolism; the toxicological literature is full of such examples (see Section 5.4). Three important and well-studied industrial pollutants will be discussed in detail to illustrate the general principles; these are: 2,3,7,8-tetrachlorodibenzo-*p*-dioxin (TCCD), industrial solvents of the benzene and chlorinated hydrocarbon types, and poly-chlorinated biphenyls (PCBs).

(a) TCDD

TCDD is a polycyclic compound (Figure 5.7) with a rigid planar structure. It is a precursor for a number of herbicides and was the toxin released in the Seveso incident in Italy recently, causing widespread chloracne and fears for the future welfare of the population exposed to the chemical.

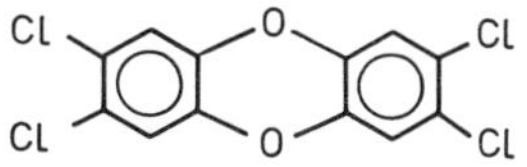

2,3,7,8-Tetrachlorodibenzo-*p*-dioxin (TCDD)

Figure 5.7 The structure of TCDD.

TCDD causes marked induction of the metabolism of polycyclic hydrocarbons and of the enzymes, UDP–glucuronyltransferase, δ-aminolaevulinic acid synthetase and ligandin; it thus can affect both phase I and II metabolism. The mechanism of action of TCDD in inducing aryl hydrocarbon hydroxylase has been particularly studied. It appears that TCDD has a specific high-affinity, low-capacity binding site in the liver cytosol (a classical receptor similar to that for the steroid hormones). Once bound to the receptor, TCDD is taken to the nucleus where it interacts with DNA and, thus, gives its induction effects (Figure 5.8). This is very similar to the activation of the 'Ah locus' and is probably the same system (see Chapter 3).

(b) SOLVENTS

Solvents are in very widespread use in industry (and in the home). Serious concern is now being expressed about their effects on the body. The two groups

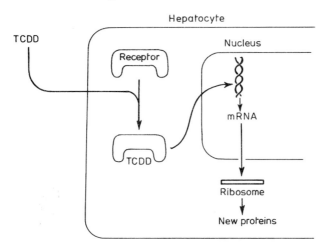

Figure 5.8 Proposed scheme for the induction of hepatic enzymes by TCDD.

of solvents of most interest in the study of drug metabolism are the benzene derivates (benzene, toluene and xylenes) and the chlorinated hydrocarbons (chloroform, trichloroethylene, dichloromethane).

The aromatic hydrocarbons (Figure 5.9) have been shown to induce cytochrome P-450-dependent enzymes in the liver but have little effect on conjugation with glucuronic acid except after long-term exposure when induction is also seen. As human exposure to these solvents is mainly by inhalation, experiments in animals tend to be inhalation experiments as well. Levels of solvent around the maximum allowed in industrial atmospheres are used so that an extrapolation of the data to Man can be attempted; species differences have, however, to be taken into account here.

Xylene has also been shown to be an inducer of cytochrome P-450 when administered by inhalation. Use of the individual components of the xylene mixture indicating that p-xylene (1,4-dimethylbenzene) was less active than the other isomers. The increases in ethoxyresorufin O-de-ethylase, n-hexane and benzo[a]pyrene hydroxylase activities were matched by elevated cytochrome P-450 levels (Table 5.13).

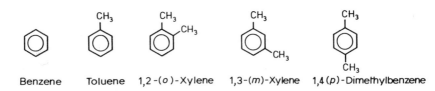

Benzene   Toluene   1,2-(o)-Xylene   1,3-(m)-Xylene   1,4(p)-Dimethylbenzene

Figure 5.9 The structure of some aromatic hydrocarbons.

Table 5.13 The effects of xylene and xylene isomers on hepatic drug metabolism in the rat

	Cytochrome P-450	7-Ethoxyresorufin O-de-ethylase	n-Hexane 2-oxidation	Benzo[a]pyrene 4,5-hydroxylation
Xylene	190*	350*	480*	1000*
o-Xylene	175*	420*	820*	620*
m-Xylene	180*	370*	650*	1200*
p-Xylene	130*	150	450	450*

Results expressed as % vs control
* $= p < 0.05$
(Data from Toftgård, R. and Nilsen, O. (1982) *Toxicology*, **23**, 197–212. Used with permission of the authors and Elsevier Biomedical Press B.V.)

Drug metabolizing activity was also induced in the kidney of these animals but, in the lung, xylene caused an inhibition of some enzymes. The overall effect on the body, however, was an increase in drug-metabolizing capacity by induction of cytochrome P-450 and, possibly, NADPH–cytochrome P-450 reductase activity. The induction was similar to that found for phenobarbitone (see Chapter 3).

The aromatic hydrocarbons, therefore, are phenobarbitone-like inducers of drug metabolism and are active by inhalation thus indicating that workers in industries using such solvents (e.g. paint industry) may have induced drug metabolism as a result of solvent exposure.

The chlorinated hydrocarbons, in contrast to the aromatic hydrocarbons discussed above, do not always show induction of drug metabolism. For example, trichloroethylene, when given chronically to rats, causes an increase in NADPH–cytochrome P-450 reductase but a decrease in cytochrome P-450 with concomitant increase in aniline 4-hydroxylation and decrease in ethylmorphine N-demethylase. An increase in 4-nitrophenol glucuronidation was also seen. Some of these effects can be explained in terms of a direct effect of trichloroethylene on the liver enzymes. Trichloroethylene competitively inhibits the metabolism of ethylmorphine when added into microsomal incubations and activates glucuronyltransferase activity *in vitro*. The increase in aniline 4-hydroxylation is thought to be due to induction of specific forms of cytochrome P-450, whereas overall cytochrome P-450 levels fall. Trichloroethylene is, therefore, an unusual compound in that it simultaneously activates, inhibits, induces and destroys various drug-metabolizing enzyme activities.

Chloroform elicits similar effects to trichloroethylene particularly with regard to the destruction of cytochrome P-450, but dichloromethane, a close relative of chloroform, when administered to rats by inhalation only caused induction of drug metabolism. There seemed to be a dose-dependent induction of a number of enzyme activities, notably biphenyl 2-hydroxylation.

Chlorinated hydrocarbons can, thus, give induction of drug metabolism as the aromatic hydrocarbons, but can also cause destruction of cytochrome *P*-450.

The ease of exposure to solvents (trichloroethylene is the solvent used for dry-cleaning and cleaning fluids; toluene is the solvent in some adhesives) means that many people are subjected to the effects noted above, and this should be considered as a severe environmental problem.

(c) POLYCHLORINATED BIPHENYLS (PCBs)

The polychlorinated biphenyls (PCBs) are a large group of compounds used in various manufacturing industries. Structurally the compounds can be split into two distinct groups: the planar and non-planar types (Figure 5.10).

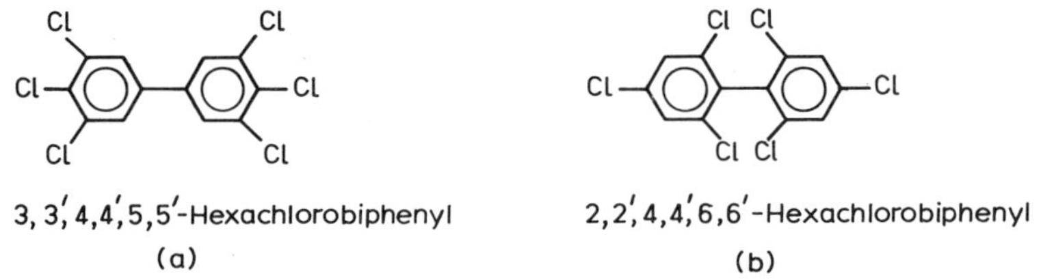

3, 3', 4,4', 5,5'-Hexachlorobiphenyl   2,2', 4,4', 6,6'-Hexachlorobiphenyl
             (a)   (b)

Figure 5.10 The structures of (a) planar and (b) non-planar polychlorinated biphenyls.

The 3,4,5-chloro-derivatives are planar whereas steric hinderance keeps the rings in the 2,4,6-chloro-derivatives at right angles to each other. These two groups of compound have different effects on drug metabolism. The planar PCBs induce hepatic drug metabolism similar to the polycyclic hydrocarbons whereas the non-planar PCBs exhibit induction of drug metabolism of the phenobarbitone type.

A mixture of PCBs (called Clophen A-50) induced cytochrome *P*-450, NADPH–cytochrome *P*-450 reductase, 4-nitroanisole *O*-demethylase, epoxide hydratase and UDP–glucuronyltransferase activities in rats within 1 week of the start of treatment. The overall induction pattern is typical of a mixed type of induction (probably due to both planar and non-planar isomers being present in the mixture). The point of interest is that a single dose of PCBs can maintain the induced level of enzymes for at least 1 month indicating that these substances persist for long periods of time in the body.

5.2.3 PESTICIDES

Pesticides of various types are prevalent environmental contaminants in air, water and food. Again, there are many different chemical types of herbicides, insecticides, etc.; only a few will be discussed here with respect to their effects on drug metabolism. The compounds to be discussed are: mirex, kepone, malathion, parathion, DDT.

Mirex and kepone are structurally similar insecticides. The effects of these compounds on drug-metabolizing capacity of rats is shown in Table 5.14. There is an indication that both of these compounds are specific inducing agents differing from each other and from the classical enzyme inducers, phenobarbitone and 3-methylcholanthrene. A novel induction profile for mirex and kepone is further substantiated by the evidence of the absorption maximum of the CO-treated cytochrome P-450 being at 449 nm (cf. 448 nm for 3-methylcholanthrene induction and 450 nm for phenobarbitone induction).

Malathion and parathion are well-known, phosphothionate-type insecticides which are converted *in vivo* and *in vitro* to the corresponding phosphates, malaoxon and paraoxon. These insecticides are inhibitors of drug metabolism both *in vivo* and *in vitro* probably due to competitive inhibition of cytochrome P-450-dependent reaction which also metabolizes the insecticides.

DDT causes induction of many drug-metabolizing enzymes but generally only affects phase I metabolism of drugs.

Pesticides can, therefore, be inducers or inhibitors of drug metabolism. Their widespread use and persistence in the body make them potentially important in determining drug metabolism both in Man and in wild and domestic animals.

5.3 Relative importance of physiological and environmental factors in determining drug-metabolizing capacity in the human population

As has been seen in the last two chapters there are numerous factors that can affect the way in which the body handles drugs, varying from the genetic make-up of the person to how much tea or coffee they drink. Attempts have been made to ascertain how much of the (sometimes quite large) inter-individual variations in drug metabolism are due to genetic differences and how much to environmental factors. Two opposing views – almost diametrically opposite to each other – have been put forward. The twin and family studies discussed earlier (see Section 4.3) seem to show that most, if not all, of the differences in drug metabolism in the population are due to genetic differences. Other research has indicated, by statistical analysis of family groups, that all of the inter-individual variations can be accounted for by environmental factors (alcohol, tea and coffee consumption and tobacco smoking) although the sex of the person has been included as an environmental factor.

Genetic sub-populations with respect to drug metabolism certainly exist (e.g.

Table 5.14 Effects of mirex, kepone, 3-methylcholanthrene and phenobarbitone on hepatic drug metabolism

Inducing agent	Cytochrome P-450 (nmoles mg^{-1} protein)	Biphenyl 4-hydroxylation (nmoles product min^{-1} mg^{-1} protein)	Biphenyl 2-hydroxylation (pmoles product min^{-1} mg^{-1} protein)	s-Warfarin 6-hydroxylation (pmoles product min^{-1} mg^{-1} protein)
Control	1.07 ± 0.01	0.54 ± 0.02	39 ± 2	0.13 ± 0.02
Mirex	$1.77 \pm 0.21^{**}$	0.56 ± 0.01	$66 \pm 1^{***}$	$0.23 \pm 0.02^{**}$
Kepone	$1.95 \pm 0.05^{**}$	0.55 ± 0.06	$56 \pm 14^{*}$	0.08 ± 0.02
3-MC	$1.98 \pm 0.17^{**}$	0.61 ± 0.03	$232 \pm 6^{***}$	$0.18 \pm 0.01^{**}$
PB				0.07 ± 0.01

Results expressed as: mean $\pm$ (standard error); $* = p < 0.05$; $** = p < 0.01$; $*** = p < 0.001$.
(From Kaminsky, L. S. *et al.* (1978) *Tox. Appl. Pharm.*, **43**, 327–38. Used with permission of Academic Press.)

isoniazid 'fast' and 'slow' acetylators, and debrisoquine 'poor' and 'extensive' metabolizers) and so a genetic component of control of drug metabolism cannot be denied. The influence of environmental factors, on top of these obvious genetic differences, then leads to the inter-individual differences seen in the general population. The different groups probably pick up different influences by virtue of different substrates used, different experimental procedures and methods of statistical analysis. Antipyrine metabolism, for instance, may be mainly controlled by environmental factors, while debrisoquine is mainly genetically controlled.

The control of drug metabolism is, thus, an extremely complex subject with many factors, some of which are interactive. A comprehensive summary of the subject is impossible but it is hoped that this chapter, together with Chapter 4, has given some idea of the factors involved and has stimulated the reader into further examination of one or more aspects of the subject, to which end a further reading list is included at the end of the chapter.

5.4 Further reading

TEXTBOOKS AND SYMPOSIA

Calabrese, E. J. (1981) *Nutrition and environmental health. The influence of nutritional status in pollutant toxicity and carcinogenicity*, Vols. I and II, Wiley, London.
Coon, M. J. *et al.* (eds) (1980) *Microsomes, drug oxidations and chemical carcinogensis*, Vols. I and II, Academic Press, New York.
Estabrook, R. W., Gillette, J. R. and Liebman, K. C. (eds) (1972) *Microsomes and drug oxidations*, Williams and Wilkins, Baltimore.
Fleischer, S. and Packer, L. (1978) *Biomembranes part C, Methods in Enzymology*, Vol. 52, Academic Press, New York.
La Du, B. N., Mandel, H. G. and Way, E. L. (1971) *Fundamentals of drug metabolism and drug disposition*, Williams and Wilkins, Baltimore.
Parke, D. V. (1968) *The biochemistry of foreign compounds*, Pergamon Press, Oxford.
Parke, D. V. and Smith, L. V. (eds) (1977) *Drug metabolism from microbe to Man*, Taylor and Francis, London.
Williams, R. T. (1959) *Detoxification mechanisms*, Chapman and Hall, London.

REVIEWS AND ORIGINAL ARTICLES

Alvares, A. P. *et al.* (1979) Regulation of drug metabolism in man by environmental factors. *Drug. Metab. Rev.*, **9**, 185–206.
Alvares, A. P. and Kappas, A. (1979) Lead and polychlorinated biphenyls: effects on heme and drug metabolism. *Drug Metab. Rev.*, **10**, 91–106.
Anderson, K. E. *et al.* (1982) Nutritional influence on chemical biotransformations in humans. *Nutrition Rev.*, **40**, 161–71.

Becking, G. C. (1978) Dietary minerals and drug metabolism. In *Nutrition and drug interrelationships* (eds J. N. Hathcock and J. Coon), Academic Press, New York.

Burns, J. J. (1962) Species differences and individual variations in drug metabolism. In *Metabolic factors controlling duration of drug action* (eds B. B. Brodie and E. G. Erdös), Pergamon, Oxford.

Caldwell, J. (1981) The current status of attempts to predict species differences in drug metabolism. *Drug Metab. Rev.*, **12**, 221–38.

Caldwell, J. (1982) Conjugation reactions in foreign-compound metabolism: definition, consequences and species variations. *Drug Metab. Rev.*, **13**, 745–78.

Campbell, T. C. (1978) Effects of dietary protein on drug metabolism. In *Nutrition and drug interrelationships* (eds J. N. Hathcock and J. Coon), Academic Press, New York.

Campbell, T. C. and Hayes, J. R. (1974) Role of nutrition in the drug-metabolizing enzyme systems. *Pharmacol. Rev.*, **26**, 171–98.

Campbell, T. C. *et al.* (1979) The influence of dietary factors on drug metabolism in animals. *Drug Metab. Rev.*, **9**, 173–84.

Colby, H. D. (1980) Regulation of hepatic drug and steroid metabolism by androgens and estrogens. *Adv. Sex Hormone Res.*, **4**, 48–91.

Conney, A. H. *et al.* (1971) Effects of environmental chemicals on the metabolism of drugs, carcinogens and normal body constituents in man. *Ann. N.Y. Acad. Sci.*, **179**, 155–72.

Davies, D. S. and Thorgeirsson, S. S. (1971) Mechanism of hepatic drug oxidation and its relationship to individual differences in rates of oxidation in man. *Ann. N.Y. Acad. Sci.*, **179**, 411–20.

Dollery, C. T. *et al.* (1979) Contribution of environmental factors to variability in human drug metabolism. *Drug Metab. Rev.*, **9**, 207–20.

Dutton, G. J. (1978) Developmental aspects of drug conjugation, with special reference to glucuronidation. *Ann. Rev. Pharm. Tox.*, **18**, 17–36.

Feuer, G. (1979) Action of pregnancy and various progesterones on hepatic microsomal activities. *Drug Metab. Rev.*, **9**, 147–72.

Fouts, J. R. (1962) Physiological impairment of drug metabolism. In *Metabolic factors controlling duration of drug action* (eds B. B. Brodie and E. G. Erdös), Pergamon, Oxford.

Gillette, J. R. (1971) Factors affecting drug metabolism. Drug metabolism in Man. *Ann. N.Y. Acad. Sci.*, **179**, 43–66.

Gustafsson, J.-Å. (1983) Sex steroid induced changes in hepatic enzymes. *Ann. Rev. Physiol.*, **45**, 51–60.

Gustafsson, J.-Å. *et al.* (1980) The hypothalamo-pituitary-liver axis: a new hormonal system in control of hepatic steroid and drug metabolism. *Rec. Prog. Hormone Res.*, **7**, 48–91.

Hänninen, O. (1975) Age and exposure factors in drug metabolism. *Acta Pharm. Tox.*, **36**, Suppl. II, 3–20.

Hodgson, E. (1979) Comparative aspects of the distribution of cytochrome *P*-450 dependent mono-oxygenase systems: an overview. *Drug. Metab. Rev.*, **10**, 15–34.

Hoyumpa, A. M. and Schenker, S. (1982) Major drug interactions: effect of liver disease, alcohol and malnutrition. *Ann. Rev. Med.*, **33**, 113–50.

Hucker, H. B. (1970) Species differences in drug metabolism. *Ann. Rev. Pharm. Tox.*, **10**, 99–118.

Idle, J. R. and Smith, R. L. (1979) Polymorphisms of oxidation at carbon centres of drugs and their clinical significance. *Drug Metab. Rev.*, **9**, 301–18.

Jondorf, W. R. (1981) Drug-metabolizing enzymes as evolutionary probes. *Drug Metab. Rev.*, **12**, 379–430.

Jusko, J. W. (1979) Influence of cigarette smoking on drug metabolism in Man. *Drug Metab. Rev.*, **9**, 221–36.

Kato, R. (1974) Sex-related differences in drug metabolism. *Drug Metab. Rev.*, **3**, 1–32.

Kato, R. (1977) Drug metabolism under pathological and abnormal physiological states in animals and Man. *Xenobiotica*, **7**, 25–92.

Krishnaswamy, K. (1983) Drug metabolism and pharmacokinetics in malnutrition. *TIPS*, **4**, 295–9.

Maines, M. D. (1979) Role of trace metals in regulation of cellular heme and hemoprotein metabolism. *Drug Metab. Rev.*, **9**, 237–58.

Marks, G. S. (1981) The effects of chemicals on hepatic heme biosynthesis. *TIPS*, **2**, 59–61.

Nebert, D. W. (1979) The Ah locus: genetic regulation of the metabolism of carcinogens, drugs and other environmental chemicals by cytochrome *P*-450-mediated monooxygenases. *CRC Crit. Rev. Biochem.*, **6**, 401–37.

Nebert, D. W. *et al.* (1981) Genetic mechanisms controlling the induction of polysubstrate monooxygenase (*P*-450) activities. *Ann. Rev. Pharm. Tox.*, **21**, 431–62.

Neims, A. H. *et al.* (1976) Developmental aspects of the hepatic cytochrome *P*-450 mono-oxygenase system. *Ann. Rev. Pharm. Tox.*, **16**, 427–46.

Netter, K. J. (1976) Developmental aspects of drug metabolism. In *Mechanisms of toxicity and metabolism* (ed. N. T. Kärki), Pergamon, Oxford.

Omaye, S. T. and Turnbull, J. D. (1980) Effect of ascorbic acid on heme metabolism in hepatic microsomes. *Life Sci.*, **27**, 441–9.

Parke, D. V. and Iaonnides, C. (1981) The role of nutrition in toxicology. *Ann. Rev. Nutr.*, **1**, 207.

Prescott, L. F. (1975) Pathological and physiological factors affecting drug absorption, distribution, elimination and response in Man. In *Handbook of experimental pharmacology*, Vol. **27** (eds J. R. Gillette and J. R. Mitchell), Springer, Berlin.

Sanvordeker, D. R. and Lambert, H. J. (1974) Environmental modification of mammalian drug metabolism and biological response. *Drug Metab. Rev.*, **3**, 201–30.

Short, C. R. *et al.* (1976) Fetal and neonatal development of the microsomal monooxygenase system. *Drug Metab. Rev.*, **5**, 1–42.

Skett, P. and Gustafsson, J.-Å. (1979) Imprinting of enzyme systems of xenobiotic and steroid metabolism. *Rev. Biochem. Tox.*, **1**, 27–52.

Sosa-Lucero, J. C. *et al.* (1973) Nutritional influences on drug metabolism. *Can. Rev. Biol.*, **32**, 69–75.

Stitzel, R. E. (1972) Effects of environmental organophosphorus insecticides on drug metabolism. *Drug Metab. Rev.*, **1**, 229–48.

Vessell, E. S. (1975) Genetically determined variations in drug disposition and response in Man. In *Handbook of experimental pharmacology*, Vol. **27** (eds J. R. Gillette and J. R. Mitchell), Springer, Berlin.

Wade, A. E. *et al.* (1978) Lipids in drug detoxification. In *Nutrition and drug interrelationships* (eds J. N. Hathcock and J. Coon), Academic Press, New York.

Walker, C. H. (1978) Species differences in microsomal mono-oxygenase activity and their relationship to biological half-lives. *Drug Metab. Rev.*, **7**, 295–324.

Walker, C. H. (1980) Species variations in some hepatic microsomal enzymes that metabolize xenobiotics. *Progress in Drug Metab.*, **5**, 113–64.

Wilkinson, G. R. and Schenker, S. (1975) Drug disposition and liver disease. *Drug Metab. Rev.*, **4**, 139–76.

Williams, R. T. (1978) Nutrients in drug detoxification reactions. In *Nutrition and drug interrelationships* (eds J. N. Hathcock and J. Coon), Academic Press, New York.

Woda, O. and Yano, Y. (1974) Adaptive responses of the liver to foreign compounds with special reference to microsomal drug-metabolizing enzymes. *Rev. Environ. Health*, **1**, 264–82.

Zannoni, V. G. (1978) Ascorbic acid and drug metabolism. In *Nutrition and drug interrelationships* (eds J. N. Hathcock and J. Coon), Academic Press, New York.

6

Pharmacological and toxicological aspects of drug metabolism

6.1 Introduction

In general, the intensity and duration of drug action is proportional to the concentration of the drug at the site of action and the time it remains there. Therefore any factor that effectively alters the drug concentration at the active site will result in a changed pharmacological response to the drug. As indicated in previous chapters, the processes of drug metabolism result in biotransformation of the drug to metabolites that are chemically different from the parent drug and would therefore be expected to have an altered affinity for the drug receptor. Thus, the processes of drug metabolism change the structure of the drug and essentially result in the production of a different chemical that often is not recognized by the relevant receptor system, and hence results in little or no pharmacological response. In this case, drug metabolism results in *pharmacological deactivation*. In contrast to the above, many drugs are pharmacologically inert and absolutely require metabolism to express their pharmacological effect. Therefore in this case, the process of drug metabolism results in *pharmacological activation*.

The above simplified picture is somewhat confounded by the fact that drug metabolites can also elicit additional biological responses that are unrelated to the pharmacological properties of the parent compound. For example, drug metabolism may result in a *change* of the pharmacological properties of the drug, enabling metabolites to interact with other receptor systems. In addition, many toxicological responses to drugs and chemicals can be rationalized by the unique biological toxicity of metabolites not shared by the parent compound – an example of *toxicological activation.*

From the above discussion it is clear that the processes of drug metabolism have to be considered as a 'double-edged sword' in that, depending on the specific drug or chemical in question, a change in the pharmacology or toxicology of the drug may arise. Accordingly, it is the purpose of this chapter to consider this concept in more detail by examining the pharmacological and toxicological aspects of drug metabolism.

6.2 Pharmacological aspects of drug metabolism

The metabolism of a drug may alter the drug's pharmacological properties in one of several ways:

(1) Pharmacological deactivation.
(2) Pharmacological activation.
(3) Change in type of pharmacological response.
(4) No change in pharmacological activity.
(5) Change in drug uptake (absorption).
(6) Change in drug distribution.
(7) Enterohepatic circulation.

6.2.1 PHARMACOLOGICAL DEACTIVATION

The concept of specific enzyme systems existing for the deactivation or detoxication of drugs is not novel. For example, many chemicals or metabolites that are produced during normal intermediary metabolism are potentially toxic to the organism, and enzyme systems are present that facilitate their inactivation. This is clearly seen in the efficient detoxication of hydrogen peroxide (arising from oxidative metabolism of endogenous substrates) by enzymes such as catalase. In a similar manner, many therapeutically used drugs and other xenobiotics are inactivated by the phase I enzymes of drug metabolism due to the substantially reduced pharmacological activity of the metabolite as compared to the parent drug (Figure 6.1).

It should be pointed out that the phase II conjugating enzymes play a very important role in the pharmacological inactivation of drugs and the further inactivation of their phase I metabolites. Although a few exceptions are known, virtually every drug conjugate is pharmacologically less active than the parent compound. This effect is achieved by gross chemical modification of the drug, thereby decreasing receptor affinity, and by enhancement of excretion and removal from the body. It is quite clear that if drug clearance

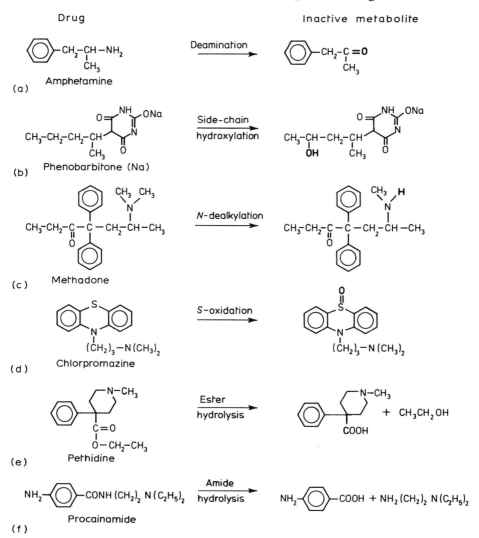

Figure 6.1 Role of phase I enzymes in the pharmacological inactivation of drugs.

from the body is enhanced by phase II conjugation, then the duration of action is curtailed.

The widely used analgesic drug paracetamol also serves as an example of phase II metabolism resulting in pharmacological inactivation of the parent drug. As shown in Figure 6.2 paracetamol undergoes glutathione, glucuronide and sulfate conjugation, and the resulting phase II conjugates are pharmacologically inactive.

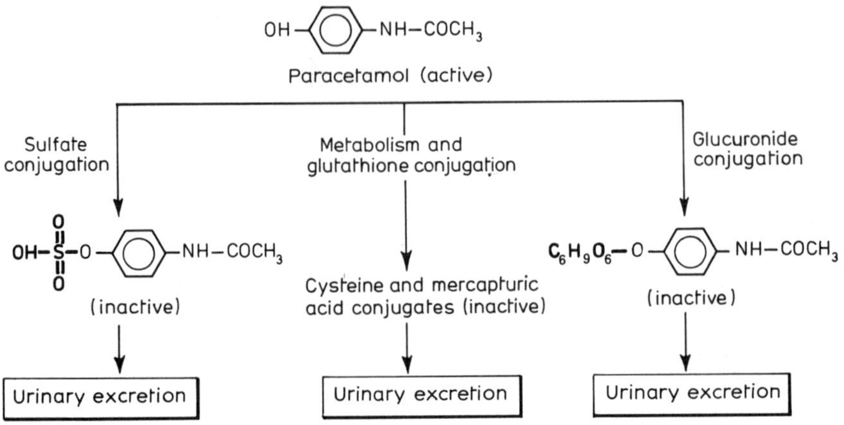

OH—⟨○⟩—NH—COCH$_3$

Paracetamol (active)

| Sulfate conjugation | Metabolism and glutathione conjugation | Glucuronide conjugation |

OH—S(=O)(=O)—O—⟨○⟩—NH—COCH$_3$

(inactive)

Cysteine and mercapturic acid conjugates (inactive)

C$_6$H$_9$O$_6$—O—⟨○⟩—NH—COCH$_3$

(inactive)

| Urinary excretion | Urinary excretion | Urinary excretion |

Figure 6.2 Role of the phase II enzymes in the pharmacological inactivation of paracetamol.

Furthermore, many drugs are pharmacologically deactivated by simultaneous phase I and phase II metabolic attack at different positions in the molecule as is observed in the metabolic inactivation of the beta-blocker, propranolol (Figure 6.3).

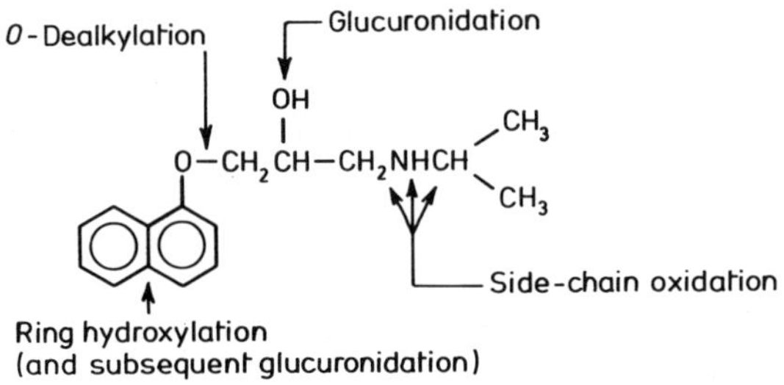

O-Dealkylation   ⌐ Glucuronidation

OH
|
O—CH$_2$CH—CH$_2$NHCH⟨CH$_3$ / CH$_3$⟩

⌐ Side-chain oxidation

Ring hydroxylation
(and subsequent glucuronidation)

Figure 6.3 Metabolic pathways resulting in the pharmacological inactivation of propranolol.

6.2.2 PHARMACOLOGICAL ACTIVATION

In contrast to the concepts discussed above, many drugs and chemicals require metabolic activation before they can exert their pharmacological action. This process of metabolic activation is usually associated with the phase I enzymes. Many of these parent drugs are essentially devoid of pharmacological activity, and this has led to the development of the so-called 'pro-drugs'. A classical example of pro-drug activation by metabolism was the early use of the dye prontosil in the 1930s to treat bacterial infections. *In vitro* studies clearly

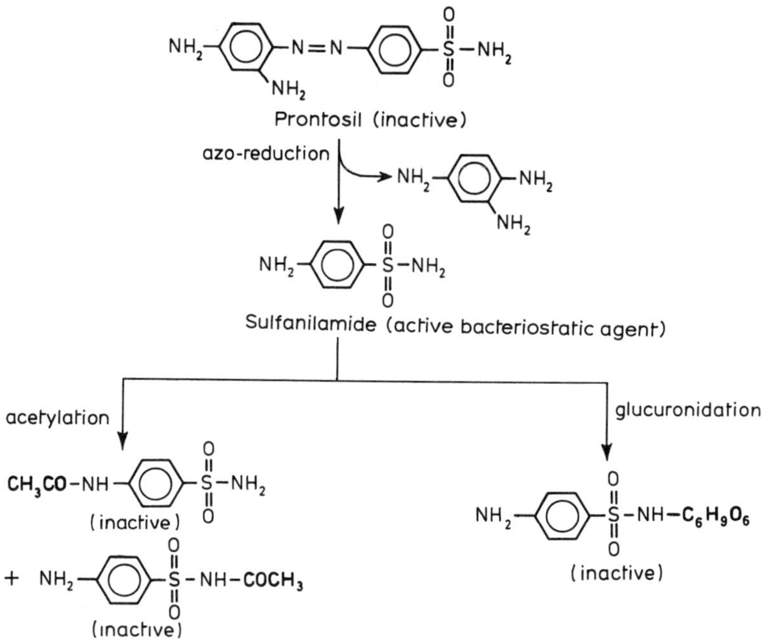

Figure 6.4 Role of metabolism in the pharmacological activation of prontosil and the pharmacological inactivation of its major metabolite, sulfanilamide.

showed that prontosil itself was inactive and required metabolic azo reduction to liberate the pharmacologically active component, sulfanilamide (Figure 6.4).

It should be noted that the active sulfanilamide is subsequently metabolically inactivated by N-acetylation at both nitrogen atoms, and by N-glucuronidation at the amide nitrogen. Accordingly, it is clear that the therapeutic effectiveness of this class of drugs is strongly influenced by the prevailing tissue balance of the azo reductase on the one hand and the acetylase and glucuronidation enzymes on the other.

The above concept of pro-drug activation has been used to target drugs to their specific site of action. For example, the anti-parkinson drug levodopa is metabolically activated in the neurone to dopamine, but the drug is given as the levodopa precursor due to its more facile uptake into the neurone.

There are many other examples of drugs whose metabolism results in pharmacological activation; some of these are given in Table 6.1.

6.2.3 CHANGE IN TYPE OF PHARMACOLOGICAL RESPONSE

In addition to modulating pharmacological responses in either a positive or negative manner as described in Sections 6.2.1 and 6.2.2 above, the process

Table 6.1 Drug metabolism reactions resulting in pharmacological activation

Pro-drug	Clinical use	Metabolic conversion	Active drug or metabolite
Azathioprine	Immunosuppressant	Thio-ether hydrolysis	Mercaptopurine
Chloral hydrate	Sedative/hypnotic	Reduction	Trichloroethanol
Clofibrate	Hypolipidaemic	Ester hydrolysis	Clofibric acid
Cyclophosphamide	Anti-tumour/immunosuppressant	Hydroxylation	4-Hydroxy-cyclophosphamide (precursor to other active metabolites)
Disulfiram	Alcohol withdrawal	Dithiol reduction	Diethylthiocarbamic acid
Glyceryl triacetate	Antifungal	Ester hydrolysis	Acetic acid
Methyldopa	Anti-hypertensive	Decarboxylation and hydroxylation	α-Methylnoradrenaline
Prednisone	Anti-inflammatory	Keto-reduction	Prednisolone
Primaquine	Antimalarial	Demethylation and oxidation	Primaquine quinone
Primidone	Anti-epileptic	Oxidation	Phenobarbitone
Proguanil	Antimalarial	Cyclization	Cycloguanil
Prontosil	Antibiotic	Azo-reduction	Sulfanilamide
Succinylsulfathiazole	Antibiotic	Amide hydrolysis	Sulfathiazole

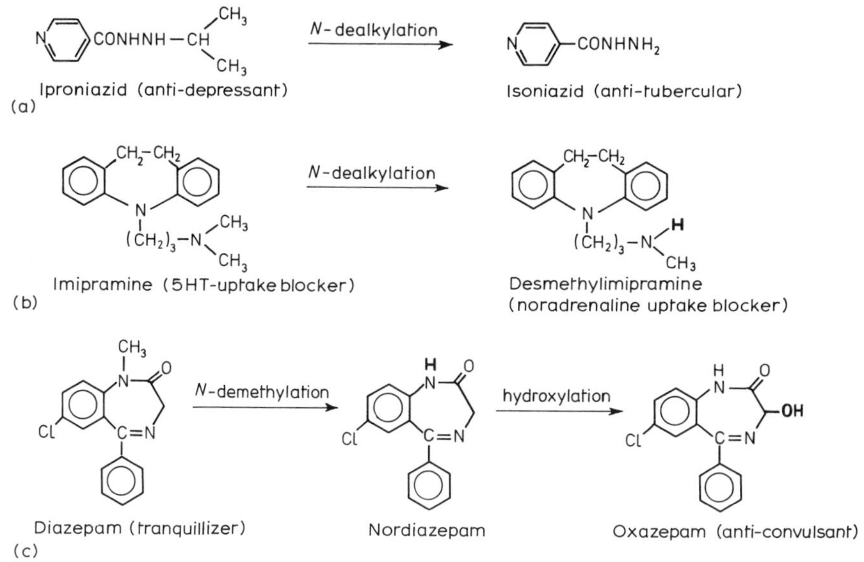

(a) Iproniazid (anti-depressant) — N-dealkylation → Isoniazid (anti-tubercular)

(b) Imipramine (5HT-uptake blocker) — N-dealkylation → Desmethylimipramine (noradrenaline uptake blocker)

(c) Diazepam (tranquillizer) — N-demethylation → Nordiazepam — hydroxylation → Oxazepam (anti-convulsant)

Figure 6.5 Drug metabolism resulting in a change in the type of pharmacological activity.

of drug metabolism can also result in a *change* in the pharmacology of the parent compound. For example, iproniazid was formerly used as an anti-depressant, but has subsequently been removed from the market because it caused severe liver toxicity. Iproniazid is metabolized by N-dealkylation resulting in the formation of the metabolite isoniazid which has pronounced anti-tubercular activity, a pharmacological activity not associated with the parent drug. Another example of this phenomenon is seen in the metabolism of the tricyclic anti-depressant drug imipramine. This drug undergoes an enzymatic N-demethylation reaction resulting in the formation of desmethylimipramine, a compound that is substantially more potent than the parent drug as an inhibitor of the neuronal uptake of noradrenaline, but less potent for the uptake of 5HT.

A third example of the ability of drug metabolism to result in a change in pharmacological response is seen in the metabolism of diazepam (valium), a benzodiazepine chiefly used as a tranquillizer. The drug undergoes N-demethylation and subsequent ring hydroxylation yielding oxazepam as a metabolite, the metabolite having pronounced anti-convulsant properties.

The metabolic pathways involved in the above reactions are summarized in Figure 6.5.

6.2.4 NO CHANGE IN PHARMACOLOGICAL ACTIVITY

Several drugs are metabolized to compounds that have the same or similar pharmacological activity. An example of this type is the N-de-ethylation of the local anaesthetic lignocaine. The N-de-ethylated metabolite (monoethyl-glycylxylidine) is as active as the parent compound and it would appear that metabolism serves no useful immediate purpose here. However it should be emphasized that metabolism may prime the substrate for subsequent phase II reactions and indirectly facilitate drug excretion and hence termination of pharmacological activity.

6.2.5 CHANGE IN DRUG UPTAKE

Changes in drug uptake by metabolism may be seen after the oral administration of drugs and is dependent on the enzymes at the site of uptake, for example the gastrointestinal tract. In most cases, drug metabolism at the site of uptake inhibits drug absorption as seen in the formation of sulfate conjugates of phenolic drugs after oral administration. As shown in Figure 6.6, isoprenaline sulfation and isoniazid acetylation by enzymes in the intestinal wall and gut flora result in more polar metabolites. The polar metabolites are less readily absorbed across the gut wall as compared to the parent drug, and are consequently preferentially excreted in the faeces.

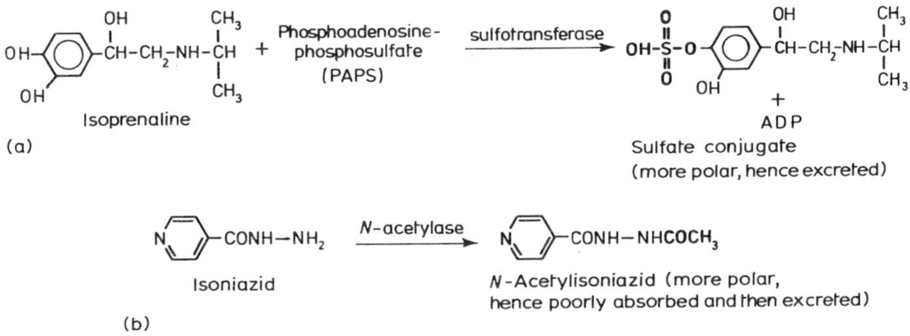

Figure 6.6 The role of drug metabolism in modifying drug uptake.

It is interesting to note that in certain cases the metabolism of a drug at the uptake site is an important factor in determining the most effective route of administration. For example, in the example of the anti-asthmatic drug, isoprenaline, given above, it is clear that oral administration is not an effective means of getting the drug to its site of action (lung) because of extensive gut metabolism. To get over this problem, isoprenaline may be given sublingually and absorbed through the buccal mucosa. Unfortunately, the circulating drug is rapidly inactivated (again by metabolism) in the liver. Isoprenaline is then best administered via aerosol inhalation – in this way, the inactivation metabolic pathways are bypassed and the drug directly reaches the lungs in sufficiently high concentration to be pharmacologically active.

In contrast to the above, gut metabolism can be used to advantage as in the oral administration of the *para*-amino-substituted sulfonamide antibiotics such as succinysulfathiazole. This drug is poorly absorbed through the gut wall and is readily hydrolysed by gut enzymes to the active sulfathiazole. This local hydrolysis in the gut ensures high, effective antibiotic concentrations, and is therefore very useful in the treatment of gut infections.

6.2.6 CHANGE IN DRUG DISTRIBUTION

Drug distribution to the various tissues in the body (and hence the site of action), is dependent on several factors including the lipid solubility of the drug. A highly lipophilic drug will be localized in highest concentrations in tissues with high fat content such as adipose tissues and the brain. As metabolism causes drugs to be less lipid-soluble in most cases, metabolism will then alter drug distribution away from the high-fat tissues and into the high-water tissues such as blood and the kidney.

A good example of the above concept is the distribution of the narcotic analgesic morphine. Morphine is highly lipophilic and is not readily excreted because it is quickly absorbed into lipid-rich tissues including the brain. However, morphine undergoes phase II conjugation with glucuronic acid in the liver, forming the morphine-3-glucuronide metabolite. This metabolite is water-soluble and does not readily enter the brain; the conjugate is then readily excreted. Thus hepatic metabolism in this instance precludes the access of morphine to the brain and thereby diminishes the pharmacological response by redistribution away from the site of action.

The lipophilicity of drugs can also radically influence the rate of onset of drug action. For example diamorphine (di-acetylmorphine, or, as it is better known, heroin) enters the brain much more rapidly than morphine because of its higher lipophilicity, and therefore has a more rapid onset of action. Once in the brain, the diamorphine is rapidly metabolized to morphine, whereupon the pharmacological effects (primarily analgesia) are observed.

6.2.7 ENTEROHEPATIC CIRCULATION

The route of drug excretion is largely influenced by its molecular weight. Drugs having a molecular weight of under approximately 300 are largely excreted in

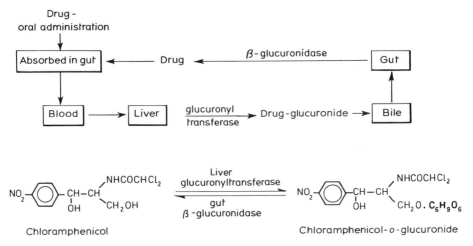

Figure 6.7 Entero-hepatic circulation of drugs.

urine, whereas drugs with a higher molecular weight are mainly excreted in the bile and hence into the intestine. Once in the intestine a drug glucuronide conjugate has two possible fates. It can either be excreted in the faeces or, additionally, the glucuronide conjugate can be hydrolysed back to the parent drug by the action of the enzyme β-glucuronidase which is present in gut bacteria. The free, de-conjugated drug is then absorbed through the gut wall and re-enters the liver via the hepatic portal vein. The free drug can then be re-conjugated with glucuronic acid, secreted into the bile and then the intestine, and the cyclic process starts again.

This cycling of drug is known as the *entero-hepatic circulation* and is outlined in Figure 6.7.

This recirculation of drugs can take place for several cycles. The overall result is that the drug is retained in the body and has a substantially increased half-life. Provided that the drug concentration is maintained high enough at the site of action, it is quite clear that this metabolism-based cycle can result in a prolongation of pharmacological activity, as is seen in the example given for chloramphenicol (Figure 6.7). The eventual excretion of the drug then arises from the faecal excretion of drug-conjugate that escapes hydrolysis in the intestine during each turn of the cycle and by other metabolic pathways.

It would appear that drugs get trapped in this cycle by accident rather than design. It is well known that conjugates of endogenous compounds such as steroids, bile salts and bilirubin undergo the same enterohepatic circulation, and therefore drugs are 'ensnared' in a normal physiological process.

In conclusion, drug metabolism can profoundly alter the uptake, distribution and pharmacological action of a particular drug as well as directing its excretion pattern. In addition, drug metabolism is of major importance in determining the method of administration, and in deciding the correct dose and frequency of drug delivery. In fact, apart from the inherent pharmacological activity of the drug itself, the metabolism of a drug is probably the most important consideration to be made in drug design and therapeutics.

6.3 Toxicological aspects of xenobiotic metabolism

As discussed above for the *pharmacological* properties of drugs and their metabolites, drug metabolism can result in either a decreased or increased *toxicity* of the parent compound, depending of course on the inherent biological potencies of the drug and its metabolite(s).

6.3.1 METABOLISM RESULTING IN INCREASED TOXICITY

As summarized in Table 6.2, many examples are known where the hepatic metabolism of drugs and chemicals results in an increased toxicity of the parent compound. The enzymes responsible for this metabolic toxification are mainly the phase I enzymes. Although some examples have been documented on the participation of phase II reactions, these latter enzymes are more often associated with detoxication reactions (see next section). This concept of metabolic toxification can be amply demonstrated by considering the following specific examples of toxic reactions to drugs and chemicals.

Table 6.2 Metabolism resulting in increased toxicity of drugs and chemicals

Compound	Metabolic pathway	Toxicity
2-Acetylaminofluorene	N-hydroxylation and sulfation	Hepatocarcinogenesis
Benzene	Epoxidation (and other pathways?)	Aplastic anaemia/ leukaemia
Cyclophosphamide	Hydroxylation (and rearrangement)	Teratogenesis
Halothane	Defluorination	Hepatitis
Isoniazid	Acetylation and hydrolysis	Hepatic necrosis
Methoxyflurane	Defluorination	Nephrotoxicity

(a) CARCINOGENESIS

As discussed previously, the polycyclic aromatic hydrocarbons represent a ubiquitous group of environmental chemicals that are well documented as causing cancer in many mammalian species. These compounds are relatively innocuous and chemically inert, but their metabolites are biologically

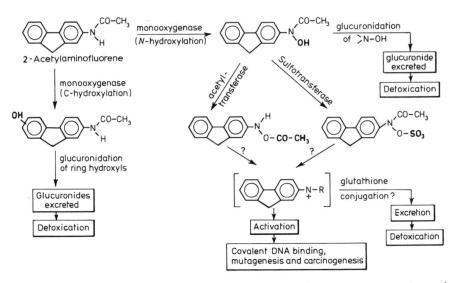

Figure 6.8 Metabolic activation and inactivation of the hepatocarcinogen, 2-acetyl-aminofluorene. (Adapted from Guenthner, T. M. and Oesch, F. (1981) *Trends in Pharmacol. Sci.*, **May**, 129–32.)

active and are potent carcinogens. The polycyclic aromatic hydrocarbons are metabolized by the cytochromes *P*-450 and epoxide hydrolase to form the electrophilic diol–epoxide metabolites which are then capable of covalent binding to nucleic acids and hence of initiating chemical carcinogenesis.

Another example of the role of metabolic activation in chemical carcinogenesis is the metabolism of the compound 2-acetylaminofluorene. This synthetic compound was originally intended for use as an insecticide. During routine safety studies prior to introduction to the market, it was discovered that it was an extremely potent hepatocarcinogen. Further studies on this carcinogen have amply documented the fact that both phase I and phase II enzymes are involved in the bioactivation of this carcinogen (Figure 6.8).

The importance of the drug-metabolizing enzymes in many types of chemical carcinogenesis cannot be overemphasized. In addition to the above examples, many other chemicals (including the aflatoxins, aromatic amines and nitrosamines) are dependent on metabolism for expression of their carcinogenicity. As a caveat to the above general description, it must be borne in mind that metabolism alone is not the sole determinant of carcinogenicity of drugs and chemicals – many other factors are important for expression of carcinogenicity including promotion and genetic predisposition. However this is a large and complex topic outside the scope of this present discussion.

(b) TERATOGENESIS

Several drugs and chemicals are known to interfere with the processes of embryo development and, if given at the critical stage of organogenesis, can result in malformations of the embryo (teratogenesis). The anti-tumour drug cyclophosphamide is a well-documented teratogen; several studies have shown that the metabolites of cyclophosphamide are much more teratogenic than the parent compound. As shown in Figure 6.9, cyclophosphamide undergoes cytochrome P-450-dependent hydroxylation at the 4-position; this hydroxy-lated metabolite serves as the precursor for the toxic metabolites, acrolein and phosphoramide mustard. Although it is not known with any degree of

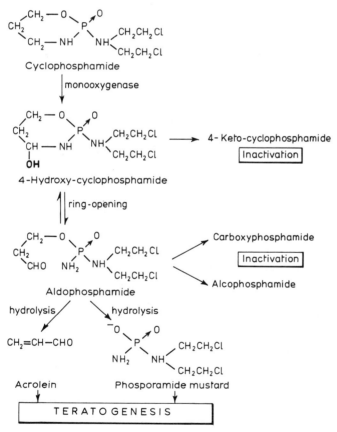

Figure 6.9 Metabolic activation of the teratogen cyclophosphamide. (Adapted from Nau, H. *et al.* (1982) *Mutat. Res.*, **95**, 105–18.)

certainty which of these two metabolites of cyclophosphamide is the major teratogen, it is quite clear that metabolism is a prerequisite for the expression of cyclophosphamide teratogenicity.

(c) PULMONARY TOXICITY

4-Ipomeanol, a furan derivative found in mouldy sweet potatoes, produces a characteristic pulmonary toxicity in several mammalian species (necrosis of the non-ciliated bronchiolar epithelial or Clara cells). Current evidence suggests that 4-ipomeanol is metabolized by a specific pulmonary cytochrome P-450, resulting in the formation of a highly biological reactive intermediate. This intermediate covalently binds to critical macromolecular targets in the Clara cell resulting in the observed necrosis in this cell type. It is interesting to note that 4-ipomeanol is selectively toxic to the lung and is relatively non-toxic in the liver, an organ very rich in xenobiotic-metabolizing enzymes. This apparent contradiction is rationalized by the observations that the liver lacks the appropriate isoenzyme of cytochrome P-450 necessary for activation, or that the liver is well-endowed with the detoxifying phase II enzymes that remove the reactive intermediate.

The above discussion emphasizes the importance of metabolism in producing toxic metabolites. Furthermore, it is clear that the presence (or absence) of phase I and phase II enzymes are an important determinant of *selective* organ toxicity of drugs and chemicals.

(d) HEPATIC TOXICITY

Many of the drugs and chemicals shown in Table 6.2 are toxic to the liver, resulting in hepatic necrosis. A well-documented example of a hepatotoxin is paracetamol, which in high doses, produces hepatic necrosis, in both experimental animals and Man. Again, as in the previous examples, paracetamol requires metabolic activation for expression of its toxicity. This is thought to occur by an initial N-hydroxylation reaction catalysed by the hepatic mixed-function oxidase enzymes (Figure 6.10), and subsequent chemical rearrangement of the hydroxylamine producing a reactive electrophile which then covalently binds to hepatic macromolecules as a prelude to liver necrosis. It must be emphasized that the reactive intermediate(s) of paracetamol may be enzymatically detoxified by conjugation with glutathione (catalysed by the glutathione-S-transferases), a concept that will be more fully developed later in this chapter.

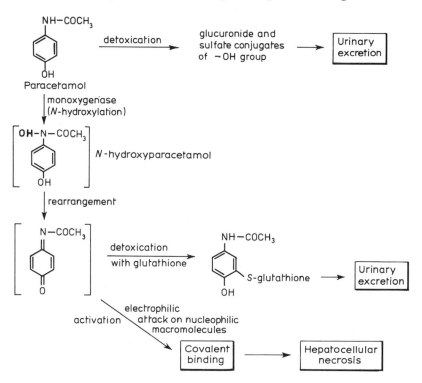

Figure 6.10 Role of metabolism in the toxicological activation of paracetamol. (Modified from Lake, B. G. and Gangolli, S. D. (1981) in *Concepts in drug metabolism* (eds P. Jenner and B. Testa), Marcel Dekker, New York, pp. 166–218.)

(e) NEPHROTOXICITY

Many drugs exhibit a selective toxicity to the kidney, including the antibiotics such as the sulfonamides. A major route of sulfonamide metabolism is by acetylation of the *para*-amino group in the molecule, a pathway that results in pharmacological inactivation. However an occasional toxic effect of the sulfonamides is crystalluria, a condition caused by precipitation of the less soluble acetylated sulfonamide metabolite in the tubular urine, especially when the urine is acidic.

In addition, the kidney has significant amounts of the mixed-function oxidase system enzymes and prostaglandin endoperoxide synthetase, two enzyme systems that have the potential to metabolically activate innocuous drugs and chemicals to toxic metabolites. Although our knowledge of the kidney metabolism of xenobiotics is not as fully developed as the equivalent system in the liver, it is becoming clearer that the kidney can also activate drugs. For example, paracetamol can be metabolized both by mixed-function oxidation and by co-oxidation in the presence of arachidonic acid and prostaglandin endoperoxide synthetase. Both of these pathways result in the production of toxic metabolites that bind to critical, cellular macromolecules, ultimately resulting in necrosis of kidney tissue in a similar fashion to the liver, as described above. In addition many urinary bladder carcinogens such as benzidine and many nephrotoxic chlorinated hydrocarbons (including chloroform, carbon tetrachloride and trichloroethylene) require metabolic activation as a necessary prelude to expression of their nephrotoxicity.

6.3.2 METABOLISM RESULTING IN DECREASED TOXICITY

From the above discussion, it is clear that many phase I reactions result in the production of toxic metabolites of xenobiotics. However this phenomenon must not be considered in isolation as many of the toxic phase I metabolites are substrates of the phase II enzymes, the resultant conjugate, in general, being considerably less toxic than the initial metabolite. For example, paracetamol is activated by the mixed-function oxidase system but, in low doses, the reactive metabolite (Figure 6.10) is conjugated with cellular glutathione and safely excreted as thiol conjugates. This protective influence of the phase II enzymes is clearly seen in experimental animals depleted of cellular glutathione by compounds such as diethyl maleate. Such glutathione-depleted animals are then rendered more susceptible to paracetamol hepatotoxicity, whereas the animals are protected against the toxicity of this analgesic by glutathione supplementation.

Another example of phase II metabolism resulting in decreased toxicity is seen in glucuronidation reactions when comparing the LD_{50} values of various compounds in species that have different abilities to form glucuronide conjugates. Whereas the rabbit is competent at glucuronidation, the cat is well known to be defective in this phase II pathway, resulting in an increased susceptibility to various compounds, as demonstrated by substantially lower LD_{50} values (Table 6.3).

6.4 Balance of toxifying and detoxifying pathways

If a drug can be metabolized either to a toxic metabolite or inactivated by metabolism, what then determines the ultimate toxicological response to the drug? An obvious answer to this question is that the *balance* of the activating and deactivating metabolic pathways is a critical determinant of the toxicity of the compound in question. A good example in this context is the hepato-carcinogen 2-acetylaminofluorene. With reference to Figure 6.8 two main

Table 6.3 Role of glucuronic acid conjugation in the toxicity of xenobiotics in the rabbit and cat

Compound	LD_{50} ($mg\,kg^{-1}$)	
	Rabbit	Cat
Phenol	250	80
Paracetamol	1200	250

(Adapted from Caldwell, J. (1980) in *Concepts in drug metabolism, Part A* (eds P. Jenner, and B. Testa), Marcel Dekker, New York.)

routes of metabolism can be seen to exist. The first is cytochrome P-450-dependent mono-oxygenation of the fluorenyl ring system and subsequent glucuronidation (detoxification); the second is cytochrome P-450-dependent mono-oxygenation of the amide nitrogen and subsequent sulfation of the hydroxylamine (activation). In the first instance, it is thought that different isoenzymes of cytochrome P-450 catalyse the above two initial oxidation reactions and therefore the relative amounts and activities of these isoenzymes will determine, in part, the ultimate biological response. In addition, Figure 6.8 shows that sulfate esterification of the N-hydroxyl metabolite is a key metabolic step in the activation of this compound to a carcinogen. Thus it is clear that the concentration and activity of the cytoplasmic sulfotransferase enzymes are a major determinant of the hepatic toxicity of 2-acetylaminofluorene. Accordingly, species, such as the guinea pig, that have low hepatic sulfotransferase activity, are resistant to 2-acetylaminofluorene-induced hepatic cancer.

As shown in Figure 6.11, the phase I metabolism of the anti-psychotic/sedative drug chlorpromazine is complex consisting of ring hydroxylation, N-demethylation, S-oxidation and N-oxidation reactions occurring in the microsomal fraction of the hepatocyte. In fact the metabolism of this drug is even more complex when the phase II glucuronidation and sulfation reactions are taken into account, resulting in the excretion of approximately 20–30

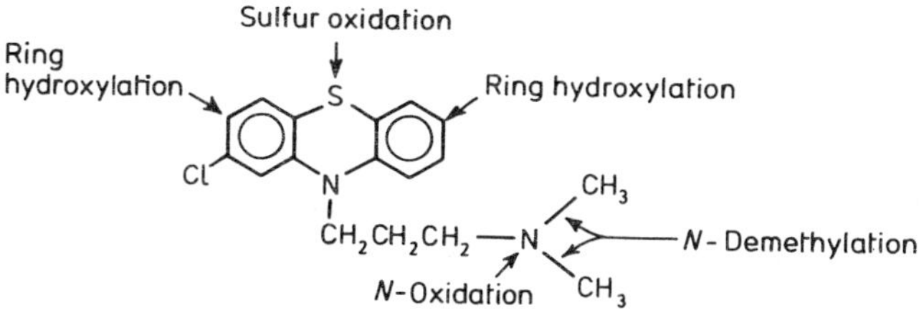

Figure 6.11 Multiple phase I metabolic pathways for chlorpromazine.

different metabolites in human urine. At present, although the pharmacological and toxicological potencies of these various metabolites have not all
been definitively characterized, it is likely that the metabolites have different
potencies and that the metabolism of this drug is another illustration of the
importance of the *balance* of metabolic pathways in determining the ultimate
biological responses.

The metabolism of the organic compound bromobenzene serves as another
excellent example of the importance of the balance between toxifying and
detoxifying enzymes. Bromobenzene is hepatotoxic and in sufficiently high
doses may result in the expression of hepatic necrosis in experimental animals
fed this compound. Many studies have shown that bromobenzene requires
metabolic activation to express its hepatotoxicity, but it must be emphasized
that other detoxifying metabolic pathways exist (Figure 6.12). Initially,
bromobenzene is metabolized to the key reactive metabolite bromobenzene-
3,4-epoxide by the cytochrome *P*-450-dependent mixed-function oxidase
system. This reaction is preferentially catalysed by a phenobarbital-induced
isoenzyme of cytochrome *P*-450, whereas epoxidation of bromobenzene is
directed towards the 2,3-positions by a polycyclic aromatic hydrocarbon-
induced variant of the haemoprotein (cytochrome *P*-448). The prevailing
balance of these cytochrome *P*-450 isoenzymes is an important determinant of
bromobenzene toxicity as the 3,4-epoxide is considerably more toxic to the liver
cell than the 2,3-epoxide. Once formed, the 3,4-epoxide may undergo several
different fates (Figure 6.12). The epoxide may be inactivated by diol formation
(catalysed by the enzyme epoxide hydrolase), by glutathione conjugation
(catalysed by the glutathione-*S*-transferases) or by covalent binding to critical
tissue macromolecules – the presumed chemico-biological interaction that
initiates cellular necrosis. It has also been postulated that the hepatotoxicity of
bromobenzene is associated with the cellular depletion of glutathione (as a
direct result of metabolism) and hence the attendant potential toxicity associated with substantial changes in cellular glutathione homeostasis. Although
the precise mechanism(s) of bromobenzene-induced hepatic toxicity have yet to
be elucidated, it should be clear from the above discussion that the balance of
the metabolizing enzymes and the availability of glutathione are important
determinants of toxicity.

One important feature of the phase II reactions is that they are quite frequently capacity-limited by the availability of the endogenous compound
required for conjugation with the parent drug or its phase I metabolite
(Table 6.4). This capacity-limited phenomenon is readily understood because
many of the endogenous conjugating molecules such as glucuronic acid,
sulfate and glutathione are additionally required for the metabolism and conjugation of endogenous substrates such as steroids and bile acids. Accordingly,

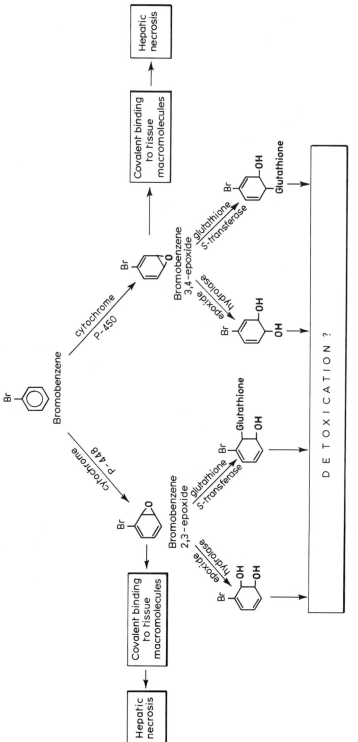

Figure 6.12 Metabolic activation and inactivation of the hepatotoxin, bromobenzene.

Table 6.4 Capacities of conjugation reactions

Capacity	Reaction
High	Glucuronidation
Medium	Amino acid conjugation
Low	Sulfation and glutathione conjugation
Variable	Acetylation

(Adapted from Caldwell, J. (1980) in *Concepts in drug metabolism,
Part A* (eds P. Jenner and B. Testa), Marcel Dekker, New York.)

when the body is challenged with high doses of drugs, higher than normal
levels of conjugating molecules are required for metabolism. If the synthesis of
the endogenous conjugating compounds is limited in any way then a predict-
able result of drug therapy in high doses would be the inability to conjugate the
drug in question. In the majority of cases, where phase II conjugation reactions
result in detoxification, failure to conjugate the drug would then result in an
overt expression of drug-induced toxicity (Table 6.5).

Table 6.5 Detoxification failure due to saturation of conjugation reactions

Compound	Species	Saturable reaction	Nature of toxicity
Paracetamol Bromobenzene	Several	glutathione conjugation	Hepatocellular necrosis
Chloramphenicol	Human neonate	glucuronidation	Agranulocytosis
Benzoic acid	Cat	glycine conjugation	Death
Phenol	Cat	sulfation	Death

(Adapted from Caldwell, J. (1980) in *Concepts in drug metabolism, Part A* (eds P. Jenner and
B. Testa), Marcel Dekker, New York.)

A good example of the capacity-limited conjugation of drugs is seen with
aspirin excretion in Man. As shown in Figure 6.13, aspirin can be conjugated
with either the amino acid glycine or with glucuronic acid. At low doses of
aspirin, glycine conjugation is the main metabolic pathway. However, on
increasing the aspirin dose, the glycine-conjugating system becomes readily
saturated and conjugation switches to glucuronide formation. At the top doses
of aspirin, the glucuronidation system also becomes saturated, and salicylic
acid becomes a major excretory product.

6.5 Conclusions

The classical viewpoint – that the process of drug metabolism is a detoxifying
pathway – must now be modified. Although many examples are known where
metabolism results in decreased pharmacological and toxicological responses,

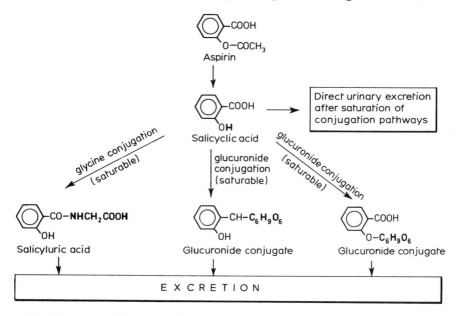

Figure 6.13 Capacity-limited metabolism of aspirin.

it must be emphasized that activation reactions have also been amply verified. This chapter has focused on specific examples of activation and inactivation, and emphasis has been placed on the critical role played by the *balance* of the drug-metabolizing enzymes in determining the ultimate biological response(s) to the drug. Accordingly, this chapter should be considered as 'integrative', i.e. consolidating the previous chapters that were descriptive of metabolic pathways and factors affecting metabolism with the responses of organisms to foreign compounds.

6.6 Further reading

TEXTBOOKS AND SYMPOSIA

Anders, M. W. (ed.) (1985) *Bioactivation of foreign compounds*, Academic Press, New York.

Bacq, Z. M. (1975) *Fundamentals of biochemical pharmacology*, Pergamon Press, Oxford.

Boobis, A. R. *et al.* (eds) (1985) *Microsomes and drug oxidations*. Taylor and Frances, London.

Bowman, W. C. and Rand, M. J. (eds) (1980) *Textbook of pharmacology*, 2nd edn, Blackwell Scientific Publications, London.

Caldwell, J. and Jakoby, W. B. (eds) (1983) *Biological basis of detoxication*, Academic Press, New York.

Goldstein, A., Aranow, L. and Kalman, S. M. (1974) *Principles of drug action*, 2nd edn, Wiley, New York.

Hodgson, E. and Guthrie, F. E. (eds) (1980) *Introduction to biochemical toxicology*, Blackwell Scientific Publications, Oxford.

Jenner, P. and Testa, B. (eds) (1980) *Concepts in drug metabolism, Part A*, Marcel Dekker, New York.

Lamble, J. W. (ed.) (1983) *Drug metabolism and distribution, Current Reviews in Biomedicine 3*, Elsevier, Amsterdam.

Mitchell, J. R. and Horning, M. G. (eds) (1984) *Drug metabolism and drug toxicity*. Raven Press, New York.

Plaa, G. L. and Hewitt, W. R. (eds) (1982) *Toxicology of the liver, target organ toxicology Series*, Raven Press, New York.

Rydström, J., Montelius, J. and Bengtsson, M. (eds) (1983) *Extra hepatic drug metabolism and chemical carcinogenesis*, Elsevier, Amsterdam.

Snyder, R., Parke, D. V., Kocsis, J. J., Jollow, D. J., Gibson, G. G. and Witmer, C. M. (eds) (1982) *Biological reactive intermediates – II, Chemical mechanisms and biological effects, Parts A and B* (*Advances in Experimental Medicine and Biology*, **Vol. 136A and 136B**), Plenum Press, New York.

REVIEWS AND ORIGINAL ARTICLES

Bakke, J. and Gustafsson, J. A. (1984) Mercapturic acid pathway metabolites and xenobiotics: generation of potentially toxic metabolites during enterohepatic circulation. *TIPS*, **5**, 517–521.

Boyd, M. R., Grygiel, J. J. and Menchin, R. F. (1983) Metabolic activation as a basis for organ-selective toxicity. *Clin. Exper. Pharmacol. Physiol.*, **10**, 87–99.

Boyd, M. R. and Statham, C. N. (1983) The effect of hepatic metabolism on the production and toxicity of reactive metabolites in extrahepatic organs. *Drug Metab. Rev.*, **14**, 35–47.

Buckpitt, A. R. and Boyd, M. R. (1983) Relationship between xenobiotic metabolism and toxicity of xenobiotics in avian species. In *Progress in drug metabolism* (eds J. Bridges and L. Chasseaud), Wiley, Sussex, pp. 397–417.

Ehrenberg, L. and Hussain, S. (1981) Genetic toxicity of some important epoxides. *Mutat. Res.*, **86**, 1–113.

Eling, T., Boyd, J., Reed, G., Mason, R. and Sivarajah, K. (1983) Xenobiotic metabolism by prostaglandin endoperoxide synthetase. *Drug Metab. Rev.*, **14**, 1023–53.

Essigmann, J. M., Croy, R. G., Bennett, R. A. and Wogan, G. N. (1982) Metabolic activation of aflatoxin B₁: Patterns of DNA adduct formation, removal and excretion in relation to carcinogenesis. *Drug Metab. Rev.*, **13**, 581–602.

Faustman-Watts, E., Greenaway, J. C., Namkung, M. J., Fantel, A. G. and Juchau, M. R. (1983) Teratogenicity *in vitro* of 2-acetylaminofluorene: role of biotransformation in the rat. *Teratol.*, **27**, 19–28.

Fishbein, L. (1983) An overview of some metabolic and modulating factors in toxicity and chemical carcinogenesis. *J. Am. Coll. Toxicol.*, **2**, 63–89.

Gelboin, H. V. (1980) Benzo[a]pyrene metabolism, activation and carcinogenesis: Role and regulation of the mixed-function oxidases and related enzymes. *Physiol. Rev.*, **60**, 1107–66.

Greim, H. A. (1981) An overview of the phenomena of enzyme induction and inhibition: their relevance to drug action and drug interactions. In *Concepts in drug metabolism, Part B* (eds P. Jenner and B. Testa), Marcel Dekker, New York, pp. 219–63.

De Groot, H. and Noll, T. (1983) Halothane hepatotoxicity: relation between metabolic activation, hypoxia, covalent binding, lipid peroxidation and liver cell damage. *Heptatol.*, **3**, 601–6.

Guengerich, F. F. and Lieber, D. C. (1985) Enzymatic activation of chemicals to toxic metabolites. *CRC Crit. Rev. Toxicol.*, **14**, 259.

Guenthner, T. M. and Oesch, F. (1981) Metabolic activation and inactivation of chemical mutagens and carcinogens. *Trends Pharmacol. Sci.*, **May**, 129–32.

Harvey, R. G. (1982) Polycyclic hydrocarbons and cancer. *Amer. Sci.*, **70**, 386–93.

Heidelberger, C. (1975) Chemical carcinogenesis. *Ann. Rev. Biochem.*, **44**, 79–121.

Hemminki, K. (1983) Nucleic acid adducts of chemical carcinogens and mutagens. *Arch. Toxicol.*, **52**, 249–85.

Hsia, M. T. S. (1983) Toxicological significance of dihydrodiol metabolites. *J. Toxicol. Clin. Toxicol.*, **19**, 737–58.

Jollow, D. J., Mitchell, J. R., Zampaglione, N. and Gillette, J. R. (1974) Bromobenzene-induced liver necrosis. Protective role of glutathione and evidence for 3,4-bromobenzene oxide as the hepatotoxic metabolite. *Pharmacol.*, **11**, 151–69.

Kriek, E. and Westra, J. G. (1979) Metabolic activation of aromatic amines and amides and interactions with nucleic acids. In *Chemical carcinogens and DNA, Vol. 2* (ed. P. L. Grover), CRC Press, Boca Raton, pp. 1–28.

Laib, R. J. (1982) Specific covalent binding and toxicity of aliphatic halogenated xenobiotics. *Rev. Drug Metab. Inter.*, **4**, 1–48.

Lake, B. G. and Gangolli, S. D. (1981) Toxification and detoxification as a result of xenobiotic metabolism. In *Concepts in drug metabolism* (eds P. Jenner and B. Testa), Marcel Dekker, New York, pp. 167–218.

Levin, W., Wood, A., Chang, R., Ryan, D. and Thomas, P. (1982) Oxidative metabolism of polycyclic aromatic hydrocarbons to ultimate carcinogens. *Drug Metab. Rev.*, **13**, 555–80.

Lock, E. A. (1982) Renal Necrosis produced by Halogenated Chemicals. In *Nephrotoxicity* (eds P. H. Bach, F. W. Bonner, J. M. Bridges and E. A. Lock), Wiley, Chichester, pp. 396–408.

Miller, E. C. and Miller, J. A. (1976) The metabolism of chemical carcinogens to reactive electrophiles and their possible mechanisms of action in carcinogenesis. In *Chemical carcinogens* (ACS Monograph 173, ed. C. E. Searle), American Chemical Society, Washington, pp. 737–62.

Mitchell, J. R., Jollow, D. J., Potter, W. Z., Davis, D. C., Gillette, J. R. and Brodie, B. B. (1973) Acetaminophen-induced hepatic necrosis: role of drug metabolism. *J. Pharmacol. Exp. Ther.*, **187**, 185–95.

Neal, R. A. and Halpert, J. (1982) Toxicology of thiono-sulphur compounds. *Ann. Rev. Pharmacol. Toxicol.*, **22**, 321–39.

Neal, R. A., Sawahata, T., Halpert, J. and Kamataki, T. (1983) Chemically reactive metabolites as suicide enzyme inhibitors. *Drug Metab. Rev.*, **14**, 49–59.

Nebert, D. W. (1983) Genetic differences in drug metabolism. Proposed relationship to human birth defects. In *Teratogenesis and reproductive toxicology, handbook of experimental pharmacology, Vol. 65* (eds E. M. Johnson and D. M. Kochhar), Springer-Verlag, Berlin, p. 49–62.

Pelkonen, O. and Nebert, D. W. (1982) Metabolism of polycyclic aromatic hydrocarbons: etiologic role in carcinogenesis. *Pharmacol. Rev.*, **34**, 189–222.

Prescott, L. F. (1983) Paracetamol overdosage: pharmacological considerations and clinical management. *Drugs*, **25**, 290–314.

Rush, G. F. and Hook, J. B. (1982) Renal drug metabolism and nephrotoxicity. In *Nephrotoxicity* (eds P. H. Bach, F. W. Bonner, J. W. Bridges and E. A. Lock), Wiley, Chichester, pp. 237–45.

Rush, G. F., Smith, J. H., Newton, J. F. and Hook, J. B. (1984) Chemically-induced nephrotoxicity: role of metabolic activation. *CRC Crit. Rev. Toxicol.* **13**, 99–160.

Sugimura, T., Wakabayashi, K., Yamada, N., Nagao, M. and Fujino, T. (1980) Activation of chemicals to proximate carcinogens. In *Mechanisms of toxicity and hazard evaluation* (eds B. Holmstedt, R. Lauwerys, M. Mercier and M. Roberfroid), Elsevier, Amsterdam, pp. 205–17.

Timbrell, J. A., Seales, M. D. C. and Streeter, A. J. (1982) Studies on hydrazine hepatotoxicity (2): biochemical findings. *J. Toxicol. Environ. Health*, **10**, 955–68.

7

Pharmacokinetics and the clinical relevance of drug metabolism

7.1 Introduction

Drug metabolism in Man is not as amenable to study as that in animals, due to the practical and ethical constraints on experimentation. There is only limited access to tissue samples (see the discussion of methods in Section 7.3) and it is very difficult to find a reasonably homogeneous group of patients on which to perform the studies. Different approaches to the study of drug metabolism have to be adopted in Man as routine procedures – the most usual of which is the measurement of drug concentrations in serum over an extended time period. Other biological fluids may also be used; these methods are discussed later. The theoretical and mathematical interpretations of tissue drug concentration data are termed *pharmacokinetics*.

Pharmacokinetics is particularly important from a clinical view as the intensity and duration of action of a drug are related to what concentration of the drug is present at the active site and how long an effective concentration is found there. The ability to calculate the concentration of drug at a particular time can be vital in assessing the dose and frequency of dosing of a drug of low therapeutic index, e.g. anticoagulants, cardiac glycosides, anti-cancer drugs (see the examples given later).

Recently, the ability to correlate *in vivo* pharmacokinetic and metabolic data with *in vitro* metabolic data has become topical. Does increased drug metabolism have any effect on elimination of drugs from the body? This question will be examined in detail later.

This chapter will deal with pharmacokinetics mainly from a physiological point of view (mathematical equations will be given where they assist in the understanding of the principles but no derivations will be given; these can be found in any standard pharmacokinetic textbook and are of little relevance here). The special relevance of the hepatic drug-metabolizing capacity to pharmacokinetics will be highlighted. The methods of obtaining clinical data related to drug metabolism will also be discussed and the correlation of *in vivo* and *in vitro* data considered. Finally, specific examples of the clinical relevance of drug metabolism will be given with a discussion of the wider implications such as induction/inhibition of drug metabolism in drug interactions and the effects of disease states on pharmacokinetic parameters.

7.2 Pharmacokinetics

Pharmacokinetics is the study of the uptake, distribution and excretion of drugs with respect to time. In practice this means measuring the concentration of drug in various tissues and body fluids over a period of time. The processes involved in the determination of pharmacokinetic patterns are illustrated in Figure 7.1.

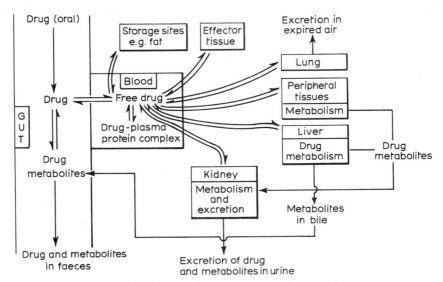

Figure 7.1 Processes involved in the determination of pharmacokinetic parameters.

7.2.1 THE ONE-COMPARTMENT MODEL

It can be appreciated that the movement of drug between different compartments of the body (blood, adipose tissue, liver etc.) is a complex, dynamic process and not readily amenable to analysis. It is therefore assumed, as a first approximation, that all body compartments are in rapid equilibrium with a central compartment (normally equated with the blood), and that the concentration of drug is constant throughout. The actual correlation of pharmacokinetic compartments with real anatomical tissues or organs is rather complex and, at times, impossible; this should be borne in mind during these discussions (for further discussion of this point see later in this chapter). Thus the therapeutic effects of a drug should be related to the concentration of drug in blood. This is not always the case and this failing of the model system should be borne in mind.

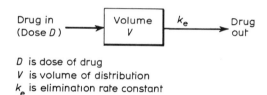

D is dose of drug
V is volume of distribution
k_e is elimination rate constant

Figure 7.2 The one-compartment model.

Using the approximation discussed above a pharmacokinetic model can be constructed where the areas in the body that the drug reaches are represented by a single compartment. Figure 7.2 shows the *one-compartment model*. It is assumed that the drug is injected directly into this compartment (e.g. intravenous injection) and distributes itself instantaneously throughout the compartment. Thus the concentration of drug at zero time (C_0) can be calculated or, conversely if C_0 is known, V can be calculated:

$$C_0 = D/V \quad \text{or} \quad V = D/C_0$$

where V is volume of distribution and D is dose of drug.

Elimination of the drug from the compartment then takes place at a rate determined by the elimination rate constant (k_e). For most drugs this elimination is a negative exponential function, i.e. a plot of log drug concentration versus time yields a straight line (Figure 7.3).

This means that the time taken for a decrease in drug concentration to half the original value (wherever on the curve the original value is taken) will always be the same. This time is referred to as the *half-life* ($t_{\frac{1}{2}}$) for the drug. The actual form of such a semi-log plot is more often similar to that shown in Figure 7.4. The deviation of the actual and theoretical curves at the start is due

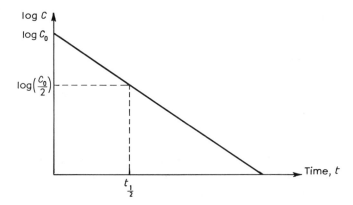

Figure 7.3 Theoretical curve for change in plasma drug concentration in the one-compartment model.

to distribution of the drug taking a finite time therefore the sampled (blood) compartment has a higher concentration of drug than the body as a whole.

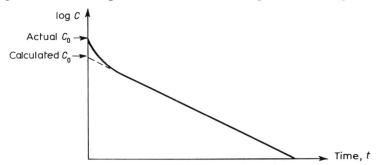

Figure 7.4 Experimental curve for change in plasma concentration of a drug approximating to the one-compartment model.

We thus have various parameters that can be measured or calculated:

$$
\begin{aligned}
V &= \text{volume of distribution;} \\
C_0 &= \text{concentration of drug at time 0;} \\
C_t &= \text{concentration of drug at various times } t; \\
t_{\frac{1}{2}} &= \text{half-life of elimination;} \\
k_e &= \text{elimination rate constant;} \\
D &= \text{dose of drug given.}
\end{aligned}
$$

The elimination rate constant (k_e) is defined as the rate of change of drug concentration at unit initial drug concentrations (or mathematically as below):

$$
dC/dt = -k_e C_0
$$

Using this equation and measurements of blood drug concentrations at various times the elimination rate constant can be calculated. The elimination rate constant is a composite figure encompassing all methods of elimination (excretion in urine, faeces, expired air, sweat etc., biotransformation and sequestration in tissues not sampled) – it is almost impossible to separate it into its components (this is important when discussing the correlations between *in vivo* and *in vitro* measures of drug metabolism – see Section 7.3.6).

If the equation above is expressed in another form:

$$\log C \; = \; \log C_0 \; - \; k_e t \log e$$

then a relationship between k_e and $t_{\frac{1}{2}}$ can be seen:

$$\log [\, C/C_0 \,] \; = \; - k_e t \log e$$

where e = the exponential function ($\log e = 0.434$).
At $t_{\frac{1}{2}}$: $C = C_0/2$

Thus $\log (\frac{1}{2}) \; = \; -0.301 \; = \; -0.434 k_e t_{\frac{1}{2}}$ and $k_e \; = \; 0.693/t_{\frac{1}{2}}$

So the elimination rate constant is inversely proportional to the half-life of the drug. This is quite logical, as the faster the elimination (greater k_e), the faster one-half of the drug will be eliminated and therefore the shorter the half-life.

So overall we have the facts that the rate at which a drug is eliminated from the body is dependent on a complex elimination rate constant, the dose of drug and the body volume through which the drug is distributed:

$$\frac{dC}{dt} \; = \; - \frac{k_e D}{V}$$

The volume of distribution of a drug is also a complex 'constant'. In physiological terms it is difficult to equate calculated volumes of distribution with actual body compartments but some aspects can be considered. The drug may only enter the blood and have a small volume of distribution, or it may enter the extracellular fluid or even permeate all cells, thus giving a large volume of distribution. In certain circumstances a volume of distribution greater than the body volume can be obtained. This is a function of the measurement of body concentration of drug (usually by blood sampling). The blood concentration of drug may be very low due to sequestration of drug in, say, adipose tissue; therefore, the volume of distribution will seem to be very large whereas in reality it is small (the drug being distributed only in adipose tissue).

This simple model shows the theoretical basis, and practical problems of interpretation, of pharmacokinetic analysis, and introduces the basic concepts that will be expanded upon in the rest of this chapter.

7.2.2 THE TWO-COMPARTMENT MODEL

The one-compartment model discussed above assumes that elimination can occur from all compartments but a glance at Figure 7.1 shows that this is not always valid: many peripheral tissues cannot excrete directly and excretions take place mainly from the blood (via urine, faeces). A refinement can be added to account for this in the form of an outer, non-excreting compartment (Figure 7.5). This is called the *two-compartment model*, where the two compartments are kinetically distinguishable and therefore different.

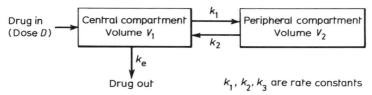

Figure 7.5 The two-compartment model.

Such a model gives a plot of log drug concentration (in the central compartment, i.e. blood) versus time as shown in Figure 7.6. There are two distinct slopes: the first (steeper) slope being related to distribution of drug from the central to the peripheral compartment, and the second (shallower) slope is the

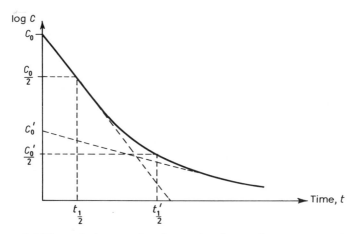

Figure 7.6 Theoretical curve for change in plasma drug concentration in the two-compartment model.

Table 7.1 Tissue groupings for pharmacokinetic
assessment

Description of group	Tissues
Plasma	Plasma
Highly perfused non-fat	Blood cells
	Heart
	Lung
	Liver
	Kidney
	Glands
Poorly perfused non-fat	Muscle
	Skin
Fatty tissues	Adipose tissue
	Bone marrow
Negligible perfusion	Bone
	Teeth
	Cartilage
	Hair

elimination of drug from the central compartment. The second half-life $t_{\frac{1}{2}}'$ is the true half-life of elimination as defined earlier. This theoretical slope more closely follows the actual plots and thus is a more realistic model.

The central compartment is generally equated with the blood, and the peripheral compartment with other tissues; but this does not always hold true as, in some instances, the extracellular space is included which can (as discussed before) be apparently larger than can possibly exist. No anatomical basis of the various compartments can thus be seen although an arbitrary subdivision of tissues has been attempted (Table 7.1). This consists of five groups ranging from the fluid which is the basis of the central compartment (the blood plasma) to a little-perfused group (of relatively minor pharmacokinetic interest). Which of these groups are included in the central and which in the peripheral compartment depends on the drug in question.

As can be imagined, mathematical analysis of a two-compartment model is more complex than that of a one-compartment model. To understand the analysis one further parameter is necessary: i.e. area under the concentration–time curve (AUC). This is exactly what its name suggests – the area under the curve when plasma drug concentration is plotted against time (Figure 7.7). The area under the curve is a measure of the total body load of drug (i.e. bioavailability) and is therefore an indirect indication of the therapeutic value of the drug.

The AUC can be measured experimentally and used to calculate the clearance of drug from the body as below. Clearance is defined as the volume of the central compartment which is cleared of drug in unit time, and this is a

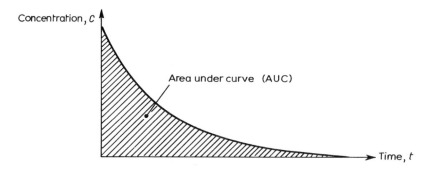

Figure 7.7 The area under the concentration–time curve.

measure of the efficiency with which a drug is eliminated from the body via all routes.

$$\text{Clearance} = D/\text{AUC} \quad \text{where } D \text{ is the dose of drug given.}$$

Clearance can also be expressed in terms of the elimination rate constant:

$$\text{Clearance} = k_e V_1$$

where k_e is the elimination rate constant; and V_1 is the volume of the central compartment.

In each case clearance appears as volume per unit time. Clearance is a very important concept in pharmacokinetics and therapeutics, as we will see later.

A number of problems arise from the use of a two-compartment model. One problem is analytical and is related to the fact that the concentration of drug in the central compartment is no longer related solely to drug elimination but also to movement of drug between the central and peripheral compartments. It depends on the relative rate constants (k_1, k_2 and k_e) whether movement of drug or elimination is the most important. A second problem is more pharmacological, and relates to the position of the receptor for the drug.

The action of the drug will be related to the concentration of drug in the same compartment as the receptor; thus analysis of drug concentrations in both compartments is strictly necessary to evaluate the relevance of pharmacokinetic data in clinical practice using a two-compartment model. The difficulty of assigning anatomical regions to the various compartments makes this somewhat suspect.

7.2.3 KINETIC ORDER OF REACTION

One final theoretical consideration to be discussed is the relationship of kinetic order-of-reaction to pharmacokinetics. All of the theory so far discussed assumes that the elimination of drug is directly related to its concentration (i.e.

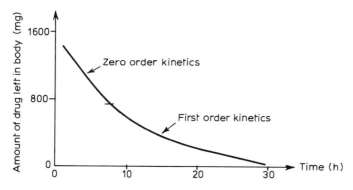

Figure 7.8 Clearance of acetylsalicylic acid in Man. (Taken from Levy, G. (1965) *J. Pharm. Sci.*, **54**, 959. Used with permission of the copyright owner.)

the elimination is first order). If, however, the processes of elimination are saturated (normally at high drug concentration when metabolism is the rate-limiting step of elimination), then the elimination rate is independent of drug concentration (i.e. zero-order kinetics). In this case a plot of drug concentration versus time is linear. This can be seen very well with higher doses of aspirin (Figure 7.8). At first, salicylate concentration falls linearly with time until a certain concentration is reached and sub-saturation is reached, when first-order kinetics reappear.

In exceptional circumstances involving two or more substances in metabolism or excretion, multi-order kinetics can be seen but such instances are rare.

7.2.4 CLINICAL APPLICATION OF PHARMACOKINETICS

In clinical practice it is unusual to give a single dose of drug and it is more usual to give a drug by a method other than intravenous injection. Consideration of multiple drug dosing and other forms of administration is therefore in order.

Let us first examine a drug administered in a way that does not give direct entry into the central compartment, i.e. involving absorption. In these cases the drug first enters another compartment, the absorption compartment. This is an extension of the one- or two-compartment models outlined above (Figure 7.9).

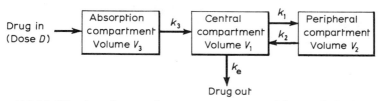

Figure 7.9 Modification of one- and two-compartment models to include the absorption compartment.

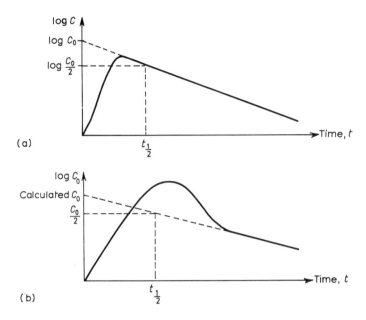

Figure 7.10 Theoretical curve for change in plasma drug concentration in the modified (a) one- and (b) two-compartment models.

The drug is subsequently distributed to the central compartment (and in the case of the two-compartment model to the peripheral compartment) and excreted. It can be seen that absorption could still be proceeding as elimination starts, and this gives the log dose response curve(s) as shown in Figure 7.10 ((a) for the one-compartment and (b) for the two-compartment model). For the one-compartment model both the absorption rate constant (k_a) and the elimination rate constant (k_e) can be calculated by extrapolation of the respective curves and by using the equations given earlier. In the two-compartment model, however, absorption, distribution and elimination are proceeding simultaneously; the early phase of the curve cannot be analysed satisfactorily. Further complications arise in oral dosing as the rate of dissolution of the drug must also be taken into account. Pharmacokinetic data from orally administered drugs are, therefore, very difficult to interpret.

Most drugs are administered for an extended period of time and it is of great interest to the clinician to know what dose and at what dosage interval to give a drug in order to achieve an effective drug concentration at its site of action. A consideration of the kinetics of multiple dosing is thus of interest.

The effect of multiple dosing depends on the relationship between the half-life of the drug and the frequency of dosing. If the dosing interval is much longer

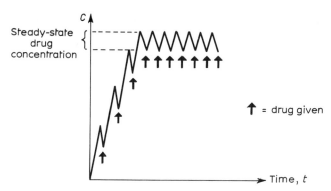

Figure 7.11 Theoretical curve for change in plasma drug concentration on multiple dosing.

than the half-life then the dose will be effectively cleared before the next is given and each dose can be considered as entirely separate. If, however, dosage interval is about $t_{\frac{1}{2}}$ or less, then accumulation of drug occurs until a steady-state concentration is reached (Figure 7.11). The steady-state concentration of drug is dependent on the dose of drug given, the fraction of drug absorbed, the half-life of the drug, the volume of distribution and the dose interval:

$$C = \frac{1.44 t_{\frac{1}{2}} FD}{Vi}$$

where C is steady state concentration; $t_{\frac{1}{2}}$ is half-life; F is fraction of drug absorbed; D is dose of drug; V is volume of distribution; and i is dose interval.

Factors affecting drug half-life, absorption and volume of distribution thus affect the steady-state concentration of drug during multiple dosing (see earlier for discussion of these parameters).

7.2.5 HEPATIC DRUG CLEARANCE

One of the major methods of removing drug from the central compartment is hepatic drug metabolism, i.e. removal by conversion to a metabolite and, probably, subsequent excretion. The ability of the liver to remove drug from the blood is related to only two variables, i.e. the intrinsic hepatic clearance Cl_{int} and the hepatic blood flow B:

$$\text{Hepatic clearance} = B\left(\frac{Cl_{int}}{B + Cl_{int}}\right) = BR_e$$

Intrinsic clearance is the maximum ability of the liver to extract drug in the absence of blood flow restrictions. The term in brackets (in the above equation) is referred to as the extraction ratio R_e.

Table 7.2 Comparison of flow- and metabolism-limited hepatic clearance

	Flow-limited	Metabolism-limited
Clearance related to	Blood flow	Intrinsic clearance
Extraction ratio	> 0.8	< 0.2
Examples	Lignocaine, propranolol	Antipyrine

When intrinsic clearance Cl_{int} is very much greater than hepatic blood flow then the extraction ratio approaches 1.0 and hepatic clearance is dependent only on blood flow, i.e. the liver extracts all of the drug presented to it. Thus, the more blood passing through the liver the more drug will be extracted. On the other hand, if Cl_{int} is very much less than blood flow, then hepatic clearance is dependent only on Cl_{int}, i.e. the liver extracts as much drug as it can from whatever blood flow is presented. These two extremes are called flow-limited and metabolism-limited extraction, respectively. The characteristics of the two conditions are summarized in Table 7.2.

Intermediate values of extraction ratio (0.2–0.8) give hepatic clearance rates that are dependent on both blood flow and hepatic intrinsic clearance to varying extents. It is obvious, therefore, that hepatic clearance of drugs may not only be related to the ability of the liver to metabolize drugs but also be dependent on factors affecting the hepatic blood flow, such as changes in cardiac output and redistribution of blood flow (e.g. during exercise or stress).

7.2.6 PHARMACOKINETICS: A SUMMARY

This has been a very brief view of the complexity of pharmacokinetics, but it is hoped that it has indicated the physiological correlation of the pharmaco-kinetic parameters where known and that it has shown the relevance of pharmacokinetic analysis to clinical practice. The usefulness of this approach must, however, be examined with respect to the failings of mathematical analysis to completely mimic the actual behaviour of the organism, due to the complexity of the processes under study.

7.3 Methods for studying drug metabolism in Man

The ability to metabolize a particular drug may be of prime importance in determining the efficacy, duration of action and, even, toxicity of the drug, particularly if the drug in question is lipophilic (fat-soluble) in nature. It is, thus, of importance to be able to assess the ability of patients to metabolize drugs, especially if the drug has a low therapeutic index and needs to be present in the body at a level close to the toxic threshold (e.g. cardiac glycosides). Many

Table 7.3 Methods of assessing drug metabolism in Man

Methods	Substrates used
In vivo clearance	Antipyrine
	Phenacetin
	Theophylline
	Hexobarbitone
	Tolbutamide
	Aminopyrine
	Amylobarbitone
	Diazepam
	Heptobarbitone
	Phenylbutazone
	Quinine
	Warfarin
Breath analysis	Aminopyrine
	Diazepam
	Caffeine
	Mephenytoin
Metabolite ratio	Sulfadimidine
	Debrisoquine
In vitro methods	Antipyrine
Non-invasive methods	
plasma γ-glutamyltransaminase	
urinary D-glucaric acid	
urinary 6β-hydroxycortisol	
plasma bilirubin	

methods have been developed to measure drug-metabolizing capacity in Man and, in this section, each method will be outlined and the relevance of the method briefly discussed together with the problems of interpreting the results obtained.

The methods are listed in Table 7.3.

7.3.1 IN VIVO CLEARANCE

The mathematical theories underlying the measurements of *in vivo* clearance have been discussed above, and study of the models reveals a number of criteria that must be fulfilled before clearance can be equated to drug metabolism. These are:

(1) The drug must be rapidly and reproducibly absorbed (preferably 100% absorbed).

2) The drug should be distributed throughout total body water (i.e. equivalent to a one-compartment model).

(3) The drug should not bind to tissue or plasma protein (only free drug is metabolized, excreted, etc.).
(4) The drug should only be metabolized by the liver with a low extraction ratio (i.e. metabolism is not flow-limited).
(5) The drug should have negligible renal clearance (i.e. hepatic clearance is the predominant method of clearance).

If all of these criteria are met then drug clearance serves as a meaningful measure of drug metabolism that is not influenced by hepatic blood flow.

The model drug which comes nearest to this ideal is antipyrine where the drug's half-life and clearance both give a good estimate of hepatic metabolism (indicating one-compartment kinetics). Antipyrine has a number of other advantages:

(1) It is easily measured in body fluids after a dose that is pharmacologically inactive.
(2) Salivary pharmacokinetics are similar to plasma pharmacokinetics, therefore saliva can be sampled instead of the more painful and potentially damaging venepuncture.

The disadvantages of antipyrine are relatively minor but should always be considered. Antipyrine clearance does not always correlate well with metabolism (clearance) of other drugs and therefore is a poor marker for certain drug-metabolizing enzyme activities. This is probably due to the existence of multiple forms of drug-metabolizing enzymes in the human liver. Antipyrine is metabolized to at least three metabolites, and the kinetics of clearance – although appearing simple – are, in fact, quite complex:

$$\text{Clearance (total)} = \text{clearance (a)} + \text{clearance (b)} + \text{clearance (c)}$$

$$+ \text{clearance (rest)}$$

where (a) = metabolite a, (b) = metabolite b, (c) = metabolite c, and (rest) = unchanged drug + non-identified metabolites.

Total clearance is a complex term, including clearance of all metabolites and unchanged drug; a change in one or more of these parameters leads to a change in total clearance, and opposite changes in two parameters can give no apparent change in total clearance, thus masking the effects. Antipyrine is also an inducer of hepatic drug-metabolizing enzymes and therefore repeated tests with the drug should be avoided to prevent misleading results being obtained.

Antipyrine is thus a suitable model drug to employ in the study of drug metabolism in Man and has had a very great deal of use. Some examples of the use of antipyrine will be given later, in Section 7.3.6.

Other model substrates have also been employed as markers of hepatic drug metabolism (see Table 7.3). Of these, phenacetin and theophylline are thought to be metabolized by a polycyclic hydrocarbon-inducible form of cytochrome P-450 (see Chapter 3) and thus act as markers of different isoenzymes than antipyrine. Theophylline is, perhaps, the better of these, as phenacetin undergoes significant metabolism in the gut wall to the O-de-ethylated product, paracetamol.

Hexobarbitone and tolbutamide are useful models as they are almost completely metabolized by the liver, tolbutamide being better as it is only metabolized to one compound, hydroxytolbutamide, and its excretion is almost entirely dependent on this biotransformation.

All of the other substrates used do not meet all of the criteria outlined earlier: phenylbutazone and amylobarbitone are not metabolized exclusively in the liver; warfarin, quinine and phenylbutazone are all to a greater or lesser extent bound to plasma proteins. The assay techniques used do not normally distinguish between free and bound drug, and, thus, an inaccurate measure of free (and, thus metabolizable and excretable) drug will be obtained.

A number of substrates can be used in the study of drug clearance, many of which are good indicators of hepatic drug metabolism. Critical use of this technique can yield useful information regarding the functioning of the liver in Man. A further discussion of the relevance of drug clearance to hepatic drug metabolism can be found in Section 7.3.6.

7.3.2 BREATH ANALYSIS

This method relies on the hepatic breakdown of aminopyrine to yield carbon dioxide (CO_2) which is excreted via the lungs. Appropriate radiolabelling (with ^{14}C) of the substrate leads to $^{14}CO_2$ being excreted which can be collected and measured (Figure 7.12). Aminopyrine is predominantly metabolized by the hepatic mixed-function oxidase system by N-demethylation and, thus, the aminopyrine breath test can be used as an indicator of the functioning of this enzyme system. Indeed the correlation between $^{14}CO_2$ excretion and *in vivo* clearance rate for aminopyrine is good, indicating the relevance of this method.

Other substrates have also been used in breath tests as aminopyrine may only be a model substrate for a limited number of the isoenzymes of the mixed-function oxidase system in the liver. Caffeine has been employed as a marker of a polycyclic hydrocarbon-induced isoenzyme.

The disadvantages of this method are that it is assumed that formation of formaldehyde (i.e. drug demethylation) is the rate-limiting step in the production of carbon dioxide (i.e. oxidation of formaldehyde to carbon dioxide is much more rapid than formaldehyde production); this has not been conclusively

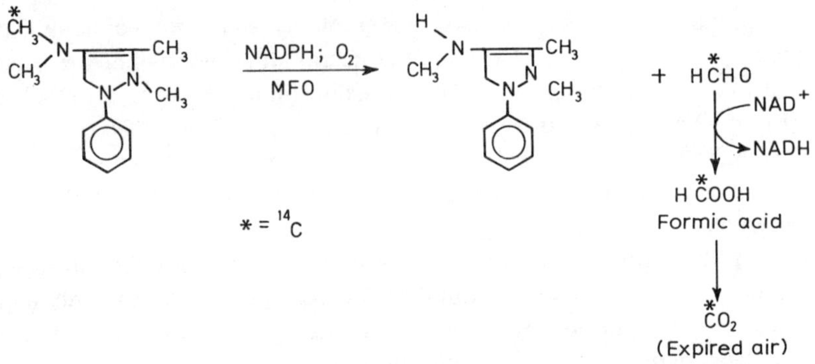

Figure 7.12 The metabolism of ^{14}C-aminopyrine showing release of $^{14}CO_2$ in expired air.

proved. The patient is also subjected to radioactivity – which is not an ideal situation; a breath test using ^{13}C (a stable non-radioactive form of carbon) is being developed which will circumvent this objection.

7.3.3 METABOLITE RATIOS

This method relies on the drug being metabolized by the liver to a compound that is released back into the blood-stream, and stays there long enough to be measured, or is excreted in the urine together with the parent compound. This, of course, is not true for all drugs, e.g. those that are excreted in bile, those metabolites that are rapidly excreted, etc. It is particularly useful, however, in the study of two reactions: N-acetylation of sulfonamides and hydrazines (e.g. isoniazid), and debrisoquine hydroxylation. This is of interest, as both of these reactions exhibit genetic polymorphism (see examples later in this chapter).

N-Acetylation is most commonly measured using sulfadimidine. The ratio of acetylated to unchanged drug in plasma is measured. The ratio gives a measure of the function of the N-acetylase in the liver and thus the so-called 'acetylator status'. The relevance of acetylator status or phenotype will be discussed later in the chapter.

Drug oxidation can also be investigated using metabolite ratios using debrisoquine as substrate; the drug is metabolized by the liver to 4-hydroxy-debrisoquine. After a single oral dose of debrisoquine, urine is collected and the ratio of 4-hydroxydebrisoquine to parent drug measured.

Another drug which has been used as a model of hepatic oxidation for metabolite ratio is sparteine. This drug has a complex metabolism leading to the formation of 2- and 5-dehydrosparteine. A method similar to that of debrisoquine is used to determine the metabolite ratio.

This method is easy to perform and does not entail any major risk to the patient. It is thought that this type of test may eventually be employed as a screening test for potential toxic reactions to drugs (see later in this chapter).

7.3.4 *IN VITRO* METHODS

It is obvious that if one wishes to investigate hepatic drug metabolism then the best model is the liver itself. Surgical removal of part (or all) of the liver and subjecting it to various tests of drug-metabolizing ability is the ideal way of gaining information on hepatic drug metabolism. This is the method most commonly employed in animal experiments and is undeniably the most logical. A number of things have to be considered, however, before such studies are initiated in Man: (1) ethical considerations; (2) sampling procedures; and (3) assay methods.

Is it ethically acceptable to take a liver sample from a healthy volunteer considering the risks involved in such a procedure? The widely held view is that it is not acceptable, and therefore most human liver material is to some extent pathological. It is only acceptable to obtain human liver biopsy material if it is suspected that something is wrong with the liver. This, of course, means that one is generally dealing with more or less diseased tissue which makes interpretation of data and extrapolation to the normal human situation difficult. The only time when 'normal' liver does become available is from individuals who have died of a non-liver-related cause, e.g. during kidney or heart transplant operations (from the donor). This procedure raises its own ethical problems of consent to removal of organs for medical research – a topic which is not within the scope of this book.

From the practical point of view, even if a sample of liver tissue is available it may not be suitable for assay of drug-metabolizing ability. Samples of liver tissue can be obtained from living patients by percutaneous needle biopsy or wedge biopsy during abdominal surgery. These methods produce fresh tissue directly from the body and are thus subject to minimum disturbance, but only small quantities (milligrams) of tissue can be taken. The size of the sample means that few tests can be performed per patient and also the relevance of the sample is suspect due to the known heterogeneity of the liver (differences in drug metabolism between the centrilobular and peripheral areas of the liver). A further complication is the risk involved in obtaining the sample, e.g. infection and internal bleeding from needle biopsy and the inherent risks of major abdominal surgery in taking a wedge biopsy.

Larger samples of liver can be obtained following death e.g. at post mortem. This method has the disadvantage that the liver starts degenerating from the moment of death even if stored cold and, thus, unless obtained relatively soon

Table 7.4 Comparison of the methods of liver sampling

Source	Amount	Ethical availability	Reliability	Background knowledge
Needle biopsy	Small	Good[†]	Fair	Good
Wedge biopsy	Small	Good[†]	Fair	Good
Post-mortem	Large	Good	Poor	Fair
Transplant	Large	Poor–fair	Good	Poor

[†]in cases of suspected liver disease; poor in other cases.

after death, the liver enzymes may not represent those found during life. Indeed a limit of 2–4 h after death is put on the liver if it is to be of any use in the study of drug metabolism. As few post mortem examinations are carried out this soon after death, this possible source of liver material is severely limited. One possibility that has been exploited is to remove the liver from clinically dead kidney donors during kidney transplant. From a practical viewpoint this is an excellent method as the liver is virtually normal and functional and so is almost the equivalent of a large biopsy sample. The ethical considerations of this approach are, however, questionable and have been discussed above. One disadvantage of transplant material is the often inadequate background knowledge of the donor (smoking and drinking habits, previous drug use etc.) which might affect drug-metabolizing capacity. A summary of the various sources of human liver material is given in Table 7.4.

Having obtained a sample of liver one has to decide the best preparation to use to assess drug-metabolizing capacity. A list of possible preparations is given in Table 7.5.

The choice is between a physiological preparation (whole perfused liver) or a biochemical preparation (cellular sub-fractions) or a compromise situation (liver slices, cubes and cells). The physiological preparation can only be used if the intact liver is available; it is difficult to set up and keep running. It does, however, give the nearest approximation to the *in vivo* situation. The preparation of subcellular fractions, mainly microsomes, derived from the endoplasmic reticulum, is the easiest method but suffers from its non-physiological nature. An attempt to reach a mid-point between physiological complexity and

Table 7.5 Liver preparations

Whole liver (perfused)
Liver slices
Liver cubes
Isolated liver cells
Liver homogenate
Isolated liver cell subfractions (e.g. microsomes)

Table 7.6 Comparison of liver preparations in assessing drug metabolism

Method	Degree of difficulty	*In vivo* relevance	Reproducibility
Perfused liver	High	Good	Poor
Liver slices	Moderate	Fair	Fair
Liver cubes	Moderate	Fair	Fair
Liver cells	Moderate	Fair	Fair
Subcellular fractions	Low	Fair–poor	Good

biochemical ease has been the use of liver slices and, more recently, cubes and isolated cells. Slices and cubes have the physiological cell–cell contact needed for liver function but are somewhat unsatisfactory due to excessive destruction of cells during preparation. Isolated liver cells can be tested for viability but lack the surface contact. Attaching the cells to beads or collagen membranes has, to a certain extent, circumvented the contact problem.

No method of using the liver material obtained is, therefore, ideal; it depends on the nature of the problem whether a more physiological or biochemical approach is required. If changes in enzyme content are under investigation then subcellular fractions may be more appropriate; whereas if hepatotoxicity is being studied then a whole liver preparation may lead to the required results. A summary of the advantages and disadvantages of the various methods is given in Table 7.6.

Recently liver banks have been set up in various hospitals where whole-liver samples and subcellular fractions of liver are stored at very low temperatures. The samples are characterized and medical researchers have access to these samples. Samples of known characteristics can thus be obtained to subject to various tests when the tests become available. A data base, of correlations between individual tests for drug-metabolizing capacity, can then be built up which can be referred back to in later experiments.

In vivo assay of drug-metabolizing capacity is the most direct method provided the techniques employed are relevant to the problem under study, and medical ethics are not contravened.

7.3.5 NON-INVASIVE METHODS

Those methods not requiring the administration of a drug are referred to as non-invasive. They rely on changes in endogenous metabolism to give a measure of changes in drug metabolism. This is not unreasonable, as much of drug metabolism is related to endogenous compound metabolism; e.g. steroid metabolism is predominantly performed by mixed-function oxidase-like enzymes, neurotransmitters are metabolized by enzymes that also metabolize drugs, and glucuronidation is related to glucose metabolism (see Chapter 1 for discussion of the inter-relationship between endogenous and xenobiotic metabolism).

The non-invasive techniques used are: measurements of plasma γ-glutamyltransferase (GGT), plasma bilirubin, urinary 6β-hydroxycortisol and urinary D-glucaric acid.

(a) γ-GLUTAMYLTRANSFERASE (GGT)

γ-Glutamyltransferase is not involved in the metabolism of drugs but rather catalyses the transfer of γ-glutamyl moieties from glutathione to other peptides. It is located in many tissues, e.g. liver, kidney, endocrine organs, and has been used for some time as a marker of liver damage.

It has been stated that hepatic enzyme induction, including induction of drug-metabolizing enzymes, is accompanied by increased plasma GGT. Other drugs, however, also cause increases in plasma GGT. Definitive studies have shown that a rise in plasma GGT is related more to a disturbance of the plasma membrane in the liver than to enzyme induction, and thus is not a good index of changes in hepatic drug metabolism.

(b) PLASMA BILIRUBIN

Bilirubin is removed from plasma by conjugation to glucuronic acid in the liver and subsequent excretion. As many drugs also rely on glucuronide conjugation for their excretion, it was thought possible that plasma bilirubin levels could be used as a measure of hepatic glucuronidation (e.g. patients with a genetically low hepatic UDP–glucuronyltransferase activity – Gilbert's disease – have raised plasma levels of unconjugated bilirubin). No direct comparisons between plasma levels of bilirubin and conjugation of drugs (e.g. chloramphenicol, morphine and oxazepam, which are cleared mainly via glucuronidation in the liver) have been made. The presence of multiple forms of UDP–glucuronyltransferases in the liver may invalidate this possible approach to studying hepatic conjugation reactions.

(c) URINARY 6β-HYDROXYCORTISOL (6β-OHC)

6β-Hydroxycortisol is produced from cortisol primarily by the hepatic mixed-function oxidase system. This is normally a minor pathway in the excretion of glucocorticoids, the major pathway being via 17-hydroxycorticosteroids (17-OHCS). Therefore the proportion of glucocorticoids excreted as the 6β-hydroxy derivatives should give a measure of the activity of the hepatic mixed-function oxidase system. A ratio of 6β-OHC/17-OHCS is a better indicator of changes in hepatic drug metabolism in Man than the simple measurement of 6β-OHC excretion. The excretion of 6β-hydroxycortisol is not, however, a general indicator of hepatic drug-metabolizing capacity as metabolite ratio studies with debrisoquine (see above) do not correlate with excretion of 6β-hydroxycortisol. This is again probably due to different isoenzymes in the liver responsible for debrisoquine and cortisol metabolism. There is also no correlation between excretion of 6β-hydroxycortisol and antipyrine clearance showing that 6β-hydroxycortisol is not an absolute indication of hepatic drug metabolsim. This test should only be used in a comparison of different groups of subjects and not as a predictive test of inter-individual variations in drug metabolism. 6β-Hydroxycortisol excretion also does not seem to be of use in assessing inhibition of drug metabolism.

(d) URINARY D-GLUCARIC ACID

D-Glucaric acid is produced in the body from glucose (Figure 7.13). Its biosynthesis is an extension of the pathway that forms glycogen and glucuronides. The measurement of urinary D-glucaric acid is somewhat complex depending

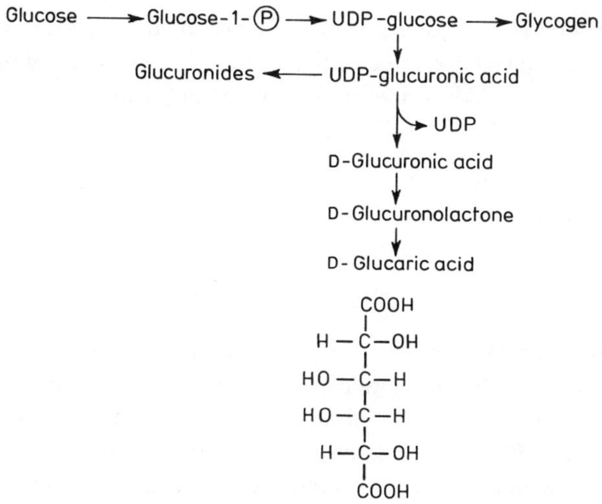

Glucose ⟶ Glucose-1-(P) ⟶ UDP-glucose ⟶ Glycogen

Glucuronides ⟵ UDP-glucuronic acid

⟶ UDP

D-Glucuronic acid

D-Glucuronolactone

D-Glucaric acid

$$
\begin{array}{c}
\text{COOH} \\
|\\
\text{H}-\text{C}-\text{OH} \\
|\\
\text{HO}-\text{C}-\text{H} \\
|\\
\text{HO}-\text{C}-\text{H} \\
|\\
\text{H}-\text{C}-\text{OH} \\
|\\
\text{COOH}
\end{array}
$$

Figure 7.13 Synthesis of D-glucaric acid.

on the conversion of the acid to the lactone (D-glucaro-1,4-lactone) and use of this compound to inhibit the breakdown of phenolphthalein glucuronide by β-glucuronidase. Very large inter-individual variation is seen which limits the use of this test and no correlation is seen between basal D-glucaric acid

Table 7.7 Comparison of non-invasive methods of assessing drug metabolism

Method	Degree of difficulty	Variation	Correlation to drug metabolism
Plasma GGT	Low	Low	Poor
Plasma bilirubin	Moderate	Moderate	Unknown
Urinary 6β-OHC	Moderate	High	Good (sometimes)
Urinary D-glucaric acid	High	High	Good (sometimes)

excretion and hepatic drug metabolism further limiting the usefulness of the test.

The major use of this test has been in looking at changes in drug metabolism. Such changes correlate with changes in D-glucaric acid excretion in many cases; but equally there are cases of marked changes in hepatic clearance of drugs that are not accompanied by changes in the excretion of D-glucaric acid. The reason for these correlations is unclear but it may be due to a co-factor link between the mixed-function oxidase system and D-glucaric acid production (NADPH is used in one and produced in the other), or that D-glucaric acid production is a measure of phase II metabolism (hence the lack of correlation with some phase I reactions). Neither of these ideas has any experimental basis as yet.

D-Glucaric acid excretion is a useful test in certain circumstances where such excretion has been shown to be correlated to the metabolism of the drug under test, but it should not be regarded as a general indicator of drug-metabolizing capacity.

A summary of the non-invasive methods of assessing hepatic drug-metabolizing capacity is given in Table 7.7.

7.3.6 *IN VIVO/IN VITRO* CORRELATIONS OF DRUG METABOLISM

In the study of human drug metabolism one problem has become topical: the relationship between drug clearance measured *in vivo* (i.e. in the whole organism) and drug metabolism measured *in vitro* (i.e. in fractions of tissues removed from the patient). This becomes relevant when it is known that the drug is predominantly cleared by hepatic metabolism. It is obviously much better to be able to check a patient's hepatic metabolism by a simple blood or urine test rather than by requiring a sample of liver tissue to examine the metabolism of the drug.

The measurement of urinary excretion of drugs has been shown to be a valid indicator of hepatic drug metabolism in certain circumstances notably the metabolism of the model drug, antipyrine. Antipyrine is metabolized by the liver to three main metabolites. All of these metabolites are also found in the urine of patients given antipyrine. A study of the relative proportions of each metabolite formed by isolated liver tissue and found in the urine showed a very good correlation. A direct comparison of the *in vivo* clearance of antipyrine metabolites with *in vitro* assessment of hepatic drug metabolism in the same patient gave good correlation for all three metabolites. In this example, therefore, *in vivo* clearance is directly related to the ability of the liver to metabolize the drug.

In order for this correlation to be true, the drug under investigation must have certain properties: (1) it must be absorbed well into the systemic circulation; (2) elimination must be first order; (3) the metabolites should be rapidly excreted in the urine without further metabolism; and (4) metabolism should be entirely in the liver. Antipyrine appears to fulfill all of these criteria although (4) is very difficult to prove.

A good correlation has also been shown between *in vivo* and *in vitro* 3-hydroxylation of amylobarbitone, but for many other drugs no correlation between *in vivo* and *in vitro* hepatic metabolism has been seen.

One such example is the clearance of the anti-diabetes drug, tolbutamide. This drug is metabolized by hydroxylation in the liver. In a study of *in vivo* clearance of tolbutamide and its hepatic metabolism *in vitro*, no correlation was found to exist, presumably because one or more of the criteria mentioned above was not satisfied. Clearance of tolbutamide varied between 0.5 and $1.31h^{-1}$ without any detectable change in maximum hepatic metabolism of the same drug. The rate-limiting step in tolbutamide clearance is thus not related to hepatic metabolism.

In other studies, the *in vivo* clearance of antipyrine has been shown to be unrelated to the *in vitro* metabolism of the precarcinogen, benzo[a]pyrene. This was thought to be a reflection of the multiple forms of the drug-metabolizing enzymes in human liver with the two compounds being metabolized by different enzymes.

In the study of human drug metabolism, therefore, *in vivo* clearance values may or may not be related to *in vitro* hepatic metabolism depending on the drug in question. Thus, *in vivo* measurements may be invalid in discussing *in vitro* drug metabolism, or vice versa. These provisos should be borne in mind when discussing such *in vivo* and *in vitro* data.

These are the methods available for the study of hepatic drug metabolism in Man. In order to put these methods into perspective, a number of examples of their use in the study of human drug metabolism will be given. It is hoped that the following examples will highlight the relevance of the study of drug metabolism in Man in deciding how best to use the drugs to get the required effects without any toxic reaction to the drug.

7.4 Clinical relevance of drug metabolism

We have now seen the methods used in measuring drug metabolism in Man, and have discussed their relevance to hepatic drug-metabolizing capacity. Hepatic drug metabolism is one of the major factors – if not the most important one – affecting the clearance and, therefore, the intensity and duration of action of drugs. It is also important in determining the toxicity of drugs.

In this section we shall be looking at some examples of drug metabolism in a clinical context: how differences in drug metabolism – caused by genetic differences (pharmaco-genetics), by induction and inhibition and by various diseases – can affect the way in which drugs act. We will also look at how the methods discussed above can be used clinically in the assessment of drug-metabolizing capacity of the liver.

7.4.1 EFFECTS OF DISEASE

Hepatic metabolism of drugs can be affected by a number of diseases, most of which logically are diseases of the liver. Early studies showed that cirrhosis of the liver caused a marked decrease in clearance of drugs from serum. Chlor-amphenicol, which is metabolized by glucuronidation, and isoniazid, metab-olized by acetylation, both exhibit longer half-lives and reduced clearance from the body. This reduced clearance approach was extended to oxidative metab-olism of drugs when it was found that cirrhotic patients had an impaired metabolism of amobarbital, although the effects of cirrhosis on tolbutamide metabolism was uncertain. Clearance of antipyrine – the most common marker of hepatic drug metabolism – was also shown to be reduced in chronic liver disease. The metabolism of other drugs, however, was unaffected by liver disease such as the hepatic clearance of clindamycin and oxazepam.

Chronic liver diseases therefore seem to have marked substrate variation in their effects on hepatic drug metabolism. This was emphasized by later studies looking at the clearance of antipyrine, aminopyrine, diazepam and indocyanine green (ICG) in the same patients. Four groups of patients were used: control, healthy volunteers, patients with hepatocellular diseases, and patients with hepatic carcinomas or cholestasis. Antipyrine clearance was measured employ-ing the saliva test, aminopyrine and diazepam metabolism were measured using the breath tests, and indocyanine green was measured in plasma samples. It is known that antipyrine, aminopyrine and diazepam are cleared from the body mainly by hepatic metabolism and have a low extraction ratio (i.e. clearance is directly related to metabolism; see Section 7.3). Indocyanine green is not metabolized, and clearance is related to hepatic blood flow. Results obtained in the above study are shown in Table 7.8.

Table 7.8 Effects of liver disease on clearance of drugs in Man

Patient group	Aminopyrine	Diazepam	Antipyrine	Indocyanine green (ICG)
Control	100 ± 21*	100 ± 21	103 ± 36	98 ± 31
Hepatocellular diseases	38 ± 21	56 ± 18	45 ± 27	44 ± 24
Hepatic carcinoma	57 ± 22	69 ± 35	62 ± 37	66 ± 24
Cholestasis	110 ± 34	120 ± 42	64 ± 14	70 ± 23

Results expressed as % vs control.
*mean ± (standard deviation)
(Adapted from Vessell, E.S. (1980) *Proc. Natl. Acad. Sci. U.S.A.*, **77**, 600–3. Used with permission of the author.)

It can be seen that the clearance of each drug is decreased by both hepatocellular diseases and hepatic carcinoma to a similar extent for each drug, whereas in cholestasis the elimination of antipyrine and ICG was markedly depressed but that of aminopyrine and diazepam was unaltered. Complex statistical analysis of these results gave the conclusion that it is misleading to extrapolate pharmacokinetic data from one drug to another even though it is thought that both drugs are cleared by the same mechanism (e.g. aminopyrine and antipyrine are cleared predominantly by hepatic metabolism but show opposite effects on clearance in cholestasis, whereas antipyrine and ICG are cleared by different mechanisms but show the same effect in cholestasis).

This study also shows the relevance of the test applied to the prediction of altered hepatic function in the various disease states studied. All tests indicate a reduction in hepatic clearance in both hepatocellular and neoplastic diseases, but the aminopyrine breath test seems to be the best at discriminating between control and diseased liver states (Table 7.9).

Benzodiazepines, of which diazepam (discussed above) is one, have been studied more extensively. Diazepam itself has been the subject of many studies which have shown marked changes in pharmacokinetics in liver disease. Liver

Table 7.9 Usefulness of clearance of various drugs in assessing liver disease

Test	Percentage outside normal range	
	Hepatocellular diseases	Hepatic neoplasia
Aminopyrine	94	67
Diazepam	31	18
Antipyrine	24	20
ICG	69	22

(Adapted from Vessell, E.S. (1980) *Proc. Natl. Acad. Sci. U.S.A.*, **77**, 600–3. Used with permission of the author.)

diseases (hepatitis and cirrhosis) increase the half-life and decrease the clearance of diazepam. In patients without liver disease, diazepam half-life increased with multiple dosing due to accumulation of a metabolite, desmethyldiazepam, which apparently inhibited diazepam clearance (product inhibition?). In cirrhotic patients the half-life of diazepam was unaffected by repeat dosing. It was suggested that reduced metabolite production was insufficient to inhibit diazepam metabolism.

These data suggest that diazepam will have a longer effect in normal patients after multiple dosing but that this dosage regimen will have little effect on cirrhotic patients although they will already show a much more marked effect of diazepam due to the impaired metabolism. It might be argued that in normal patients a steadily decreasing dose of diazepam is necessary to maintain serum concentrations whereas in cirrhotic patients a lower but constant dose is needed.

In studies on benzodiazepines metabolized by the liver to form glucuronides (e.g. oxazepam and lorazepam), no significant effect of liver diseases could be found. There seems to be a marked difference between the effects of hepatic diseases on oxidative and conjugative metabolism.

The data shown above are linked to increased possibility of drug-induced coma in patients treated with benzodiazepines who also have liver diseases. Impairment of psychomotor function has also been seen.

Changes in hepatic drug clearance also occur in other diseases not directly affecting the liver, such as thyroid disorders, pituitary dwarfism, acromegaly and diabetes mellitus. These are all hormonal disorders and have indirect effects. Thyroid hormones generally stimulate hepatic drug metabolism; therefore hypothyroidism leads to diminished clearance of antipyrine whereas hyperthyroidism gives increased antipyrine clearance. Pituitary dwarfism and acromegaly are lack of, and excess of, growth hormone, respectively. Growth hormone inhibits drug metabolism, particularly in children. Insulin, the hormone missing in some forms of diabetes mellitus, has recently been implicated as an inducer of drug metabolism; lack of this hormone, therefore, leads to reduced capacity of the liver to metabolize drugs. The relevance of the effect of these diseases on drug treatment has not yet been assessed.

Disease states are, thus, a major influence on the ability of the body to clear drugs from the body by metabolism. The clinical relevance of altered drug metabolism in disease states is of great importance in the treatment of these diseases.

7.4.2 GENETIC POLYMORPHISM IN HUMAN DRUG METABOLISM

A genetic factor in determining the often large inter-individual variations in drug metabolism in Man has been suspected for a long time since the

Table 7.10 Drug metabolism phenotypes

Group	Drugs affected
Acetylator phenotype	Isoniazid
	Sulfonamides
Pseudocholinesterase phenotype	Succinylcholine
Drug oxidation phenotype	Debrisoquine
	Sparteine
	Phenacetin
	Phenytoin

metabolism of antipyrine in homozygous twins (identical twins) was shown to be almost the same, whereas in heterozygous (fraternal) twins there was as much variation as in the general population.

The existence of genetic control of drug metabolism has been strengthened by the discovery of a number of metabolic phenotypes (see Table 7.10).

The acetylator phenotypes, named 'slow' and 'fast' acetylators, are related to toxicity of, for example, isoniazid. Isoniazid is normally cleared from the body by N-acetylation, but in the 'slow' acetylator group, the therapeutic dose of the drug is sufficient to cause marked build-up of unchanged drug and, thus, the toxic side-effects of central stimulation and peripheral neuritis. 'Fast' acetylators are, however, more susceptible to drug-induced hepatic damage. In studies using a single blood sample following oral isoniazid treatment, over half of the subjects tested showed 'slow' acetylator status, and genetic investigation revealed that control is via two autosomal alleles, **R** for 'fast' acetylation and **r** for 'slow' (**R** being dominant and **r** recessive). The high incidence of the recessive trait indicates a selective advantage for the 'slow' acetylators which is not related to drug metabolism.

The most common test for acetylator status is the acetylation of sulfadimidine (see Section 7.3.3) which can be used to type a patient before isoniazid is given. The likely side effects of the drug will then be known. Interaction with other drugs can also be predicted, as 'slow' acetylators develop toxicity when isoniazid and phenytoin are given together, probably due to the higher blood levels of isoniazid inhibiting phenytoin metabolism, thus giving phenytoin toxicity. In these cases, knowing the acetylator status of the patient, toxicity can be avoided by modifying the dose of the drugs.

Pseudocholinesterase phenotype is characterized by a marked sensitivity to the muscle relaxant, succinylcholine, which is normally metabolized by the serum pseudocholinesterase. Succinylcholine is of particular use in conjunction with general anaesthetics, tetanic seizures and in electroconvulsive therapy because of its extremely short half-life (about 2 min). Patients with atypical pseudocholinesterase, however, show a half-life of effect of the drug of about 2–3 h. Total paralysis (including the respiratory muscles) for this length of time is obviously not advisable. The atypical reaction to succinylcholine has been shown to be controlled by an autosomal recessive gene and to be related to a structurally altered pseudocholinesterase in serum: the enzyme is not absent as in some other inherited defects of metabolism but is sufficiently altered to make it unable to metabolize succinylcholine.

About 1 in every 3000 individuals will have atypical pseudocholinesterase; this can be tested by inhibition studies on the serum enzyme. The normal enzyme is inhibited to 80% by 10^{-5} M dibucaine whereas the atypical enzyme is only inhibited to 20%; heterozygotes show an inhibition of 50–70%. The percentage inhibition is referred to as the 'dibucaine number' or 'DN'. The rarity of the recessive trait suggests that little selective advantage can be gained from having the atypical pseudocholinesterase.

Another atypical pseudocholinesterase has also been found with a higher activity towards succinylcholine. This is a very rare occurrence and again appears to be genetically controlled. The presence of this highly active pseudocholinesterase confers succinylcholine resistance on the individual.

All early drug metabolism polymorphism was related to drug hydrolysis (succinylcholine) or drug conjugation (isoniazid and sulfonamides) and no polymorphism of drug oxidation was observed although large inter-individual differences in drug oxidations were seen. Recently, however, drug oxidation polymorphism has been seen, notably with debrisoquine.

Debrisoquine is an adrenergic blocking drug (used in the treatment of hypertension) which is metabolized by the liver mixed-function oxidase system mainly to 4-hydroxydebrisoquine. Marked inter-individual variation in excretion pattern and pharmacological effect of the drug was noted with maintenance doses ranging from 20–400 mg d^{-1} and urinary excretion of 8–70% as unchanged drug. A good correlation between dose needed and unchanged drug excreted was seen. Investigation of the metabolite pattern in urine of volunteers given debrisoquine gave a clue to the nature of the variation (Table 7.11).

Table 7.11 Urinary excretion patterns of debrisoquine

Metabolite	Percentage dose excreted as metabolite			
	Subject 1	Subject 2	Subject 3	Subject 4
Debrisoquine	45	28	27	40
4-Hydroxydebrisoquine	30	37	39	2
Others	2.7	4.8	13.7	5.3

(Data from R. L. Smith, personal communication.)

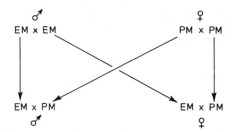

Figure 7.14 Family study of debrisoquine 4-hydroxylation. EM is extensive-metabolizer gene (dominant); PM is poor-metabolizer gene (recessive). (Data from R. L Smith, personal communication.)

One subject (no. 4) had a very low conversion of parent drug to 4-hydroxy derivative. This subject was also very sensitive to the anti-hypertensive effects of debrisoquine. A larger study based on this chance finding revealed that there were, indeed, two populations of debrisoquine metabolizers, and they could be classified according to the ratio of

$$\frac{\% \text{ dose excreted as debrisoquine}}{\% \text{ dose excreted as 4-hydroxydebrisoquine}}.$$

The major section of the population had a low ratio (about 1) and were termed 'extensive metabolizers' (EM); a much smaller section, with high ratios (about 20), were termed 'poor metabolizers' (PM). Over 90% belonged to the EM group.

Family studies indicated that extensive metabolism is a dominant and poor metabolism a recessive trait. The genetic control is via a single gene pair, i.e. the offspring of a homozygous EM and a homozygous PM will all be heterozygous (Figure 7.14). All of the offspring will therefore be extensive metabolizers. Two heterozygous parents can thus produce a homozygous recessive child; this has been seen in practice (see Figure 7.15). It should be noted that heterozygous extensive metabolizers have higher ratios than homozygotes, indicating that the dominance of the extensive trait is not complete.

We therefore have a drug oxidation polymorphism that can relatively easily be measured by examining the metabolite ratio of debrisoquine in urine. This

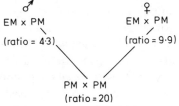

Figure 7.15 Family study of debrisoquine 4-hydroxylation showing the appearance of a child with poor-metabolizer status. (Data from R. L. Smith, personal communication.)

Table 7.12 Drugs whose metabolism is related
to debrisoquine 4-hydroxylation

Nortryptiline	Metoprolol
Phenacetin	4-Methoxyamphetamine
Phenformin	Carbocysteine
Phenytoin	Bufanolol
Sparteine	Encainide
Perhexiline	Guanoxan
Metiamide	

would be merely of academic interest, however, if it were not for the fact that the debrisoquine polymorphism turns out to be a model for many other clinically used drugs where a genetic component controlling the drug's metabolism has been suspected. A list of drugs whose metabolism is associated with debrisoquine 4-hydroxylation is shown in Table 7.12.

The list is expanding rapidly and debrisoquine 4-hydroxylation may be a very good model drug for a test of metabolic status. Not all drug metabolism, however, is similar to that of debrisoquine: the metabolism of tolbutamide, antipyrine, acetanilide, cortisol and amylobarbitone does not follow debrisoquine 4-hydroxylation.

The genetic polymorphism discussed above can be referred back to a number of unexplained sensitive groups of individuals, e.g. unusual sensitivity to phenytoin – where sensitive individuals develop toxic side effects (e.g. nystagmus and ataxia) at much lower doses of the drug. This sensitivity was related to reduced 4-hydroxylation of phenytoin, and has now been identified with the poor-metabolizer status.

Phenacetin metabolism is also related to debrisoquine metabolizer status. In some patients, phenacetin is hydroxylated rather than the usual route of de-ethylation. This unusual route of metabolism was thought to be the cause of the toxic side effects seen (methaemoglobinaemia). Impaired metabolism of phenacetin to paracetamol, and subsequent conversion of the remaining phenacetin to the 2-hydroxylated products, is correlated to poor-metabolizer status for debrisoquine.

The metabolism of guanoxan is also correlated with debrisoquine 4-hydroxylation so that poor metabolizers of debrisoquine are also poor metabolizers of guanoxan (Table 7.13). Guanoxan is, like debrisoquine, used as an antihypertensive and has side effects similar to debrisoquine – poor metabolizers are, therefore, more susceptible to the central effects and hepatotoxicity of guanoxan.

The simple debrisoquine metabolite ratio test can therefore be used as a routine test for susceptibility of patients to the toxic effects of a number of clinically important drugs, and it has useful predictive value in this respect. Using this test it has been shown that different racial groups exhibit different

Table 7.13 The effect of debrisoquine phenotype on the metabolism of guanoxan

Phenotype	% dose excreted as		Ratio $\left(\dfrac{\text{parent drug}}{\text{metabolite}}\right)$
	Guanoxan	OH-guanoxan	
EM	1.5 ± 0.3[†]	29 ± 5	0.06 ± 0.02
PM	48 ± 12	6.2 ± 1.4	7.8 ± 0.2

[†]mean $\pm$ (standard deviation)
(Data from R. L. Smith, personal communication.)

proportions of poor and extensive metabolizers (Table 7.14). Egyptians show the lowest incidence (about 1%) whereas West Africans show a high incidence (about 13%). Caucasians are intermediate between these two groups. This is a good example from the developing discipline of ethnopharmacology.

Table 7.14 Incidence of 'poor' metabolizer (PM) phenotype in different ethnic groups

Ethnic group	Number studied	Number PM	Percentage incidence of PM
Caucasian	106	5	5
Egyptian	72	1	1.5
Nigerian	34	5	15
Ghanaian	27	3	12

(Data from R. L. Smith, personal communication.)

The existence of at least two sub-populations with markedly different drug-metabolizing capacities has far-reaching and important correlates, particularly where drug oxidation is concerned and especially considering the high incidence of individuals with impaired drug-oxidizing capacity. From the examples given above, it becomes obvious that drugs linked to the debrisoquine phenotype should be given in lower doses to PM individuals than to EM, so reducing the risk of overdose and subsequent toxic effects. It is, in fact, possible that drugs have been withdrawn from clinical use due to a high incidence of toxic side-effects, when a reduction in dosage after a debrisoquine test may have been all that was required. Phenformin, for example, has been restricted due to build-up of lactic acid (lactoacidosis) in certain individuals. Phenformin metabolism is known to be correlated to debrisoquine 4-hydroxylation but no information is available as to whether lactoacidosis is correlated to PM status. If such a correlation was found, phenformin could be re-introduced on a wider scale following a debrisoquine test of prospective recipients.

The setting-up of a volunteer panel of known EM- or PM-status people would also be useful to the drug industry as it would enable them to investigate the effect of debrisoquine metabolism status on the effects of their compounds under test. At present no such attempt is performed to ascertain the range of effect a drug can have.

7.4.3 INDUCTION AND INHIBITION OF DRUG METABOLISM

The use of multiple drug therapy in the treatment of many diseases has led to problems with drug interactions. Many drug interactions are the result of interference of one drug with the metabolism of another and the subsequent increase or decrease in the clearance of the latter drug.

Interaction of drugs with phenobarbitone is, perhaps, the most studied example of this phenomenon as phenobarbitone is an inducer of the metabolism of many other drugs (see Chapter 3) and numerous clinical interactions with this drug are seen. Table 7.15 lists some of the drugs that interact with phenobarbitone at a metabolic level.

Table 7.15 Drugs which interact with phenobarbitone on a metabolic level

Phenytoin	Chlorpromazine
Warfarin	Phenylbutazone
Bishydroxycoumarin	Pethidine
Lignocaine	Cyclophosphamide
Digitoxin	Griseofulvin
Fenoprofen	Cortisol
DDT	

Of particular interest is the interaction of phenobarbitone and phenytoin which are both used in the treatment of epilepsy. Treatment of patients already given phenytoin with phenobarbitone reduced the steady-state serum concentration of phenytoin markedly (Figure 7.16). Withdrawal of phenobarbitone treatment returned serum concentrations of phenytoin to control levels.

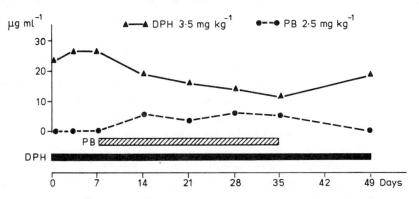

Figure 7.16 Effect of phenobarbitone pre-treatment on the steady-state serum concentration of phenytoin in Man. (Taken from Cucinelli, S. A. (1972) in *Anti-epileptic drugs* (eds D. M. Woodbury, J. K. Penry and R. P. Schmidt), Raven Press. Used with permission.)

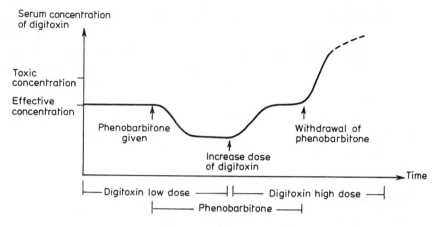

Figure 7.17 Changes in serum concentration of digitoxin following treatment with, and
withdrawal of, phenobarbitone.

Control of seizures by phenytoin can thus be greatly influenced by the presence
of phenobarbitone, itself a drug used to control seizure. The complex interactions theoretically available make the use of phenytoin and phenobarbitone
in combination a somewhat unpredictable and therefore dangerous therapy.

The interaction of phenobarbitone with digitoxin (a drug with low therapeutic index) is also of major concern to the clinician. Digitoxin is a cardiac
glycoside used in the treatment of heart failure, but with major side-effects at
slightly above clinical doses (toxicity includes anorexia, CNS disturbances,
atrial fibrillation and tachycardia). Steady-state concentrations of digitoxin fell
to about half following treatment with phenobarbitone, with a marked fall in
plasma half-life of digitoxin from about 8 to 4 days. Polar metabolites of
digitoxin increased in urine following phenobarbitone treatment. It thus
appears that phenobarbitone increased the metabolism of digitoxin, thereby
reducing its serum concentration and effectiveness. Increasing the dose
of digitoxin to counter this effect will lead to excess, toxic concentrations
of digitoxin being present in serum when phenobarbitone is withdrawn
(Figure 7.17).

A very similar effect is seen with warfarin (this has been discussed in
Chapter 3).

The use of phenobarbitone to increase drug-metabolizing capacity in liver
diseases has been attempted. For instance patients with liver disease metabolize
phenylbutazone very slowly (plasma $t_{\frac{1}{2}}$ of about 100 h) and this can be
shortened to about 50–55 h by treatment with phenobarbitone. Patients suffer-
ing from unconjugated hyperbilirubinaemia (caused by a relative deficiency of
UDP–glucuronyltransferase in the liver, whether the mild Gilbert's disease or

the more severe Crigler–Najjar syndrome) can be treated with phenobarbitone to relieve the symptoms. Dramatic reductions in serum bilirubin levels can easily be achieved by this method which probably relies on the ability of phenobarbitone to induce hepatic UDP–glucuronyltransferase activity, as there is a linear relationship between hepatic UDP–glucuronyltransferase activity and bilirubin clearance.

Other barbiturates such as barbitone, hexobarbitone and amylobarbitone show similar effects to phenobarbitone and should, perhaps, be viewed as a group.

Of the other drugs that are considered to be inducers of drug metabolism, the majority are seen to induce their own metabolism. Tolerance to glutethimide, meprobamate and diazepam, for instance, develops partly due to the increased metabolism of the drug owing to induction. Carbamazepine is a drug recently investigated in terms of induction of metabolism of itself, other exogenous compounds and endogenous compounds. The clearance of antipyrine, measured by the saliva test, increased after two weeks' treatment while carbamazepine half-life, measured in plasma, decreased from a control level of 32.3 h to 19.1 h during the same period.

Increases in enzymes involved in endogenous metabolism were also found in this study, with 6β-hydroxylation of cortisol (see Section 7.3) increased, and the level also raised of leucocyte δ-aminolaevulinic acid synthetase (the rate-limiting enzyme in the biosynthesis of haem). Carbamazepine has also been shown to induce the metabolism of phenytoin and warfarin.

Oral contraceptives containing estrogens and/or progestins have been reported to inhibit hepatic drug metabolism, probably by competitive inhibition. Steroids are metabolized in the liver by the same enzyme systems as drugs and therefore such inhibitory interactions are not unlikely. Aminopyrine clearance is significantly lower in women taking an oral contraceptive pill but there is no effect on paracetamol clearance. Another known inhibitor of drug metabolism is ethanol which again shares a common breakdown enzyme with drugs and steroids. The mixture of ethanol and many drugs is thus more toxic than the drug alone. Repeated administration of ethanol, however, can act as an inducer of drug metabolism – e.g. the half-lives of tolbutamide, warfarin and phenytoin are reduced in alcoholic patients. Therapy with these drugs in alcoholics is thus fraught with problems, as the patients, when sober, metabolize the drugs more quickly than usual but, when intoxicated, metabolize the drugs more slowly.

It can be seen from these examples that drug–drug interactions involving induction or inhibition of drug metabolism can be of great importance in determining the action and toxicity of drugs. Induction and inhibition is, however, important in another respect and that is the interaction of environmental factors with hepatic drug metabolism.

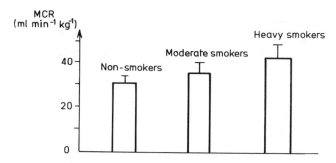

Figure 7.18 Relationship between daily cigarette consumption and clearance of anti-pyrine. MCR = mean clearance rate. (Taken from Vestal, R. E. *et al.* (1975) *Clin. Pharm. Ther.*, **18**, 425–32.)

One major group of compounds, widespread in our environment, which have a major effect on hepatic drug metabolism are the polycyclic hydro-carbons (e.g. benzo[*a*]pyrene). These are found in cigarette smoke and in any food cooked over open heat (e.g. charcoal-broiled meat). Much work has been done on the effects of polycyclic hydrocarbons on drug metabolism and their relationship to the intake of tobacco smoke and charcoal-broiled meat.

The clearance of antipyrine and paracetamol is greatly increased by smoking (Figure 7.18). It is seen that there is a graded response to the number of cigarettes smoked.

The effect of cigarette smoking on the plasma concentrations of phenacetin is even more dramatic (Figure 7.19). The area under the concentration curve is seen to be much less in smokers, indicating that the bioavailability of phenacetin is lower, but half-life is similar in both groups. Animal studies have shown that benzo[*a*]pyrene – a major constituent of tobacco smoke – induces mixed-function oxidase activity in the small intestine and the increased first-pass effect caused by such induction may be the explanation of the reduced bioavailability without increased hepatic metabolism seen in Man.

Other drugs, however, are unaffected by smoking with respect to their metabolism; a list of drugs known to be affected and unaffected by tobacco smoking is shown in Table 7.16.

In drug therapy it is therefore important to know the smoking habits of patients particularly if the drug to be used is metabolized by a polycyclic hydrocarbon-sensitive pathway.

If we now turn and look at polycyclic hydrocarbon inducers in food, we find that any meat cooked over open heat (i.e. any browning of food) causes build-up of such compounds. These have been shown to be potent inducers of drug metabolism in a very similar manner to cigarette smoking.

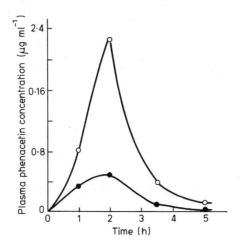

Figure 7.19 Mean plasma concentration of phenacetin in smokers (●) and non-smokers (○), as a function of time following oral administration of a 900 mg dose. (Taken from Pantuck, E. *et al.* (1972) *Science*, **175**, 1248–50. Used with the permission of the author and the American Association of Science. © 1972 AAAS.)

Table 7.16 The effect of smoking on drug metabolism

Metabolism affected	Metabolism unaffected
Nicotine	Ethanol
Phenacetin	Pethidine
Antipyrine	Diazepam
Paracetamol	Phenytoin
Theophylline	Nortryptiline
Imipramine	Warfarin
Pentazocine	

Plasma levels of phenacetin are markedly reduced in subjects on a charcoal-broiled meat diet – the subjects in this case acting as their own controls so cutting down problems from inter-individual variations (Table 7.17). As with tobacco smoking the area under the curve is significantly reduced (Figure 7.20) indicating a lack of bioavailability of phenacetin in subjects eating charcoal-broiled meat. No effect on plasma levels of the metabolite, paracetamol, were seen – showing that hepatic metabolism was little affected by the treatment. It is seen that at least 75% of phenacetin never enters the plasma in subjects on a charcoal-broiled meat diet. This has obvious clinical relevance for treatment with this drug: a patient may need four times the dose to achieve the same effect simply because of eating charcoal-broiled meat.

Table 7.17 The effect of a diet containing charcoal-broiled meat on the plasma concentration of phenacetin in Man

Time after administration (h)	Plasma phenacetin concentration $(ng\,ml^{-1})$	
	Control diet	Charcoal diet
1	$1328 \pm 481^\dagger$	319 ± 90
2	925 ± 166	163 ± 32
3	313 ± 60	74 ± 17
4	149 ± 27	34 ± 9
5	66 ± 14	15 ± 4

†mean $\pm$ (standard deviation)
(Data from Pantuck, E. *et al.* (1972) *Science*, **175**, 1248–50. Used with permission of the author and the American Association for the Advancement of Science. © 1972 AAAS.)

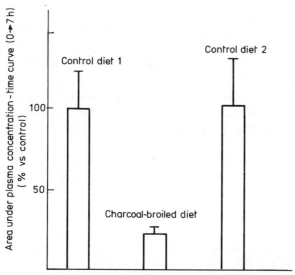

Figure 7.20 Effect of feeding a charcoal-broiled meat diet on the area-under-curve for phenacetin. (Taken from Pantuck, E. *et al.* (1972) *Science*, **175**, 1248–50. Used with permission of the author and the American Association for the Advancement of Science. © 1972 AAAS.)

If antipyrine and theophylline plasma half-life and clearance are examined in subjects on a charcoal-broiled meat diet a different picture emerges. For both antipyrine and theophylline, plasma half-life is decreased and total clearance increased. As antipyrine and theophylline are both predominantly cleared by hepatic metabolism, it seems reasonable to suggest that the effect of charcoal-broiled meat, in this instance, is on the liver and that we are seeing induction of hepatic mixed-function oxidases by the polycyclic hydrocarbons in the diet. This is similar to the effect of tobacco smoke seen earlier.

Induction and inhibition of drug metabolism – whether by other drugs, environmental or dietary chemicals – can be important factors in the action of drugs; changes in metabolism caused by such factors should be taken into account when treating patients.

7.5 Summary

Using as a theoretical basis the mathematical interpretation of drug concentrations in the body and drug elimination from the body (i.e. pharmacokinetics), we can measure various parameters of the drugs used in modern medicine. These parameters (such as half-life, clearance, etc.) can be related to the duration and intensity of action of a drug to give a meaningful measure of a drug's usefulness and possible toxicity.

The methods used in measuring these parameters have been discussed and examples, of how these methods can be used, have been given. The clinical relevance of the examples chosen has been explained where known.

It is hoped that this chapter has given some insight into the usefulness of pharmacokinetics and drug metabolic measurements in Man but that, at the same time, it has also pointed out the weaknesses of the methods and, perhaps, stimulated some thought as to how these techniques could be improved or better used.

7.6 Further reading

BOOKS AND SYMPOSIA

Creasey, W. A. (1979) *Drug disposition in humans*, Oxford University Press, Oxford.
Curry, S. H. (1974) *Drug disposition and pharmacokinetics*, Blackwell, London.
Curry, S. H. and Whelpton, R. (1983) *Manual of laboratory pharmacokinetics*, J. Wiley & Sons, Chichester.
Dost, F. H. (1968) *Grundlagen der pharmakokinetic*, Thieme, Stuttgart.
Gibaldi, M. and Perrier, D. (1980) *Pharmacokinetics*, Dekker, New York.
Gillette, J. R. and Mitchell, J. R. (eds) (1977) *Concepts in biochemical pharmacology, Part 3, handbook of experimental pharmacology*, Vol. 28, Springer-Verlag, Berlin, pp. 1–34, 35–85, 169–212, 234–258, 272–314, 359–382, 383–461.
Okita, G. T. and Acheson, G. H. (eds) (1973) *Pharmacology and the future of man*, **Vol. 3**, *Problems of Therapy*, S. Karger, Basel, pp. 34–55, 139–149, 165–73, 174–81, 182–90.
Omenn, G. S. and Gelboin, H. V. (eds) (1984) *Genetic variability in responses to chemical exposure*. Banbury Report 16, Cold Spring Harbor Laboratory.

Parke, D. V. and Smith, R. L. (eds) (1977) *Drug metabolism from microbe to Man*, Taylor and Francis Ltd., London, pp. 123–46, 357–68, 369–92, 393–430.

Siest, G. (ed.) (1985) *Drug metabolism: molecular approaches and pharmacological implications*, Pergamon Press, Oxford.

Wagner, J. G. (1971) *Biopharmaceutics and relevant pharmacokinetics*, Drug Intelligence, Hamilton.

REVIEWS AND ORIGINAL ARTICLES

Alvares, A. P. *et al.* (1979) Regulation of drug metabolism in Man by environmental factors. *Drug Metab. Rev.*, **9**, 185–206.

Atkinson, A. J., Jnr. and Kushner, W. (1979) Clinical Pharmacokinetics. *Ann. Rev. Pharm. Tox.*, **19**, 105–28.

Boxenbaum, H. G. *et al.* (1979) Influence of gut microflora on bioavailability. *Drug Metab. Rev.*, **9**, 259–80.

Caranasos, G. J. *et al.* (1985) Clinically desirable drug interactions. *Ann. Rev. Pharmacol.*, **25**, 67–95.

Dollery, C. T. *et al.* (1979) Contribution of environmental factors to variability in human drug metabolism. *Drug Metab. Rev.*, **9**, 207–20.

Eriksson, M. and Yaffe, S. J. (1973) Drug metabolism in the newborn. *Ann. Rev. Med.*, **24**, 29–40.

Green, T. P. *et al.* (1979) Determinants of drug disposition and effects in the fetus. *Ann. Rev. Pharm. Tox.*, **19**, 285–322.

Hoyumpa, A. M. *et al.* (1978) The disposition and effects of sedatives and analgesics in liver disease. *Ann. Rev. Med.*, **29**, 205–18.

Hunter, J. and Chausseaud, L. F. (1974) Clinical aspects of microsomal enzyme induction. In (eds J. W. Bridges and L. F. Chausseaud) *Prog. Drug Metab.*, **1**, 129–92.

Idle, J. R. and Smith, R. L. (1979) Polymorphisms of oxidation at carbon centres of drugs and their clinical significance. *Drug Metab. Rev.*, **9**, 301–18.

Israili, Z. H. (1979) Correlation of pharmacological effects with plasma levels of antihypertensive drugs in Man. *Ann. Rev. Pharm. Tox.*, **19**, 25–52.

Jusko, W. J. (1979) Influence of cigarette smoking on drug metabolism in Man. *Drug Metab. Rev.*, **9**, 221–36.

Mucklow, J. C. (1980) Environment, diet and drug metabolism. *Topics in Therap.*, **6**, 103–110.

Park, B. K. (1981) Assessment of urinary 6β-hydroxycortisol as an *in vivo* index of mixed-function oxygenase activity. *Brit. J. Clin. Pharm.*, **12**, 97–102.

Park, B. K. (1982) Assessment of the drug metabolism capacity of the liver. *Brit. J. Clin. Pharm.*, **14**, 631–51.

Park, B. K. and Breckenridge, A. M. (1981) Clinical implications of enzyme induction and enzyme inhibition. *Clin. Pharmacokin.*, **6**, 1–24.

Perrier, G. D. and Gibaldi, M. (1974) Clearance and biologic half-life as indices of intrinsic hepatic metabolism. *J. Pharm. Exptl. Ther.*, **191**, 17–24.

Powell, J. R. *et al.* (1977) The influence of cigarette smoking and sex on theophylline disposition. *Am. Rev. Respir. Dis.*, **116**, 17–24.

Raisfeld, I. H. (1973) Clinical pharmacology of drug interactions. *Ann. Rev. Med.*, **24**, 385–418.

Rawlins, M. D. (1980) Methods for studying drug metabolism in Man. In (ed. H. F. Woods) *Topics in Therap.*, **6**, 86–94.

Reidenburg, M. M. and Drayer, D. E. (1978) Effects of renal disease upon drug disposition. *Drug Metab. Rev.*, **8**, 293–302.

Routledge, P. A. and Shand, D. G. (1979) Presystemic drug elimination. *Ann. Rev. Pharm. Tox.*, **19**, 447–68.

Scheline, R. R. (1973) Metabolism of foreign compounds by gastrointestinal microorganisms. *Pharmacol. Rev.*, **25**, 451–523.

Sjöquist, F. and von Bahr, C. (1973) Interindividual differences in drug oxidation: clinical importance. *Drug. Metab. Disp.*, **1**, 469–82.

Smolen, V. F. (1978) Bioavailability and pharmacokinetic analysis of drug responding systems. *Ann. Rev. Pharm. Tox.*, **18**, 495–522.

Timbrell, J. A. (1979) The role of metabolism in the hepatotoxicity of isoniazid and iproniazid. *Drug Metab. Rev.*, **10**, 125–48.

Vessell, E. S. (1977) Genetic and environmental factors affecting drug disposition in man. *Clin. Pharm. Ther.*, **22**, 659–79.

Vessell, E. S. (1978) Disease as one of the many variables affecting drug disposition and response: alterations of drug disposition and response: alterations of drug disposition in liver disease. *Drug Metab. Rev.*, **8**, 265–92.

Vessell, E. S. (1979) The antipyrine test in clinical pharmacology. Conceptions and misconceptions. *Clin. Pharm. Ther.*, **26**, 275–86.

Wilkinson, G. R. and Shand, D. G. (1975) A physiological approach to hepatic drug clearance. *Clin. Pharm. Ther.*, **18**, 377–90.

Zaffaroni, A. (1978) Therapeutic systems: the key to rational drug therapy. *Drug Metab. Rev.*, **8**, 191–222.

8

Techniques and experiments illustrating drug metabolism

8.1 Introduction

This chapter is designed to illustrate experimentally some of the concepts discussed in this book. The experiments described herein are derived from undergraduate practicals that have been running in the authors' laboratories for several years. The design of adequate experiments illustrating drug metabolism is not an easy task. For example, practical classes can suffer from time constraints in that the experiments usually have to be completed in one day. In addition, experimental design must also take account of practical constraints such as availability of reagents or analytical instrumentation. Accordingly, we have described a series of experiments that are flexible and can be tailored to suit either the size of a practical class, the time available or access to specific instrumentation.

This chapter is sub-divided into the following four sections:

8.2: *In vitro* assays for drug-metabolizing enzymes.

8.3: Factors affecting drug metabolism, including co-factor requirements, species differences, tissue differences, sex differences and temperature of incubation.

8.4: Induction of drug metabolism and a correlation of *in vivo* drug action with *in vitro* hepatic drug-metabolizing activity.

8.5: Excretion of paracetamol in Man.

239

Section 8.2 provides a spectrum of methods and analytical techniques that, depending on availability, can be used to illustrate the experiments described in detail in Sections 8.3, 8.4 and 8.5. In certain experiments, particular assays of drug metabolism are described, but it must be emphasized that alternative assays can be used, and these are usually indicated in each experiment.

8.2 *In vitro* assays for drug metabolizing enzymes

8.2.1 PREPARATION OF TISSUE HOMOGENATES

One of the most widely used methods to study *in vitro* drug metabolism is the use of tissue homogenates, particularly liver homogenates. It should be noted that in the preparation of tissue homogenates, all apparatus and solutions should be cooled and stored on ice (or at 4 °C) prior to the start of the experiment. In addition, to minimize degradation of tissue enzymes, it is important that the tissue does not exceed 4 °C during any stage of preparation and isolation.

The animals are killed in an appropriate manner (for example cervical dislocation), remembering that no chemical or drug should be used as this may influence the activity or content of the drug-metabolizing enzymes. (Thus, sacrificing animals by treatment with ether, chloroform or barbiturates should be avoided.)

The tissue(s) to be used are rapidly excised and immediately placed in ice-cold 0.25 M sucrose to wash off excess blood and to cool the tissue. The tissue is then blotted dry, weighed and added to four times its weight of 0.25M sucrose, i.e. a 20% w/v homogenate. The tissue is finely chopped with scissors and homogenized such that no large pieces of tissue are evident. The amount of homogenization required depends on the tissue being used, some tissues being more difficult to disrupt and homogenize than others. The recommended homogenizer is the Potter–Elvehjem type consisting of a teflon pestle and a glass homogenizer tube. Normally four passes of the homogenizer are sufficient to disrupt the tissue; the homogenizer tube should be immersed in an ice bucket, and excessive 'frothing' avoided (a sure sign that protein (enzyme) denaturation is occurring).

Having obtained a tissue homogenate as above, the homogenate is centrifuged in a refrigerated centrifuge to isolate sub-cellular fractions. Two main sub-cellular fractions are routinely used in the study of drug metabolism – namely the post-mitochondrial supernatant and the endoplasmic reticulum (microsomal) fraction. The choice of sub-cellular fraction used depends on several factors including time constraints in tissue preparation or the availability of a refrigerated ultracentrifuge.

For preparation of the post-mitochondrial supernatant, the tissue homogenate is centrifuged at 12 500 g for 15 min to pellet intact cells, cell debris, nuclei and mitochondria. The resultant supernatant (the post-mitochondrial supernatant) is *carefully* decanted – it contains the microsomal plus soluble (cell sap) fractions of the cell. Clearly this method of preparation is rapid and is useful when tissue homogenates are quickly required.

Microsomal tissue fractions can be prepared from the post-mitochondrial supernatant by one of two centrifugation techniques, one involving the use of an ultracentrifuge and the other involving a calcium precipitation method.

(i) *Ultracentrifugation method*

Aliquots (approximately 10–12 ml) of the post-mitochondrial supernatant are transferred to ultracentrifuge tubes and centrifuged at 100 000 g for 45 min in a refrigerated ultracentrifuge. After centrifugation, the supernatant (cell sap fraction) is decanted and discarded, and the microsomal pellet rinsed with three 5 ml washes of 0.25 M sucrose, transferred to a small homogenization vessel, and gently re-suspended in 5 ml of 0.1 M tris buffer, pH 7.4. This procedure yields the final microsomal suspension.

(ii) *Calcium precipitation method*

This method is based on the calcium-dependent aggregation of endoplasmic reticulum fragments and subsequent 'low-speed' centrifugation of the aggregated microsomal particles. The advantages of this method are that it is less time-consuming and does not require an ultracentrifuge. Aliquots (approximately 10–12 ml) of post-mitochondrial supernatant are mixed with 88 mM calcium chloride solution, such that 0.1 ml of 88 mM $CaCl_2$ solution is added per ml of supernatant (final $CaCl_2$ concentration is 8 mM). It is then left to stand on ice for 5 min, with occasional gentle swirling. The mixture is then centrifuged at 27 000 g for 15 min, the supernatant discarded and the pellet re-suspended by homogenization in 5 ml of 0.1 M tris buffer, pH 7.4, yielding the microsomal suspension.

If time permits, the microsomal fractions prepared by both of the above methods may be further washed by re-suspending the microsomal pellet in 0.1 M tris buffer, pH 7.4, containing 0.15 M KCl to remove either adventitious protein or excess $CaCl_2$. The microsomal pellet is then precipitated, as above, and re-suspended in 5 ml of 0.1 M tris buffer, pH 7.4. It is not mandatory to re-suspend the final microsomal preparations in tris buffer; other buffers such as phosphate may be used. It should be noted that the yield of microsomal protein per g liver is usually around 20 mg g^{-1} liver for both methods.

Table 8.1 Preparation of sub-cellular tissue fractions

---

(1) Kill animal and remove tissue as rapidly as possible.

(2) Blot tissue dry and weigh.

(3) Make a 20% w/v homogenate in 0.25 M sucrose.

(4) To prepare a post-mitochondrial supernatant, centrifuge the homogenate at 12 500 g for 15 min, decant and reserve the supernatant, and discard the pellet.

(5) To prepare microsomal fractions by the ultracentrifugation method, centrifuge the post-mitochondrial supernatant at 100 000 g for 45 min, discard the supernatant and resuspend the microsomal pellet in 5 ml of 0.1 M tris buffer, pH 7.4.

(6) To prepare microsomal fractions by the calcium chloride precipitation method, take an aliquot of the post-mitochondrial supernatant, add calcium chloride (8 mM final), swirl occasionally for 5 min and centrifuge at 27 000 g for 15 min.

The final post-mitochondrial supernatant prepared as above can then be used to study drug metabolism. It is preferable to use the tissue fractions fresh on the day of preparation, but in some cases this may not be possible. Accordingly, the tissue fractions may be stored frozen (-20 to $-80\,^{\circ}$C) for several weeks without appreciable loss of activity if glycerol (20%, v/v) is added to the final preparation.

An abbreviated version of preparation of sub-cellular homogenates is given in Table 8.1.

(a) REAGENTS REQUIRED

Sucrose, 0.25 M: 256.8 g to 3 l water.

Calcium chloride solution, 88 mM: 1.93 g $CaCl_2$ to 100 ml water.

(b) OTHER MATERIALS

Experimental animals.

Surgical instruments.

Potter–Elvehjem homogenizers (50 ml and 10 ml).

Appropriate refrigerated centrifuge, rotor, tubes.

8.2.2 INDUCTION OF HEPATIC DRUG-METABOLIZING ENZYMES

As described in earlier chapters, the activity or specific content of the hepatic drug-metabolizing enzymes may be induced by pre-treatment of experimental animals with drugs and other xenobiotics, the most commonly used being phenobarbital or β-naphthoflavone.

(i) *Phenobarbital induction*

Experimental animals are given three daily intraperitoneal injections of $80\,\text{mg}\,\text{kg}^{-1}$ (sodium salt, dissolved in saline), and sub-cellular fractions prepared on the fourth day as described above. Control animals should receive an equivalent volume of saline. Alternatively, sodium phenobarbital may be administered in the drinking water as a 0.1% w/v solution over a period of 5 days, normal drinking water being returned to the animals overnight before sacrifice.

(ii) *β-Naphthoflavone induction*

Animals are given an intraperitoneal injection of $80\,\text{mg}\,\text{kg}^{-1}$ β-naphthoflavone (dissolved in corn oil) once daily for 3 days, prior to sacrifice. Control animals are given corn oil (equivalent volume to the test group) as an intraperitoneal injection according to the same schedule.

If an experiment is designed to investigate the influence of xenobiotic induction on hepatic (or other tissue) drug biotransformation, other inducing agents may be used. These additional inducers include isosafrole (Ryan *et al.*, 1980), pregnenolone-16α-carbonitrile (Elshourbagy and Guzelian, 1980), ethanol (Ohnishi and Lieber, 1977) and clofibrate (Gibson *et al.*, 1982). The animal doses and pre-treatment schedules are given in the cited references (see Section 8.7).

8.2.3 PROTEIN DETERMINATION

When comparing tissue fractions for their ability to catalyse drug biotransformation, a measure of the tissue protein is required. Protein is readily determined by the colorimetric method of Lowry *et al.* (1951), with reference to a standard curve of bovine serum albumin. The coloured complex is thought to arise as a result of a complex between the alkaline copper–phenol reagent used and tyrosine and tryptophan residues of the protein. For each tissue sample, determine the protein present (in duplicate) and a standard curve (in duplicate) as described in Table 8.2.

(a) REAGENTS REQUIRED

Sodium carbonate, 2% w/v, in 0.1 M NaOH.
Copper sulfate (hydrated), 1% w/v, in water.
Sodium potassium tartrate, 2% w/v, in water.

Table 8.2 Determination of tissue protein content by the Lowry method

---

(*a*) *Tissue sample*

(1) Dilute the tissue sample 1 : 100 with 0.5 M NaOH.

(2) Take 0.2, 0.4, 0.6, 0.8 and 1.0 ml of the diluted tissue sample and make up to a final volume of 1 ml with 0.5 M NaOH. Prepare a blank containing 1.0 ml of 0.5 M NaOH instead of the tissue sample.

(3) Add 5 ml of 'copper' reagent to all samples (including the blank), mix thoroughly by vortexing or inversion, and allow to stand for 10 min.

(4) Add 0.5 ml of 1 N Folin reagent, mix immediately and completely and stand for 30 min.

(5) Read absorbance at 750 nm on a spectrophotometer, after zeroing the instrument on the blank.

(6) The tissue protein content can then be directly interpolated from the standard curve below.

(*b*) *Bovine serum albumin standard curve*

(1) Make a stock solution of bovine serum albumin ($100 \, \mu g \, ml^{-1}$) in 0.5 M NaOH.

(2) Take 0, 0.2, 0.4, 0.6, 0.8 and 1.0 ml of the above stock solution (equivalent to 0, 20, 40, 60, 80 and 100 μg protein ml^{-1} respectively) and make up to a final volume of 1 ml with 0.5 M NaOH.

(3) Process the standard curve as described in (a) above starting from (3) and continuing to (5).

(4) Construct the standard curve by plotting absorbance against bovine serum albumin (μg) per assay.

Notes

(1) Prepare the stock bovine serum albumin and 'copper' reagent fresh on day of use.

(2) If the tissue protein content absorbance values read higher than the standard curve range, further dilute the tissue sample to 1 : 500 and repeat the determination.

(3) If a spectrophotometer is not available to read 750 nm, absorbances can also be read at 540 nm.

(4) If tissue samples have been stored in glycerol, an appropriate correction must be made in the blank, as glycerol gives a positive reaction with the 'copper' reagent.

(Copper reagent is prepared fresh by mixing the above sodium carbonate, copper sulfate and sodium potassium tartrate solutions in the ratios of 100 : 1 : 1 by volume respectively.)

Bovine serum albumin, $100 \, \mu g \, ml^{-1}$ in 0.5 M NaOH.

(b) OTHER MATERIALS

Vortex mixer.

Spectrophotometer capable of reading absorbances at either 750 nm or 540 nm.

8.2.4 COFACTOR SOLUTIONS

Reduced nicotinamide adenine dinucleotide phosphate (NADPH) is a necessary cofactor for many drug biotransformation reactions, and it serves as a source of reducing equivalents in the reaction (particularly hydroxylation and de-methylation reactions). When studying drug metabolism reactions, NADPH can be added directly to the incubation mixture, but this suffers from the drawback that it is relatively expensive to use on a large scale. However, if NADPH is used, a final concentration of 1 mM in the incubation mixture is usually sufficient to support drug metabolism.

An alternative method is frequently used to generate NADPH and this involves the use of an auxilliary enzymatic reaction as follows:

$$\text{Isocitrate} + \text{NADP}^+ \xrightarrow[\text{isocitrate dehydrogenase}]{\text{Mg}^{2+}} \alpha\text{-ketoglutarate} + \text{NADPH} + \text{H}^+ + \text{CO}_2$$

Accordingly, an NADPH generating system is easily made up as shown in Table 8.3.

Table 8.3 Preparation of an NADPH-generating cofactor solution

The following components are mixed:	
Tris buffer, 0.1 M, pH 7.4	8.5 ml
Magnesium chloride solution, 0.15 M	1.0 ml
Nicotinamide, 0.5 M	1.0 ml
Trisodium isocitrate	40 mg
Isocitrate dehydrogenase	2 Units
NADP$^+$	8 mg

Notes

(1) The above components should be thoroughly mixed and dissolved just prior to use.
(2) It is particularly important that this mixture is not left to stand for more than a few minutes, otherwise the generated NADPH will break down. Accordingly, it is recommended to make up the above solution, and add the NADP$^+$ immediately prior to use.
(3) The nicotinamide is included to prevent the destruction of pyridine nucleotide by tissue nucleosidases.
(4) For drug metabolism reactions, 1 ml of the above co-factor solution is usually required per assay. Therefore the above solution is sufficient for ten assays.

An alternative NADPH generating system may be used taking advantage of the following reaction:

$$\text{Glucose-6-phosphate} + \text{NADP}^+ \xrightarrow[\text{dehydrogenase}]{\text{glucose-6-phosphate}} \text{6-phospho-gluconolactone} + \text{NADPH} + \text{H}^+$$

When this regenerating system is used, the isocitrate and isocitrate dehydrogenase (Table 8.3) is substituted by glucose-6-phosphate (4 μmol ml^{-1} in final mixture) and glucose-6-phosphate dehydrogenase (20 Units ml^{-1} in final mixture). It should be noted that when the post-mitochondrial supernatant is used as a source of tissue enzymes, the glucose-6-phosphate dehydrogenase may be omitted from the cofactor solution, as this fraction already contains the enzyme. A more detailed discussion of the cofactor requirements and cofactor solution preparation is to be found in Chapters 26 and 27 of La Du *et al.* (1972).

(a) REAGENTS REQUIRED

Magnesium chloride solution, 0.15 M: 15.25 g of $MgCl_2 \cdot 6H_2O$ to 500 ml water.

Nicotinamide, 0.5 M; 30.5 g to 500 ml water.

NADPH, NADP$^+$, isocitrate, isocitrate dehydrogenase, glucose-6-phosphate and glucose-6-phosphate dehydrogenase, as supplied.

8.2.5 SPECTRAL DETERMINATION OF CYTOCHROME *P*-450

Cytochrome *P*-450 is a haemoprotein and use is made of the fact that when the haem iron is reduced and complexed with carbon monoxide, a characteristic absorption spectrum results. The reduced, carbon monoxide difference spectrum of cytochrome *P*-450 absorbs maximally at around 450 nm (hence the name), and the extinction coefficient for the wavelength couple 450–490 nm has been accurately determined to be 91 NM^{-1} cm^{-1}, thus allowing quantitative determination of this haemoprotein.

Because of the turbidity of tissue homogenates containing cytochrome *P*-450, spectrophotometric determination of the haemoprotein must be carried out in a split-beam instrument, i.e. one containing both a sample and reference compartment to offset the high turbidity. The spectrophotometric assay is described in Table 8.4.

The cytochrome *P*-450 content is calculated as in the following example:

$$\text{Absorbance difference (450–490 nm)} = 0.22$$

$$\text{Extinction coefficient (450–490 nm)} = 91 \text{ mM}^{-1} \text{ cm}^{-1}$$

Therefore, using Beer's Law and assuming a cuvette path length of 1 cm, the cytochrome *P*-450 concentration is given by

$$\frac{0.22 \times 1000}{91} \text{ nmol ml}^{-1} \text{ diluted sample} = 2.4 \text{ nmol ml}^{-1} \text{ diluted sample.}$$

The *specific* content of cytochrome *P*-450 in the original tissue sample is then calculated knowing the dilution factor used and the protein content of the

Table 8.4 Spectrophotometric determination of cytochrome *P*-450

---

(1) Tissue samples are diluted in 0.1 M tris buffer, pH 7.4 containing 20% v/v glycerol to approximately $2\,mg\,ml^{-1}$.
(2) The diluted sample, 2 ml, is then added to both matched sample and reference cuvettes, and a baseline recorded between 400 and 500 nm.
(3) A few grains of solid sodium dithionite are added to both sample and reference cuvettes with gentle stirring, and the sample cuvette *only* is gently bubbled with carbon monoxide for approximately 1 min.
(4) The spectrum is then re-scanned from 400 nm to 500 nm.

Notes

(1) Glycerol is included in the buffer to minimize conversion to the inactive cytochrome *P*-420.
(2) Use only a few grains of dithionite as excess reductant will destroy the haemoprotein.
(3) Gas the sample with carbon monoxide as soon after dithionite addition as possible, as the reduced ferrous form of cytochrome *P*-450 is relatively unstable.
(4) When gassing with carbon monoxide, the gas flow rate should be approximately one bubble per second. Excessively high flow rates will result in frothing and protein denaturation.
(5) If a prominent peak is observed at 420 nm after gassing with carbon monoxide, this is indicative of the presence of inactive cytochrome *P*-420, and is to be avoided.

---

original sample. For example, if the dilution was 1 : 10 and the original tissue protein was $26\,mg\,ml^{-1}$, then the cytochrome *P*-450 specific content is given by

$$\frac{2.4 \times 10}{26}\;nmol\,mg^{-1}\;protein \;=\; 0.92\,nmol\,mg^{-1}\;protein.$$

This value will vary depending on the tissue examined, animal pre-treatment with inducers and the species, strain, age and sex of the animal used. As a general rule of thumb, for un-induced (control), male adult rats, this value will usually fall in the range 0.4–$1.0\,nmol$ cytochrome *P*-450 mg^{-1} microsomal protein derived from hepatic tissue.

It should be noted that the tissue content of cytochrome b_5 can also be analysed using the same sample. If both cytochrome *P*-450 and cytochrome b_5 concentrations are required from the same sample, the cytochrome b_5 must be determined first as in the method given below.

(a) REAGENTS

Tris buffer, 0.1 M, pH 7.4, containing 20% v/v glycerol.
Solid sodium dithionite.
Carbon monoxide.

(b) OTHER MATERIALS

Two matched glass or quartz cuvettes (3 ml capacity).
Split-beam recording spectrophotometer.
Tissue homogenate.

8.2.6 SPECTRAL DETERMINATION OF CYTOCHROME b_5

This is achieved by determining the absorbance difference spectrum of NADH-reduced versus oxidized cytochrome b_5. The reduced, ferrous form of cytochrome b_5 has an absorbance maximum at 424 nm in difference spectrum, and the extinction coefficient for the wavelength couple 424–490 nm is $112 \, \text{mM}^{-1} \, \text{cm}^{-1}$. NADH is used as the reductant because of the presence of the flavoprotein enzyme NADH–cytochrome b_5 reductase in tissue preparations, an enzyme that relatively specifically and quantitatively reduces cytochrome b_5. The spectral determination of cytochrome b_5 is summarized in Table 8.5.

Table 8.5 Spectrophotometric determination of cytochrome b_5

---

(1) Tissue samples are diluted to approximately 2 mg protein ml^{-1} as for cytochrome P-450 determination and split between a sample and reference cuvette as in Table 8.4.
(2) A baseline is recorded between 400 nm and 500 nm.
(3) NADH solution (2% w/v), 25 μl, is added to the sample cuvette only, the cuvette contents gently stirred and the spectrum re-recorded between 400 nm and 500 nm.
(4) The absorbance difference between 424 nm and 490 nm (relative to the baseline) is then determined and the cytochrome b_5 concentration determined as described in the text.

Notes

When the cytochrome b_5 has been determined as above, the same sample may be analysed for cytochrome P-450 by proceeding from step (3) in Table 8.4.

The tissue cytochrome b_5 content is then calculated as in the following example:

$$\text{Absorbance difference (424–490 nm)} = 0.11$$

$$\text{Extinction coefficient (424–490 nm)} = 112 \, \text{mM}^{-1} \, \text{cm}^{-1}$$

Applying Beer's Law for a 1 cm cuvette, the cytochrome b_5 concentration is given by

$$\frac{0.11 \times 1000}{112} \, \text{nmol ml}^{-1} \text{ diluted sample} = 0.98 \, \text{nmol ml}^{-1} \text{ diluted sample.}$$

In a similar manner to the example given for the cytochrome P-450 calculation above, the *specific* content of cytochrome b_5 is given by (assuming a $1:10$ dilution and an original tissue protein concentration of 26 mg ml^{-1})

$$\frac{0.98 \times 10}{26} \text{ nmol mg}^{-1} \text{ protein } = 0.38 \text{ nmol mg}^{-1} \text{ protein}$$

Again, as for cytochrome P-450, the value of the specific content is dependent on various factors. In general, for hepatic microsomal fractions derived from adult, male rats (non-induced), the specific content of cytochrome b_5 is in the region of $0.2–0.5$ nmol mg^{-1} protein, i.e. approximately one-half of the cytochrome P-450-specific content in the same tissue.

(a) REAGENTS

NADH, 2% w/v: 10 mg to 0.5 ml water (sufficient for twenty assays) – prepared fresh.

(b) OTHER MATERIALS

Two matched glass or quartz cuvettes (3 ml capacity).
Split-beam recording spectrophotometer.
Tissue homogenate.

8.2.7 SPECTRAL DETERMINATION OF SUBSTRATE BINDING TO HEPATIC MICROSOMAL CYTOCHROME P-450

As described in Chapter 2, many drugs and xenobiotics can bind to cytochrome P-450, resulting in characteristic perturbations of the absorbance of the haem iron. The absorbance changes can be utilized to quantitatively describe drug binding to the haemoprotein, resulting in the determination of the apparent spectral dissociation constant K_s and the maximum spectral change elicited by the drug (ΔA_{max}). These two parameters are formally similar to the K_m and V_{max} values described by Michaelis–Menten kinetics for enzyme-catalysed reactions. In the broadest sense, K_s is a measure of drug affinity for cytochrome P-450 and ΔA_{max} is the maximum spectral change. These two spectral parameters are therefore of use in comparing drug interaction with various forms of cytochrome P-450 or in comparing the interactions of different drugs with the same form of cytochrome P-450.

The method for determining hexobarbital-induced spectral changes of cytochrome P-450 is given in Table 8.6, and results of a typical experiment are given in Figure 8.1. As can be seen from this figure, increasing concentrations of hexobarbital result in increasing spectral changes as judged by the difference in absorbance between 390 and 420 nm ($\Delta A_{390-420}$). The shape of the 'titration' is hyperbolic in nature (Figure 8.2(a)), indicating saturation of

Table 8.6 Quantitative spectral interactions of hexobarbital with cytochrome *P*-450

(1) Rat liver microsomes are diluted to 2 mg protein ml^{-1} in 0.1 M tris buffer, pH 7.4.
(2) Samples, 2 ml, of the diluted microsomes are placed in both a sample and a reference cuvette of a split-beam recording spectrophotometer, and a baseline recorded between 350 nm and 500 nm.
(3) Aliquots of a stock solution of 50 mM sodium hexobarbital are then added to the sample cuvette *only* as follows: 1.7 μl (micro syringe) of the stock hexobarbital is added to the sample cuvette and gently, but thoroughly, stirred. The spectrum is re-scanned from 350 nm to 500 nm.
(4) Further additions of 1.7, 7.0 and 30 μl of hexobarbital are added to the sample cuvette and the spectrum re-recorded between 350 nm and 500 nm after each addition.

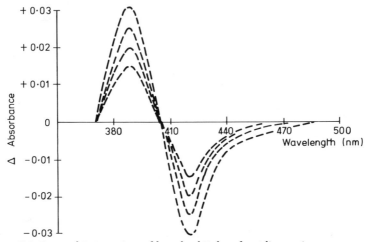

Figure 8.1 Spectral interaction of hexobarbital and rat liver microsomes.

cytochrome *P*-450 at high substrate concentrations. When the data are analysed by the double-reciprocal plot procedure (Lineweaver–Burk plot), a straight line is usually obtained (Figure 8.2(b)).

The K_s and ΔA_{max} parameters are derived from the Lineweaver–Burk plot from the axis intercepts as shown in Figure 8.2(b). In this example

$$-\frac{1}{K_s} = -21.2$$

Therefore $\qquad K_s = 0.047 \, \text{mM}$

and $\qquad \dfrac{1}{\Delta A_{max}} = \dfrac{1}{16}$

Hence $\qquad \Delta A_{max} = 0.063.$

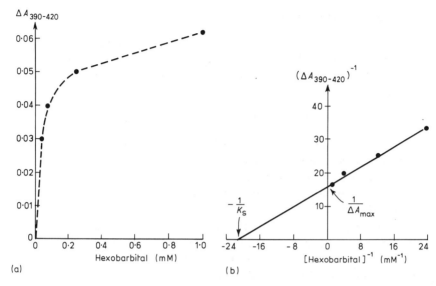

Figure 8.2 Determination of K_s and ΔA_{max} for the interaction of hexobarbital with rat liver microsomal cytochrome *P*-450. (a) Titration curve; (b) Lineweaver–Burk plot.

It should be noted that hexobarbital usually gives a type I spectral change with an absorbance maximum and minimum at approximately 390 nm and 420 nm respectively, with an isosbestic point around 407 nm. Other type I substrates may be used including those described in Table 2.4, which also includes type II and reverse type I substrates. Although the spectra of type II and reverse type I substrates are different from that described for hexobarbital above, the methodology and data analysis are the same.

For a more detailed analysis of the interaction of drugs and xenobiotics with cytochrome *P*-450, the reader is referred to the review by Schenkman *et al.* (1981) and the original paper of Schenkman *et al.* (1967), the latter containing many valuable experimental details for a variety of drugs and xenobiotics.

(a) REAGENTS

Tris buffer, 0.1 M, pH 7.4.
Sodium hexobarbital, 50 mM, 13 mg to 1 ml.

(b) OTHER MATERIALS

Two matched glass or quartz cuvettes (3 ml capacity).
Split-beam recording spectrophotometer.
Hepatic microsomes.

8.2.8 NADPH-CYTOCHROME C (*P*-450) REDUCTASE

NADPH–cytochrome c (*P*-450) reductase is a flavoprotein enzyme (localized in the microsomal fraction of the liver) that transfers the necessary reducing equivalents from NADPH to cytochrome *P*-450 during certain drug metabolism reactions as

NADPH $\longrightarrow$ NADPH–cytochrome c (*P*-450) reductase $\longrightarrow$ cytochrome *P*-450.

As the reduction of cytochrome *P*-450 is relatively difficult to assay directly, a simplified determination of enzyme activity is widely used, utilizing exogenous cytochrome c (oxidized, ferric form) as an artificial electron-acceptor. According-ly, the reduction of cytochrome c by NADPH–cytochrome c (*P*-450) reductase mirrors the reduction of cytochrome *P*-450.

The principle of the method is that oxidized (ferric) cytochrome c has a characteristic absorption spectrum as does the reduced (ferrous) form. How-ever, the reduced form has a characteristic absorption band at 550 nm, a band that is absent in the oxidized form. Therefore the enzyme activity can be

Table 8.7 Spectrophotometric determination of NADPH–cytochrome c (*P*-450) reductase activity in hepatic microsomal fractions

---

(1) Mix 250 μl cytochrome c (ferric form, 5 mg ml^{-1}), 2.15 ml of 0.1 M tris buffer, pH 7.4, and 0.1 ml of a liver microsomal preparation (10 mg ml^{-1}) in a 3 ml spectro-photometer cuvette.
(2) Place the cuvette in the spectrophotometer and initiate the reaction by the addition of 25 μl of a 2% (w/v) NADPH solution; mix well and as rapidly as possible.
(3) Record the absorbance change at 550 nm as a function of time for the linear period of the reaction.

Note

For tissue samples that have a high turbidity, this can be offset by using a split-beam spectrophotometer and proceeding as in (1) above but with cytochrome c, buffer and microsomes in both a sample and a reference cuvette. The reaction is initiated by the addition of NADPH as in (2) above, the NADPH being added to the sample cuvette *only*.

Calculation of enzyme activity

Protein concentration in cuvette   = 0.4 mg ml^{-1}
Extinction coefficient for reduced (ferrous) cytochrome c at 550 nm
                                                                                    = 19.6 mM^{-1} cm^{-1}
Absorbance change (550 nm) per minute (linear portion)   = 0.784

Therefore, using Beer's Law and assuming a cuvette pathlength of 1 cm, then the specific activity of NADPH–cytochrome c (*P*-450) reductase is given by

$$\text{Specific activity} = \frac{0.784}{19.6 \times 0.4} \ \mu\text{mol cytochrome c reduced per min per mg protein}$$

$$= 0.1 \ \mu\text{mol cytochrome reduced per min per mg protein}$$

---

conveniently assayed by measuring the increase in absorbance at 550 nm as a function of time. The detailed method for determination of this enzyme activity is given in Table 8.7.

(a) REAGENTS

NADPH, 2% w/v: 10 mg to 0.5 ml water (sufficient for forty assays) – prepared fresh.
Cytochrome c, 5 mg ml^{-1}: 50 mg to 10 ml water (sufficient for forty assays) – prepared fresh or stored frozen.
Tris buffer, 0.1 M, pH 7.4.

(b) OTHER MATERIALS

Two 3 ml glass or quartz cuvettes.
Recording spectrophotometer, to read at 550 nm.
Liver microsomal preparation (10 mg ml^{-1}).

8.2.9 ASSAY OF ANILINE 4-HYDROXYLASE ACTIVITY

Many drugs are hydroxylated in the liver by the cytochrome *P*-450-dependent, mixed-function oxidase system and the 4-hydroxylation of aniline is a convenient, reproducible assessment of this reaction as

$$C_6H_5-NH_2 \xrightarrow[\text{NADPH, O}_2]{\text{Mixed-function oxidation}} HO-C_6H_4-NH_2$$

The 4-aminophenol metabolite produced is chemically converted to a phenol–indophenol complex with an absorption maximum at 630 nm, and is based on the method of Schenkman *et al.* (1967). It should be borne in mind that this assay only measures 4-aminophenol and therefore can give an underestimate of *total* aniline hydroxylation, which can also occur at the 2- and 3-positions. It has been suggested that haemoglobin can catalyse the 4-hydroxylation of aniline and it is therefore important to remove as much blood from the tissue (during preparation) as is possible.

The detailed method is given in Tables 8.8 and 8.9. Calculation of enzyme activity is as follows. The amount of metabolite formed can be calculated by direct reference to the standard curve and should be expressed as nmol product formed (4-aminophenol) per min per mg protein *or* per g wet weight of tissue as appropriate.

Absorbance of unknown sample	=	0.2
Incubation time	=	30 min
Protein content	=	2.5 mg ml^{-1}
Concentration of product from standard curve	=	2 nmol ml^{-1}
∴ Amount of product in incubation (2 ml)	=	4 nmol

Table 8.8 The 4-hydroxylation of aniline by rat liver homogenates

(1) Mix 1 ml of co-factor solution (Table 8.3) with 0.5 ml of 10 mM aniline HCl solution in suitable flasks or test tubes at 37 °C for 2 min in a water bath. A suitable blank is prepared by replacing aniline with 0.5 ml water.
(2) Initiate the enzyme reaction by adding 0.5 ml of microsomes or post-mitochondrial supernatant (containing 10 mg protein per ml) and continue incubation at 37 °C for 30 min.
(3) Stop the reaction with 1 ml of ice-cold 20% trichloroacetic acid and stand on ice for 5 min, then transfer to centrifuge tubes.
(4) Centrifuge to give a clear solution (5 min in a bench centrifuge at maximum speed is usually sufficient).
(5) Take 1 ml of the supernatant fluid and add to 1 ml of 1% phenol in a separate test tube, mix well and add 1 ml sodium carbonate. Mix well.
(6) Stand for 30 min at room temperature and read the absorbance at 630 nm, after zeroing the instrument on the blank.
(7) Construct a standard curve using known concentrations of 4-aminophenol, as in Table 8.9.

Notes

(1) All incubations should preferably be done in triplicate, or at least in duplicate.
(2) If the final solution to be read in (6) above is at all turbid or cloudy, clarify by centrifugation in a bench centrifuge.
(3) Under the above conditions, the final aniline concentration in the incubation mixture is 2.5 mM ($2.5 \, \mu\mathrm{mol \, ml^{-1}}$), and the protein concentration is $2.5 \, \mathrm{mg \, ml^{-1}}$.

Table 8.9 Standard curve for 4-aminophenol

(1) Make a stock solution of 10 μM 4-aminophenol.
(2) Take 0, 0.2, 0.4, 0.6, 0.8 and 1.0 ml of 10 μM 4-aminophenol stock solution and make up to a constant volume of 1 ml with 6% trichloroacetic acid.
(3) Proceed as in Table 8.8 (step (5)), replacing the supernatant fluid with the standard curve samples.
(4) Construct a standard curve for 4-aminophenol by plotting the absorbance value at 630 nm against the known 4-aminophenol concentration.

$$\therefore \text{Enzyme activity} = \frac{4}{(\text{time}) \times (\text{total protein in 2 ml})} \, \text{nmol min}^{-1} \, \text{mg}^{-1} \, \text{protein}$$

$$= \frac{4}{30 \times 5} = 0.027 \, \text{nmol min}^{-1} \, \text{mg}^{-1} \, \text{protein}.$$

(a) REAGENTS

Co-factor solution (see Table 8.3).
Aniline hydrochloride, 10 mM: 93 mg to 100 ml water – stored in dark bottle.
Trichloroacetic acid, 6% w/v: 60 g to 1 litre water.

Trichloroacetic acid, 20% w/v: 200 g to 1 litre water.
Phenol, 1% w/v: 20 g phenol and 40 g NaOH to 2 l water.
Sodium carbonate solution, 1 M: 200 g Na$_2$CO$_3$ (anhydrous) to 2 l water.
4-Aminophenol, 10 μM: 36.5 mg of 4-aminophenol made up to 10 ml with water. Take 0.1 ml of this solution, add to 15 g trichloroacetic acid and make up to 250 ml with water.

(b) OTHER MATERIALS

Ehrlenmeyer conical flasks (10 ml or 25 ml) or test tubes (10 ml), for incubation.
Thermostatted shaking water bath.
Liver microsomal or post-mitochondrial supernatant fraction.
Bench centrifuge and centrifuge tubes.
Spectrophotometer to read at 630 nm.
Vortex mixer or parafilm.

8.2.10 ASSAY OF AMINOPYRINE N-DEMETHYLASE ACTIVITY

N-Demethylation of drugs is a common metabolic pathway and proceeds by initial hydroxylation at the α-carbon atom and subsequent breakdown of the carbinolamine intermediate liberating formaldehyde (Figure 8.3(a)). Therefore if the formaldehyde produced could be measured, this would then yield an appropriate assay for the N-demethylase activity. Formaldehyde may be trapped in solution as the semicarbazone and measured by the colorimetric procedure of Nash (1953), based on the Hantzsch reaction (Figure 8.3(b)).

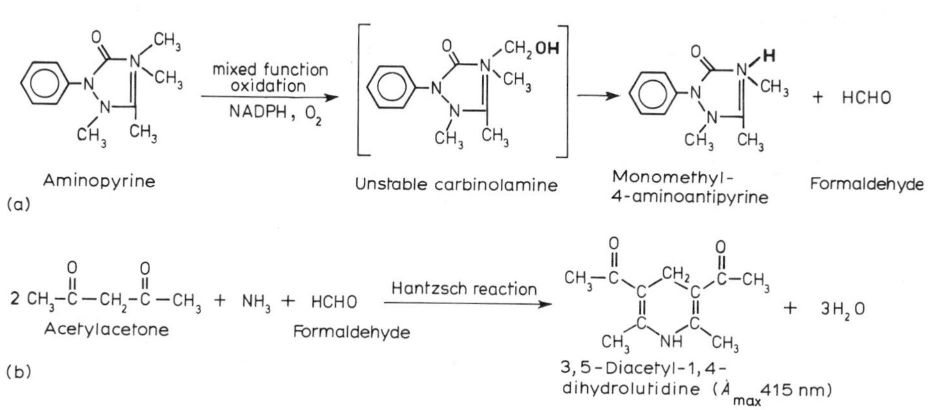

Figure 8.3 (a) Metabolic N-demethylation of aminopyrine and (b) colorimetric determination of formaldehyde.

Table 8.10 Assay for aminopyrine N-demethylase activity

(1) Prepare a *modified* co-factor solution – to include semicarbazide – as follows. Replace the 1.0 ml of 0.15 M MgCl$_2$ in Table 8.3 with 1.0 ml of 0.15 M MgCl$_2$/0.1 M semicarbazide.

(2) Mix 1 ml of modified co-factor solution and 0.5 ml of 20 mM aminopyrine, and incubate in a shaking water bath at 37 °C for 2 min. A suitable blank is prepared by replacing aminopyrine with 0.5 ml water.

(3) Initiate the enzyme reaction by adding 0.5 ml microsomes or post-mitochondrial supernatant (containing 10 mg protein per ml) and continue the incubation for 30 min.

(4) Terminate the incubation by the addition of 0.5 ml of 25% zinc sulfate, thoroughly mix and stand on ice for 5 min.

(5) Add 0.5 ml of saturated barium hydroxide solution, mix again, stand for 5 min and centrifuge to a clear supernatant on a bench centrifuge (maximum speed for 5 min).

(6) Take 1 ml of the clear supernatant (from (5)), add 2 ml Nash reagent and incubate at 60 °C for 30 min. Cover tubes with marbles to prevent water loss and hence inaccuracy.

(7) Cool the tubes and read the absorbance at 415 nm. If the tubes show any cloudiness, centrifuge briefly before reading. Zero the instrument on the blank.

(8) Construct a standard curve for formaldehyde as in Table 8.11.

Notes

(1) Under the above conditions, the final concentrations of protein and aminopyrine in the incubation medium are 2.5 mg ml^{-1} and 5 mM (5 μmol ml^{-1}) respectively.

(2) All incubations should be done in triplicate or duplicate.

(3) This assay can be used for other substrates that undergo N-demethylation including ethylmorphine, benzphetamine and p-chloro-N,N-dimethylaniline.

It should be noted that both aminopyrine and monomethyl-4-aminoantipyrine are metabolized by other pathways (including additional demethylation reactions), and therefore this particular assay does not reflect the *overall* metabolism of the substrate.

The specific procedures for this N-demethylase assay are given in Tables 8.10 and 8.11.

Table 8.11 Standard curve for formaldehyde

(1) Prepare stock solution of 0.1 mM formaldehyde.

(2) Take 0, 0.2, 0.4, 0.6, 0.8 and 1.0 ml of stock, 0.1 mM formaldehyde solution and make up to 1 ml with distilled water.

(3) Proceed as in Table 8.10, from step (6), replacing the supernatant fluid with the standard curve samples.

(4) Construct a standard curve for formaldehyde by plotting the absorbance values at 415 nm versus the known formaldehyde concentration.

Note

Prepare all tubes in triplicate or duplicate.

The rate of product formation (i.e. enzyme activity) can be calculated by direct reference to the formaldehyde standard curve and should be expressed as nmol formaldehyde formed per min per mg protein or per g wet tissue weight, as appropriate. The calculations of enzyme activity are as described before for aniline-4-hydroxylase.

(a) REAGENTS

Magnesium chloride solution (0.15 M)/semicarbazide (0.1 M): 15.25 g $MgCl_2 \cdot 6H_2O$ and 3.75 g semicarbazide to 500 ml water.
Modified co-factor solution see Table 8.10.
Aminopyrine, 20 mM: 1.16 g to 250 ml water (stored in dark bottle).
Zinc sulfate solution, 25% w/v: 125 g $ZnSO_4$ to 500 ml water.
Saturated barium hydroxide solution: excess $Ba(OH)_2$ is added to boiling water and stirred for at least 2 h. Cool the mixture and filter to remove excess solute.
Nash reagent: 30 g ammonium acetate and 0.4 ml acetylacetone made up to 100 ml with water.
Formaldehyde, 0.1 mM: take 0.75 ml of stock 40% formaldehyde solution and make up to 100 ml with water. Take 0.25 ml of this dilution and make up to 250 ml with water. Prepare fresh formaldehyde solution and keep in a tightly stoppered bottle.

(b) OTHER MATERIALS

Rat liver microsomal or post-mitochondrial supernatant.
Thermostatted, shaking water bath.
Marbles.
Spectrophotometer to read at 415 nm.
Ehrlenmeyer conical flasks (10 ml or 25 ml) *or* test tubes (10 ml) for incubation.
Bench centrifuge.
Vortex mixer or parafilm.
Centrifuge tubes.

8.2.11 ASSAY OF 4-NITROANISOLE *O*-DEMETHYLASE ACTIVITY

In a similar manner to the *N*-demethylation of xenobiotics, many drugs can undergo *O*-demethylation reactions, catalysed by the microsomal, cytochrome *P*-450-dependent, mixed-function oxidase system. A useful substrate to

Table 8.12 Assay for 4-nitroanisole *O*-demethylase activity

---

(1) Mix 1 ml cofactor solution (Table 8.3) and 1 ml of microsomes *or* post-mitochondrial supernatant (containing 10 mg protein per ml), and incubate at 37 °C for 2 min in a shaking water bath.

(2) Initiate the reaction with 10 μl (micro syringe) of 500 mM 4-nitroanisole solution and continue incubation for 15 min.

(3) Blank incubations should be prepared as above, but by substituting a tissue homogenate previously heated to 70–100 °C for 10 min to denature the enzymes. This is necessary as the 4-nitroanisole has some yellow colour of its own.

(4) Terminate the enzyme reaction by the addition of 1 ml of ice-cold 20% trichloroacetic acid solution and allow to stand on ice for 5 min.

(5) Centrifuge the mixture to obtain a clear supernatant (bench centrifuge, maximum speed for 5 min).

(6) Take 1 ml of the supernatant and add 10 M NaOH until the pH is approximately 10–11. Add distilled water to give a final volume of 1.5 ml, mix well, and read the absorbance at 400 nm.

(7) Construct a standard curve for 4-nitrophenol, as in Table 8.13.

Notes

(1) Under the above conditions, the final concentrations of protein and 4-nitroanisole in the incubation medium are 5 mg ml^{-1} and 2.5 mM (2.5 μmol ml^{-1}) respectively.

(2) Carry out all incubations in duplicate or triplicate.

---

monitor *O*-demethylation reactions is 4-nitroanisole which is converted to 4-nitrophenol as

$$NO_2-C_6H_4-OCH_3 \xrightarrow[\text{NADPH, } O_2]{\text{Mixed-function oxidation}} NO_2-C_6H_4-OH + HCHO$$

The 4-nitrophenol thus produced forms an intense yellow colour at pH 10, with an absorbance maximum at 400 nm. Hence the activity of the enzyme system can be followed spectrophotometrically as described in detail in Tables 8.12 and 8.13.

Table 8.13 Standard curve for 4-nitrophenol

---

(1) Prepare a stock 0.1 mM solution of 4-nitrophenol.

(2) Take 0, 0.2, 0.4, 0.6, 0.8 and 1.0 ml of stock 0.1 mM 4-nitrophenol solution and make up to a constant volume of 1 ml with appropriate volumes of 6% trichloroacetic acid.

(3) Proceed as in Table 8.12 from step (6), replacing the supernatant with the standard curve samples.

(4) Construct a standard curve for 4-nitrophenol by plotting the absorbance values at 400 nm against the known 4-nitrophenol concentration.

Note

Prepare tubes in triplicate or duplicate.

The amount of product formed is calculated by reference to the 4-nitrophenol standard curve. Express the activity as nmol product formed per min per mg protein or per g wet tissue weight as appropriate. Calculation is similar to that for aniline-4-hydroxylase activity, above.

(a) REAGENTS

Co-factor solution: see Table 8.3.
4-Nitroanisole, 500 mM: 765 mg to 10 ml of acetone (keep solution in a dark, air-tight bottle).
Trichloroacetic acid, 20% w/v: 200 g to 1 litre water.
Trichloroacetic acid, 6% w/v: 60 g to 1 litre water.
Sodium hydroxide solution, 10 M: 400 g NaOH to 1 litre water.
4-Nitrophenol, 0.1 mM: 3.5 mg 4-nitrophenol and 15 g trichloroacetic acid made up to 250 ml with water.

(b) OTHER MATERIALS

Rat liver microsomes or post-mitochondrial supernatant.
Thermostatted, shaking water bath.
Spectrophotometer to read at 400 nm.
Ehrlenmeyer conical flasks (10 ml or 25 ml) *or* test tubes (10 ml) for incubation.
Centrifuge tubes and bench centrifuge.
Vortex mixer or parafilm.

8.2.12 ASSAY FOR GLUCURONYLTRANSFERASE ACTIVITY

The glucuronyltransferase family of enzymes is important in phase II drug conjugation reactions; many examples are known where glucuronic acid is conjugated with the hydroxyl, carboxyl or amino groups of the substrates. A useful compound to assess glucuronyltransferase activity is 2-aminophenol, because this phenol readily forms an O-linked glucuronide conjugate in the presence of microsomal fractions and UDP–glucuronic acid.

The assay for glucuronidation of 2-aminophenol is based on the colorimetric diazotization method for free primary amino groups, originally developed by Bratton and Marshall (1939) for the estimation of sulfonamides. The principle of the analytical method is based on the observation that, when an aqueous solution of sodium nitrite is added to a cold, acidified solution of an aromatic amine, a diazonium salt is formed. Excess nitrite is removed by the addition of ammonium sulfamate, and the diazonium salt is finally reacted with a complex aromatic amine (N-naphthylethylene diamine), to produce a brightly-coloured

Table 8.14 Assay for glucuronyltransferase activity

(1) Mix 1 ml co-factor solution with 0.5 ml of 1 mM 2-aminophenol and initiate the reaction with either 0.5 ml microsomal or post-mitochondrial fraction (containing 10 mg protein per ml) at 37 °C in a shaking water bath.
(2) A suitable blank is prepared by adding 0.5 ml water instead of 2-aminophenol.
(3) Continue the incubation for 30 min.
(4) Stop the reaction with 1 ml of ice-cold 20% trichloroacetic acid in 0.1 M phosphate buffer, pH 2.7, stand on ice for 5 min and clarify the supernatant by centrifugation (bench centrifuge).
(5) To 1 ml of the supernatant fluid, add 0.5 ml (*fresh*) 0.1% sodium nitrite, mix well and stand for 2 min.
(6) Add 0.5 ml of 0.5% ammonium sulfamate, mix well and stand for 3 min.
(7) Add 0.5 ml of 0.1% N-naphthylethylene diamine, mix well and allow to stand at room temperature *in the dark* for 60 min.
(8) Read the absorbance at 540 nm against the substrate blank.
(9) Prepare a standard curve (aniline) as described in Table 8.15.

Notes
(1) Under the above conditions, the concentrations of protein and 2-aminophenol in the incubation mixture are 2.5 mg ml^{-1} and 0.25 mM (0.25 μmol ml^{-1}) respectively.
(2) Prepare incubations in triplicate or duplicate.
(3) 2-Aminophenol is one of the many substrates used to monitor glucuronyl transferase activity. Many other substrates may be used (both endogenous and exogenous substrates); the reader is referred to the articles by Burchell (1974) and Falany and Tephly (1983) for more detailed descriptions.

azo compound that can be analysed spectrophotometrically. This method, therefore, detects the amino group of the 2-aminophenyl glucuronide. The method is relatively specific because excess substrate (2-aminophenol) is destroyed under the assay conditions (at pH 2.7) and therefore does not take part in the diazotization reaction.

As the glucuronyltransferases usually exhibit enzyme latency in the microsomal membrane, the assay is carried out in the presence of the detergent Triton X-100 to offset the latency. Ascorbic acid is included as an anti-oxidant. Because the cofactor requirement for glucuronyltransferase activity is different to that for cytochrome *P*-450-dependent, mixed-function oxidase activity described earlier in this section, the following cofactor solution is required.

0.1 M tris buffer, pH 8.0	8.0 ml
Magnesium chloride solution, 0.15 M	1.0 ml
Triton X-100, 1% w/v	0.5 ml
Ascorbic acid, 0.02 M	1.0 ml
UDP–glucuronic acid	10 mg

and is sufficient for ten assays. The assay procedure is given in Table 8.14, and the standard curve procedure in Table 8.15.

Table 8.15 Standard curve for 2-aminophenol glucuronide

(1) Prepare a stock solution of 0.1mM aniline in 6% trichloroacetic acid. (Aniline is used in the standard curve because it produces a chromophore of similar properties to 2-aminophenol glucuronide, which is not routinely available.)

(2) Take 0, 0.2, 0.4, 0.6, 0.8 and 1.0 ml of 0.1 mM aniline stock solution and make up to a constant volume of 1 ml with appropriate volumes of 6% trichloroacetic acid in 0.1M phosphate buffer, pH 2.7.

(3) To each tube of the standard curve, add 0.5 ml (*fresh*) 0.1% sodium nitrite, mix well and stand for 2 min.

(4) Proceed as in Table 8.14 from step (6).

(5) Construct a standard curve for aniline by plotting the absorbance values at 540 nm against the aniline concentration.

Note

Prepare the standard curve in triplicate or duplicate.

The amount of product formed is calculated by reference to the standard curve (see Table 8.15). Express the activity as nmol product formed per min per mg protein or per g wet tissue weight, as appropriate.

(a) REAGENTS

2-Aminophenol, 1 mM: 11 mg to 100 ml.

Trichloroacetic acid, 20% w/v: 200 g to 1 litre.

Trichloroacetic acid, 6% w/v: 60 g to 1 litre.

Magnesium chloride solution, 0.15 M: 15.25 mg $MgCl_2 \cdot 6H_2O$ to 500 ml.

Triton X-100, 1% w/v: 100 mg to 10 ml.

Ascorbic acid, 0.02 M: 180 mg to 50 ml.

Trichloroacetic acid, 20% w/v, buffered: 200 g to 1 litre of 0.1 M phosphate buffer, pH 2.7.

Trichloroacetic acid, 6% w/v, buffered: 60 g to 1 litre of 0.1 M phosphate buffer, pH 2.7.

Sodium nitrite, 0.1% w/v: 100 mg to 100 ml (make-up just prior to use).

Ammonium sulfamate, 0.5% w/v: 500 mg to 100 ml.

N-Naphthylethylene diamine, 0.1% w/v: 100 mg to 100 ml.

Aniline, 0.1 mM, in 6% w/v trichloroacetic acid. Aniline (HCl salt), 13 mg, plus trichloroacetic acid, 6 g, to 100 ml.

(b) OTHER MATERIALS

Rat liver microsomes or post-mitochondrial supernatant.

Thermostatted, shaking water bath.

Spectrophotometer to read at 540 nm.

Ehrlenmeyer conical flasks (10 ml or 25 ml) *or* test tubes (10 ml) for incubation.
Centrifuge tubes and bench centrifuge.
Vortex mixer or parafilm.

8.2.13 ASSAY FOR GLUTATHIONE-*S*-TRANSFERASE ACTIVITY

The glutathione-*S*-transferases are a family of isoenzymes that function to catalyse the conjugation of the endogenous tripeptide glutathione (γ-glutamyl-cysteinyl-glycine) with a large number of structurally diverse, electrophilic xenobiotics or their metabolites. As discussed earlier, the glutathione-*S*-transferases consist of two sub-units each of which is inducible by many drugs or xenobiotics. Although some exceptions are known, their prime function is in detoxication of biologically reactive electrophiles.

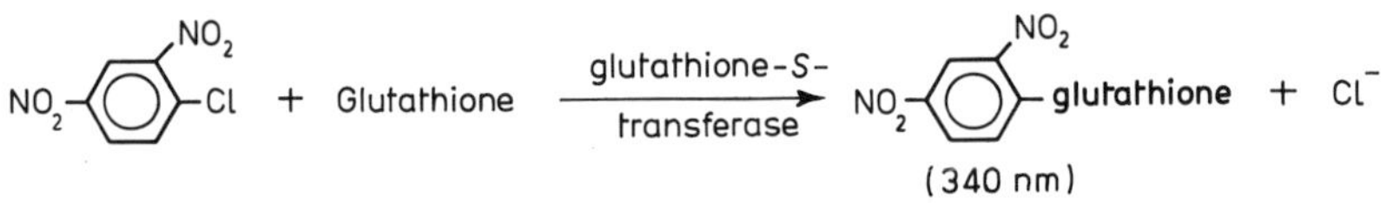

Figure 8.4 Conjugation of 1-chloro-2,4-dinitrobenzene and glutathione as catalysed by glutathione-*S*-transferase.

A convenient spectrophotometric method has been developed for the analysis of glutathione-*S*-transferase activity based on the enzyme-catalysed condensation of glutathione with the model substrate 1-chloro-2,4-dinitrobenzene (Figure 8.4). The product formed (2,4-dinitrophenyl-glutathione) absorbs light at 340 nm, and the extinction coefficient of this product is known to be $9.6 \text{ mM}^{-1} \text{ cm}^{-1}$, thus facilitating the analysis of enzyme activity based on product formation. It should be pointed out that the glutathione-*S*-transferase isoenzymes have similar but overlapping substrate specificities for the electrophilic substrate to be conjugated. Therefore one substrate which is readily reactive with a particular isoenzyme may not be a substrate for another isoenzyme. With this limitation in mind, dinitrochlorobenzene is a good substrate for most of the glutathione-*S*-transferase isoenzymes, but still it must be remembered that the observed activity is a composite result of the activity of each isoenzyme present in the tissue preparation.

Conditions for the assay are given in Table 8.16 and a simple calculation of enzyme activity is as follows:

Protein concentration in cuvette $= 2 \text{ mg ml}^{-1}$
Extinction coefficient for glutathione adduct $= 9.6 \text{ mM}^{-1} \text{ cm}^{-1}$
Absorbance change (340 nm) per min (linear portion) $= 0.4$

Table 8.16 Assay for glutathione-*S*-transferase activity

(1) To each of two 3 ml spectrophotometer cuvettes, add 0.1 ml of 30 mM glutathione, 0.1 ml of 30 mM dinitrochlorobenzene and 2.2 ml of 100 mM potassium phosphate buffer, pH 6.5.
(2) Place the cuvettes in the sample and reference compartment of a split-beam recording spectrophotometer.
(3) Initiate the reaction by adding 0.6 ml of a post-mitochondrial supernatant (or 100 000 g supernatant) from liver (10 mg protein ml^{-1}) and balance the reference cuvette volume by adding 0.6 ml of the appropriate buffer or medium (i.e. the medium in which the tissue homogenate was prepared). Mix both cuvettes thoroughly. Carry out this step as rapidly as possible.
(4) Record the increase in absorbance at 340 nm with time over a 5 min period.

Notes
(1) A split-beam recording spectrophotometer is not essential; the essay may be carried out in a single-cuvette instrument, remembering to subtract the enzyme blank from the test value. In addition, a recording spectrophotometer is not essential – in this case, record absorbance changes timed with a clock.
(2) Depending on the activity of the tissue under study, the linearity period of the reaction may vary. If the linear period is short, then use less of the enzyme preparation (for example 0.1 ml). If the reaction is slow, then extend the observation period.
(3) Many other substrates (in addition to dinitrochlorobenzene) may be used; the reader is referred to the original article by Habig *et al.* (1974) for additional substrates and for a detailed discussion of the glutathione-*S*-transferase assay procedure.

Therefore, using Beer's Law and assuming a cuvette path length of 1 cm, then the specific activity of the glutathione-*S*-transferase is given by

$$\text{Specific activity} = \frac{0.4}{9.6 \times 2} \ \mu\text{mol product formed per min per mg protein}$$

$$= 0.02 \ \mu\text{mol product formed per min per mg protein}$$

(a) REAGENTS

Dinitrochlorobenzene, 30 mM: 62 mg to 10 ml ethanol.
Glutathione, 30 mM: 16 mg to 2 ml water. This is sufficient for ten assays.
Potassium phosphate buffer, 100 mM: pH 6.5.

(b) OTHER MATERIALS

Post-mitochondrial supernatant, or 100 000 g supernatant from rat liver.
Split-beam recording spectrophotometer to read at 340 nm.
Cuvettes (3 ml).

8.2.14 ADDITIONAL *IN VITRO* ASSAYS FOR DRUG METABOLISM

The above *in vitro* assays have been chosen and described in detail because they are easy to perform, give reproducible results, are rapid to perform and involve the use of a relatively widely available analytical end-point, i.e. a spectrophotometer. However, many other analytical techniques may be used to assay the activity of drug-metabolizing enzymes including fluorimetry and radiochemical methods for example. Unfortunately these latter techniques are either time-consuming or require more expensive or less readily available instrumentation. On the other hand, fluorimetry and radiochemical methods are generally more sensitive than spectrophotometry, and – dependent on the substrate investigated – may provide more incisive information about a particular metabolic pathway. Some of these assays are outlined in Tables 8.17 and 8.18, and references are also given to the detailed methodologies and analytical techniques required.

8.3 Factors affecting drug metabolism

8.3.1 EXPERIMENT 1: COFACTOR REQUIREMENTS OF DRUG METABOLISM

The cytochrome *P*-450-dependent oxidation of xenobiotics in hepatic microsomes uses an electron-transport pathway to deliver reducing equivalents from NADPH to the terminal electron-acceptor, cytochrome *P*-450. Two electrons are required in this reaction, the first of which must be supplied by NADPH via NADPH–cytochrome *P*-450 reductase. The second electron can be supplied either from NADPH as above or from NADH via NADH–cytochrome b_5 reductase and cytochrome b_5 as described earlier in Chapter 2.

According to the above scheme, NADH alone only poorly supports drug metabolism reactions, but if the second electron transfer is rate-limiting, then the addition of NADH to an NADPH-driven reaction will increase the rate of product formation. Accordingly, the following experiment is designed to show the validity of this scheme for the hepatic oxidative metabolism of drugs. It should be noted that some substrates show an increase in metabolism in the presence of NADH added to NADPH-fortified liver homogenates (termed NADH synergism), whereas other substrates do not. Aniline is a classical substrate for displaying NADH synergism, whereas the aminopyrine response is variable. Accordingly, the following experiment is designed to investigate NADH synergism for the metabolism of both aniline and aminopyrine. This experiment can easily be completed in one day (8 h).

Table 8.17 Additional assays of *in vitro* phase I drug metabolism

Enzyme involved	Metabolic pathway	Substrate	Analytical technique	Reference
Cytochrome *P*-450	Ring hydroxylation	Coumarin	Fluorimetric	Jacobson *et al.* (1974)
Cytochrome *P*-450	O-De-ethylation	7-Ethoxycoumarin	Fluorimetric	Jacobson *et al.* (1974)
Cytochrome *P*-450	O-De-ethylation	Ethoxyresorufin	Fluorimetric	Burke and Mayer (1975)
Cytochrome *P*-450	Ring hydroxylation	Benzo[*a*]pyrene	Fluorimetric	Nebert and Gelboin (1968)
Cytochrome *P*-450	Alkyl hydroxylation	Lauric acid	TLC/radiochemical	Parker and Orton (1980)
Cytochrome *P*-450	Alkyl hydroxylation	Lauric acid	HPLC/radiochemical	Gibson *et al.* (1982)
Cytochrome *P*-450 and NADPH–cytochrome *P*-450 reductase	Azoreductase	Amaranth	Spectrophotometric	Mallet *et al.* (1982)
Cytochrome *P*-450	Epoxidation	Aldrin	GLC	Wolff *et al.* (1979)
Cytochrome *P*-450	Ring hydroxylation	Testosterone or androstenedione	HPLC	Wood *et al.* (1983) and Tredger *et al.* (1984)
Cytochrome *P*-450	Ring- and N-hydroxylation	2-Acetylaminofluorene	HPLC	Astrom *et al.* (1982)
Cytochrome *P*-450	N-Hydroxylation	2-Acetylaminofluorene	TLC	Lotlikar *et al.* (1974)
Cytochrome *P*-450 and microsomal oxidases	N-Oxidation	N,N-Dimethylaniline	Spectrophotometric	Ziegler and Pettit (1964)
Cytochrome *P*-450	Ring and benzylic hydroxylation	Warfarin	HPLC	Kaminsky *et al.* (1983)
Cytochrome *P*-450	De-ethylation	Phenacetin	Radiochemical	Guengerich and Martin (1980)
Cytochrome *P*-450	Ring and side-chain oxidation	Propranolol	HPLC	Bargar *et al.* (1983)
Epoxide hydrase	Epoxide hydration	Styrene oxide	Radiochemical	Oesch *et al.* (1971)
Epoxide hydrase	Epoxide hydration	Benzo[*a*]pyrene-4,5-oxide	Radiochemical	Schmassmann *et al.* (1976)
Epoxide hydrase	Epoxide hydration	Various epoxides	Spectrophotometric	Guengerich and Mason (1980)

Note
Additional information on *in vitro*, phase I drug metabolism assays (and purification of the enzymes) can be found in Guengerich (1982).

Table 8.18 Additonal assays of *in vitro* phase II drug metabolism

Enzyme involved	Metabolic pathway	Substrate	Analytical technique	Reference
UDP–glucuronyltransferase	Glucuronidation	Morphine	Radiochemical	Sanchez and Tephly (1974)
UDP–glucuronyltransferase	Glucuronidation	4-Nitrophenol	Colorimetric	Tukey *et al.* (1978)
UDP–glucuronyltransferase	Glucuronidation	4-Methylumbelliferone	Fluorimetric	Aitio (1974)
Glutathione–S-transferase	Glutathione conjugation	Various	Spectrophotometric	Habig *et al.* (1974)

(a) SOLUTIONS (sufficient for two groups, each using one substrate)

Sucrose, 0.25 M: 85.6 g to 1 litre water.
Calcium chloride solution, 88 mM (if using CaCl$_2$-precipitated microsomes): 1.93 g CaCl$_2$ to 100 ml water.
NADPH, 5 mM: 21 mg to 5 ml water. Make up immediately prior to use and store on ice.
NADH, 5 mM: 18 mg to 5 ml water. Make up immediately prior to use and store on ice.
Tris buffer, 0.3 M: pH 7.4: 1 litre.
Aniline, 50 mM: 465 mg aniline HCl salt to 100 ml water.
Aminopyrine, 100 mM: 272 mg to 10 ml water.
Magnesium chloride solution, 0.15 M: 15.25 mg MgCl$_2$ · 6H$_2$O to 500 ml water.
Nicotinamide, 0.5 M: 3.05 g to 50 ml water.
Solutions for protein assay (Section 8.2.3), aniline hydroxylase assay (Section 8.2.9) and aminopyrine N-demethylase assay (Section 8.2.10).

(Note that NADPH and/or NADH replaces the cofactor solution in this instance.)

(b) APPARATUS (for two groups, each using one substrate)

Test tubes, 120 mm × 15 mm: 200.
Bench centrifuge tubes, 50 ml: 20.
Ultracentrifuge tubes (if needed for microsome preparation): 20.
Beakers, 25 ml, 50 ml and 250 ml: as required.
Homogenization vessels, 15 ml and 50 ml: 1 of each.
Cuvettes (disposable), 3 ml: 50.
Cuvettes (disposable), 1 ml: 50.
Balance (up to 30 g): 1.
Timers: 2.
Ice buckets: 5.
Automatic pipettes, 10–100 μl, 200–1000 μl, 1–5 ml: 2 of each.
Shaking water bath: sufficient to take 28 tubes.
Refrigerated centrifuge: 1, capable of 27 000 g.
Ultracentrifuge: 1, capable of 100 000 g. (Only required if microsomes are prepared by ultracentrifugation.)
Spectrophotometer, UV–visible: 1.

(c) METHOD

All apparatus and solutions needed for the tissue preparation should be pre-cooled on ice before the start of the experiment. It is important that the tissue does not exceed $+4\,°C$ during preparation.

Experimental animals are killed and hepatic microsomal fractions prepared, as in Section 8.2.1 – either by the $CaCl_2$ aggregation method or by ultra-centrifugation. Ten male rats ($100–200\,g$ body weight) are sufficient for this experiment. Determine the microsomal protein content (Section 8.2.3) and dilute to $10\,mg$ protein ml^{-1}.

Test tubes are set up (in duplicate for both substrates) as described in Table 8.19. Tube 1 is a blank containing no NADPH or NADH and should be incubated in addition to the substrate blank as described under the appropriate substrate. Tube 2 contains only NADH as co-factor, and tube 3 only NADPH. Tubes 4–7 contain differing proportions of NADH and NADPH. Tubes 2 and 3 will show the requirement for NADH and NADPH respectively when compared to the experimental blank (tube 1). Tubes 4–7 will show if any NADH synergism is evident.

The tubes are placed in a shaking water bath at $37\,°C$ for $2\,min$ and the reaction started by adding $0.1\,ml$ of *either* $50\,mM$ aniline *or* $100\,mM$ amino-pyrine. Incubation is continued at $37\,°C$ for $30\,min$ for both substrates. The reaction is stopped, and assay is carried out for aniline hydroxylase activity or aminopyrine N-demethylase activity as indicated in Tables 8.8 and 8.10 respectively.

Both enzyme activities are expressed as nmol product formed per min per mg protein, and the data tabulated to show the co-factor requirements. With reference to the results, the following questions should be answered.

(1) Is NADH or NADPH required for microsomal drug metabolism?
(2) Can NADH alone as co-factor support drug metabolism? If so, how does this fit in with the accepted theory of oxidative metabolism.
(3) Was NADH synergism observed with either substrate? If not, why?
(4) If NADH synergism was observed, was there any difference in the degree of synergism seen at different ratios of NADH/NADPH?

8.3.2 EXPERIMENT 2: FACTORS AFFECTING DRUG METABOLISM

Many factors can affect the rate of metabolism of drugs by the liver including the species, sex and age of the animal, its genetic make-up and state of health. There are also major effects of hormonal, nutritional and environmental factors. These aspects of drug metabolism are discussed in more detail in

Table 8.19 Incubations to investigate the co-factor requirements of drug metabolism

Tube no.	Magnesium chloride solution, 0.15 M (ml)	Nicotinamide 0.5 M (ml)	NADPH, 5 mM (ml)	Tris buffer, 0.3 M pH 7.4 (ml)	Microsomes, 10 mg ml^{-1} (ml)	NADH, 5 mM (ml)	Water (ml)
1	0.1	0.1	0	0.5	0.5	0	0.7
2	0.1	0.1	0	0.5	0.5	0.2	0.5
3	0.1	0.1	0.2	0.5	0.5	0	0.5
4	0.1	0.1	0.2	0.5	0.5	0.05	0.45
5	0.1	0.1	0.2	0.5	0.5	0.10	0.4
6	0.1	0.1	0.2	0.5	0.5	0.20	0.3
7	0.1	0.1	0.2	0.5	0.5	0.40	0.1

Note that after substrate addition, the final incubation volume is 2 ml.

Chapters 4 and 5. The ability of different tissues to metabolize drugs is also of interest, particularly in terms of tissue selective toxicity, and in cases where hepatic metabolism may be low as in liver disease.

From a biochemical viewpoint, the temperature and pH of the buffer being used in the assay can also be of importance in determining the enzyme activity measured.

(a) OUTLINE

In this experiment, a number of the variables mentioned above are tested for their effect on drug metabolism using some of the assays described in Section 8.2. In order to keep the experiment within one day (8 h), it is necessary to restrict the number of parameters investigated to around four per group, and for each group to use two substrates. The groups given in Table 8.20 can be used as a single experiment to illustrate the effects of species, tissue, sex and temperature on drug metabolism. The large number of tissue samples used means that metabolism by post-mitochondrial supernatants must be measured – unless access to a number of ultracentrifuges is available, or the class is relatively small.

Table 8.20 Outline of experiments to illustrate some factors influencing drug metabolism

Animal	Groups
Male rat	Liver preparations incubated at 0, 20, 30, 37, 45 and 60 °C
Male rat	Preparations from liver, kidney, brain and lung incubated at 37 °C
Female rat	Liver preparations incubated at 37 °C
Male frog	Liver preparations incubated at 0, 20, 30, 37, 45 and 60° C

(b) METHOD

(1) Prepare post-mitochondrial supernatants from male and female rats and from the male frog, for the tissues indicated in Table 8.20, following the method in Section 8.2.1.
(2) Determine the protein content of each tissue preparation as in Section 8.2.3.
(3) Split the class into appropriate groups and assign each group a particular experiment (Table 8.20). For each group determine the drug-metabolizing activity (in duplicate) for two substrates, and ensure that all groups investigate the same two substrates.
(4) Express drug-metabolizing activity as both activity per mg protein and activity per g original wet tissue weight.
(5) Collate the results from all groups and use them to answer the following questions:

Are the effects of the various factors investigated the same for both substrates? If not, why?

How do the temperature curves for enzyme activity compare between the male rat liver and male frog liver? If they are different, why?

Do the male and female rat metabolize the two chosen substrates to the same extent. If not, why?

In the male rat, place the ability of each tissue to metabolize both substrates in descending order. If the enzyme activity is expressed as per mg protein or per g original wet tissue weight, does this make any difference to the order of activity?

Discuss the importance of the various factors studied in the *regulation* of drug metabolism.

Discuss the relevance of the various factors studied in the *clinical use* of drugs.

(c) SOLUTIONS

Sucrose, 0.25 M: 256.8 g to 3 l water.

Calcium chloride solution, 88 mM (if using $CaCl_2$-precipitated microsomes): 1.93 g $CaCl_2$ to 100 ml water.

Appropriate amounts of the solutions required for assay of the metabolism of two substrates, as in Section 8.2.

(d) APPARATUS (sufficient for ten students/groups)

Test tubes, 120 mm × 15 mm: 400.
Centrifuge tubes, 50 ml: 100.
Ultracentrifuge tubes (if required): 100.
Beakers, 25 ml, 50 ml and 250 ml: as required.
Homogenization vessels, 50 ml: minimum of 3.
Homogenization vessels, 15 ml: minimum of 3.
Cuvettes (disposable), 3 ml: 100.
Cuvettes (disposable), 1 ml: 100.
Balance, up to 30 g: 1.
Timers: 10.
Ice-buckets: 10.
Automatic pipettes, 10–100 μl, 200–1000 μl and 1–5 ml: 10 of each, although a smaller number can be shared if necessary.
Thermostatted, shaking water-baths: 5.
Refrigerated centrifuge, up to 27 000 g: 1.
Refrigerated ultracentrifuges (if required): as many as are available to cut down on tissue processing time.
Spectrophotometer, UV–visible: 1.

8.4 Induction and inhibition of drug metabolism and a correlation of *in vivo* drug action with *in vitro* hepatic drug-metabolizing activity

8.4.1 INTRODUCTION

The duration and intensity of action of many drugs is critically influenced by the rate of their metabolism. As previously discussed in Chapter 3, the rate of drug metabolism can be substantially altered (either increased or decreased) by the prior treatment of animals with various compounds, some of which may be structurally unrelated to the drug metabolized.

The following two experiments are designed to demonstrate the effects of a compound that stimulates (induces) the liver drug-metabolizing enzymes (phenobarbital), or inhibits (destroys) these enzymes (carbon tetrachloride) on:

(1) The *in vivo* duration of action of the hypnotic drug pentobarbital;
(2) The drug-metabolizing activity of the 12 500 g liver supernatant as measured by the *in vitro* N-demethylation of aminopyrine;
(3) The levels of cytochrome *P*-450 in the hepatic microsomal fraction.

It is then possible to compare the duration of action of a drug *in vivo* with both the activities of the drug-metabolizing enzymes *in vitro* and the levels of cytochrome *P*-450.

Note that the experiments can easily be completed in one day provided that the class is large enough (around 20) and the class is split into groups. However, if the class is small (around 6–10) the the two experiments may have to be attempted on separate days.

8.4.2 EXPERIMENT 1: THE DURATION OF ACTION OF THE HYPNOTIC DRUG PENTOBARBITAL

Pentobarbital is a hypnotic drug whose duration of action can be measured in rats by the sleeping time (i.e. the time from when the animal falls asleep to when it regains its 'righting reflex'). Therefore, because pentobarbital is metabolized by the hepatic microsomal cytochrome *P*-450 enzyme action (Figure 8.5), its duration of action can be altered by inducing agents or by inhibitors.

(a) ANIMAL PRE-TREATMENT

Male rats, initially weighing 80–100 g and fed a standard laboratory diet are used in groups of ten per treatment. It is important that the rat body weights are as close together as possible at the start of the pre-treatment, in view of the

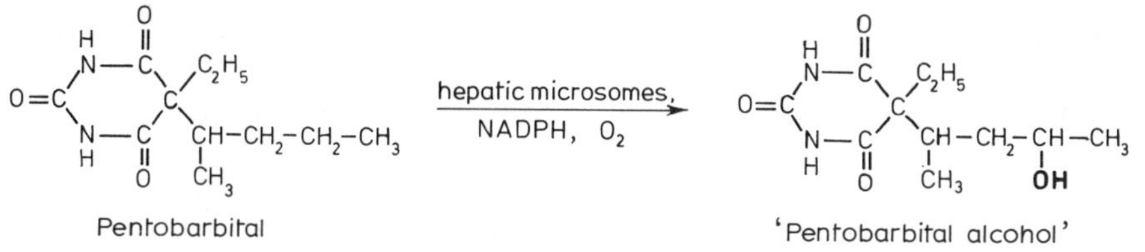

Figure 8.5 The cytochrome *P*-450-dependent metabolism (side-chain hydroxylation) of pentobarbital.

well-documented age differences in drug metabolism and drug response. Ten rats are injected intraperitoneally once daily for 3 d prior to the experiment with either sodium phenobarbitone, $80 \, mg \, kg^{-1}$ (in saline), or an equivalent volume of saline – the latter saline-treated group serving as vehicle controls. In addition, a third group of ten rats are injected on the third day only with a *single*, intraperitoneal injection of carbon tetrachloride, $1.25 \, ml \, kg^{-1}$ (in corn oil). Although a corn oil, vehicle control group of rats should ideally be used, previous experience indicates that the corn oil control is not significantly different from the saline control, and hence the latter group serves as a control group for both pre-treatments.

If the above protocol is followed, then all groups of rats will be ready for the start of the experiment on the fourth day, i.e. 24 h after the last injection.

(b) METHOD

Three groups of rats (10 in each group) are now available to study the influence of animal pre-treatment on the *in vivo* duration of action of pentobarbital. It is advisable to start this experiment in the morning so that when the sleeping times are being monitored, the tissue homogenates are being simultaneously prepared for use in the afternoon.

Every rat, in all three groups, is then given an intraperitoneal injection of pentobarbitone at a dose of $30 \, mg \, kg^{-1}$. The rats can be separately caged or appropriately marked to monitor individual sleeping times. Note the times at which each rat is

(1) Injected;
(2) Falls asleep, as measured by its loss of the righting reflex;
(3) Wakes up, as measured by regaining the righting reflex, twice within a period of ten s.

The righting reflex is easily monitored by gently placing the rat on its back: if the righting reflex is still present, the animal will 'right' itself. If the reflex has been abolished, the animal will attempt to get up but will be unable to do so.

Clearly, from the above discussion, the 'sleeping time' is the difference between (2) and (3).

It should be noted that, dependent on the rat strain used, the drug response may vary. In our experience, for the stated dose in male Wistar rats, the control group will sleep for around 1 h, the CCl_4-treated group for about 3 h and the phenobarbital-treated group for much less than an hour.

(c) TREATMENT OF DATA

The mean sleeping time, plus/minus standard error and standard deviation, for each group of rats should be calculated and compared statistically with the control group to determine if the pre-treatment has had a statistically significant effect in either increasing or decreasing the sleeping time.

8.4.3 EXPERIMENT 2: INFLUENCE OF PRE-TREATMENT ON THE *IN VITRO* N-DEMETHYLATION OF AMINOPYRINE AND MICROSOMAL CYTOCHROME P-450 CONTENT

The purpose of this experiment is to determine the ability of rat liver to N-demethylate aminopyrine, to determine the hepatic microsomal cytochrome P-450 content and to investigate the influence of pre-treatment with either phenobarbital or carbon tetrachloride on these two parameters. Because the animal pre-treatment involves the same two compounds used to assess the influence on the sleeping time in the previous experiment, then the two experiments can be finally compared to determine if modulation of *in vitro* drug-metabolizing activity is reflected in any change in drug action *in vivo*.

(a) ANIMAL PRE-TREATMENT

In order to compare the results of this experiment with the previous one, the pre-treatment schedules are *identical* to that described for the sleeping times, with the only exception that smaller groups of animals are used. This is largely because of constraints of available centrifuge space and time of preparation of individual tissue homogenates. Accordingly, it is recommended to use only five animals per group, with the same three groups of control, phenobarbital-treated, and CCl_4-treated rats. The treatment should start on the same day as for the sleeping time experiment.

(b) METHOD

The rats are killed, the livers removed, blotted dry and weighed; a 12 500 g supernatant is made from each individual liver in all groups, as described in

Section 8.2.1. Remove 12 ml of each of the 12 500 g supernatant preparations and determine the protein content of each sample, as in Section 8.2.3. This preparation is then used for the aminopyrine N-demethylase determination, as described in Section 8.2.10.

The remainder of the 12 500 g supernatant is then centrifuged at 100 000 g (as in Section 8.2.1), to prepare microsomal fractions. Alternatively, microsomal fractions may be prepared by the $CaCl_2$-aggregation method (Section 8.2.1). Determine the protein content (Section 8.2.3) and cytochrome P-450 content (Section 8.2.5) of each of the microsomal preparations.

(c) TREATMENT OF DATA

(1) Calculate the aminopyrine N-demethylase specific activity of each sample, expressing your results both as activity per mg of 12 500 g supernatant protein and as activity per g wet liver weight. For each pre-treatment group, calculate the mean specific activity for aminopyrine N-demethylation, and the standard error and standard deviation. Statistically compare the influence of both phenobarbital and CCl_4 pre-treatments on drug metabolism activity as compared to the control (saline-treated) group of rats.

(2) Calculate the cytochrome P-450 specific content of each microsomal preparation, expressed as nmol cytochrome P-450 per mg microsomal protein (Section 8.2.5). For each pre-treatment group, determine the mean ($\pm$ s.e. and s.d.) cytochrome P-450 content, and statistically test if the pre-treatment has influenced the results obtained, by comparison to the control group.

(3) Finally, compare the results of experiments 1 and 2 (Sections 8.4.2 and 8.4.3) to determine if modulation of *in vitro* drug-metabolizing enzyme activity is mirrored by appropriate changes in the *in vivo* sleeping times.

The following solutions and materials are required, assuming that both experiments are completed in the one day.

(d) SOLUTIONS

Phenobarbital ($20\,mg\,ml^{-1}$).
Pentobarbital ($6\,mg\,ml^{-1}$).
Carbon tetrachloride (undiluted).
Corn oil (undiluted).
Saline, 0.9% w/v: 900 mg NaCl to 100 ml water.
Sucrose, 0.25 M: 85.6 g to 1 litre water.
Calcium chloride solution, 88 mM (if using $CaCl_2$-precipitated microsomes): 1.93 g $CaCl_2$ to 100 ml water.

Sufficient solutions for protein determination (Section 8.2.3), aminopyrine-N-demethylation (Section 8.2.10) and cytochrome *P*-450 determination (Section 8.2.5).

(e) APPARATUS AND OTHER MATERIALS

Male rats, 80–100 g body weight: 45.
All other materials are as given in the apparatus section of experiment 2 (Section 8.3.2).

8.5 Urinary excretion of paracetamol in Man

Paracetamol (acetaminophen) in normal therapeutic doses is generally considered one of the safest of all the minor analgesics, although it should be pointed out that large overdoses of paracetamol may produce hepatic necrosis in Man and other animals. After administration, paracetamol is eliminated from the body by the apparent, first-order processes of metabolism and, to a small extent, excretion, the principal metabolites in Man being the glucuronide and sulfate conjugates (Figure 8.6).

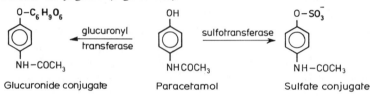

Figure 8.6 The *in vivo* metabolism of paracetamol.

The elimination of paracetamol may be rationalized mathematically according to the method of Cummings *et al.* (1967). Using this approach, it has been shown that a plot of the log rate of excretion of 'total' drug will ultimately become a straight line, of slope equal to

$$- \frac{k_e}{2.303}$$

where k_e is the elimination rate constant. Thus in this experiment, the log excretion rate of 'total drug' ($mg\,h^{-1}$) is plotted at the mid-point of each time interval of urine collection. As discussed in Chapter 7, the elimination rate constant k_e is estimated from the slope of the above plot and the half-life $t_{\frac{1}{2}}$ of paracetamol can be calculated from

$$t_{\frac{1}{2}} = \frac{0.693}{k_e}$$

(a) HUMAN SUBJECTS

In normal, healthy individuals, the dose of paracetamol used in this experiment is entirely without side-effects, and is a dose taken routinely as an analgesic for headaches. However, it must be emphasized that this drug should not be taken by people who:

(1) Have a history of hepatic or kidney disease of any type;
(2) Habitually take paracetamol;
(3) Exhibit allergic or hypersensitivity reactions to this drug;
(4) Are under current therapy with other drugs;
(5) Are generally in poor health.

If the subject is in *any doubt at all* about whether or not to take paracetamol, they should seek professional advice *prior* to participating in the experiment. Furthermore, if the experiment is being conducted as a class practical, it is the *organizer's* responsibility to ensure that the experimental protocol is in agreement with the local ethical and safety guidelines laid down by the appropriate institutional body.

(b) PRELIMINARY NOTES

(1) This experiment can be conducted in pairs, one member of each pair taking the drug. This protocol then gives the advantage that the excretion of paracetamol can be compared from subject to subject.
(2) In view of the fact that urine samples have to be collected over a 6-h period, it is convenient for the subject to take the drug and collect urine samples the day prior to being analysed. The urine samples can be stored overnight at 4 °C without appreciable decomposition and analysed the following day.

(c) PARACETAMOL ADMINISTRATION AND COLLECTION OF URINE

(1) In order to maintain a reasonable urine flow, the subject should initially drink about 200 ml of water. After 30 min, the bladder should be voided into a suitable container; this sample represents the blank urine.
(2) Paracetamol (500 mg) is ingested with 200 ml of water and a clock started; this is time zero.
(3) After 1 h, the bladder is voided again, the volume of urine measured, the sample is annotated and an additional 100 ml of water taken.
(4) The same procedure as in (3) is repeated every hour for 2 h, 3 h, 4 h, 5 h and 6 h.
(5) The 'total drug' in each urine sample is measured (in duplicate) as below.

(d) ANALYTICAL METHOD

The urine samples will be analysed for 'total paracetamol' by treatment of urine samples with acid. In this method, paracetamol and its sulfate and glucuronide conjugates present in urine are hydrolysed in the presence of acid to 4-amino-phenol. This compound is subsequently coupled with phenol in the presence of hypobromite to form an indophenol dye whose concentration is determined spectrophotometrically with reference to a standard curve as follows:

(1) The standard curve is obtained by initially preparing a stock solution of paracetamol ($1 \, \text{mg ml}^{-1}$) in water. Dilutions of this stock are made with water giving standard paracetamol solutions of 50, 100, 200, 400, 600 and $800 \, \mu\text{g ml}^{-1}$.

(2) Blank urine, 1 ml, is pipetted (in duplicate) into a test-tube followed by 4 ml of 4 M HCl and 1 ml of each standard paracetamol solution. Mix thoroughly. A suitable blank is prepared (in duplicate) in which 1 ml of water is added instead of the standard paracetamol solution.

(3) The tubes are covered with marbles and placed in a boiling water bath (in a fume cupboard) for 1 h.

(4) The tubes are cooled and the volume in each made up accurately to 10 ml with water.

(5) After thorough mixing, a 1 ml aliquot is pipetted from the (10 ml) hydrolysed urine sample into a separate test tube, and 10 ml of the 'colour-forming solution' is added. After mixing gently, the solution is allowed to stand for 40 min.

(6) The absorbance of each solution is measured at 620 nm in a spectrophotometer, zeroing the instrument on the drug-free, blank urine sample.

(7) Starting from (2) above, each collected urine sample is treated (in duplicate, preferably at the same time) in a similar manner, substituting the timed urine sample for the blank urine. In addition, the 1 ml standard paracetamol solution is replaced with 1 ml of water.

(e) TREATMENT OF RESULTS

(1) A calibration curve is plotted of absorbance at 620 nm versus the known concentration of paracetamol (in $\mu\text{g ml}^{-1}$).

(2) The 'total drug' in each urine sample is then determined from the calibration curve, and hence the amount per hour is determined, knowing the volume of each urine sample.

(3) A graph of the log rate of excretion (mg h^{-1}) is plotted against the mid-point of each time interval.

(4) From the plot in (3), estimates can be made of the elimination rate constant k_e and the half-life $t_{\frac{1}{2}}$ for paracetamol excretion.
(5) The class results are compared, and any substantial differences noted in the kinetic parameters for paracetamol excretion from subject to subject. If a substantial variation in k_e or $t_{\frac{1}{2}}$ is noted, reason(s) should be suggested why this is so.

(f) SIMPLE QUALITATIVE TESTS ON URINE TO DETERMINE THE NATURE OF THE METABOLITES

These, following, tests should be carried out on all the urine samples, including the blank.

(i) *Naphthoresorcinol test for glucuronide conjugates*

Urine (0.5 ml), solid naphthoresorcinol (approx. 2 mg) and concentrated HCl (1 ml) are boiled (in a fume cupboard) for 3 min, then cooled. Ethyl acetate (3 ml) is added and the mixture shaken. A purple coloration in the organic layer indicates the presence of glucuronic acid or a glucuronide; comparison should be made with a control of normal urine. This is a sensitive test; it cannot be used for biliary metabolites owing to the large amounts of bilirubin glucuronide present.

Further information on the glucuronide may be obtained by carrying out Benedict's test on the urine. Glucuronides of carboxyl groups (ester glucuronides) and N-glucuronides will give a positive test, as they are hydrolysed by the alkaline conditions of the test. Glucuronides of hydroxyl groups (ether glucuronides) will not react as this glycosidic linkage is stable to alkali.

(ii) *Barium chloride test for sulfate conjugates*

A urine sample (0.5 ml) is adjusted to pH 4–6 and 2 ml of 2% $BaCl_2$ solution added. The $BaSO_4$ precipitate, which is formed from the inorganic sulfate present, is then centrifuged. Two drops of concentrated HCl are added to the supernatant, and the solution is boiled (in a fume cupboard) for 3 min. The formation of a further precipitate or turbidity suggests the presence of a sulfate conjugate; comparison should be made with a control of normal urine. This test is rather insensitive.

(iii) *Ferric chloride test for phenols*

To a urine sample (0.5 ml) adjusted to pH 7, 2% $FeCl_3$ solution is added dropwise. The first few drops produce a precipitate of ferric phosphate which may be centrifuged if necessary. Further dropwise addition of FeCl$_3$ may produce a purple or green coloration if a phenol is present. The sensitivity of this test varies for different phenols – many do not produce a colour at all.

(g) SOLUTIONS (sufficient for ten pairs/groups)

Paracetamol, 1 mg ml^{-1}: 100 mg to 100 ml water.

HCl, 4 M: 2 l.

Sodium hydroxide solution, 0.2 M: 32 g NaOH to 4 l (for colour-forming reagent).

Phenol, 1% w/v: 5 g to 500 ml (for colour-forming reagent) – freshly made-up.

Sodium carbonate (2 M)–bromine solution: 53 g anhydrous sodium carbonate dissolved in water, and diluted to 500 ml. Add 75 ml of bromine-saturated water solution to 500 ml of the sodium carbonate solution (used in colour forming reagent) – freshly made-up.

Colour-forming reagent: mixture of 4 l of 0.2 M NaOH, 500 ml of 1% phenol and 500 ml of the carbonate–bromine reagent – freshly made-up.

Naphthoresorcinol, solid.

Concentrated HCl: 200 ml.

Ethyl acetate: 600 ml.

Barium chloride solution, 2% w/v: 8 g BaCl$_2$ to 400 ml.

Ferric chloride solution, 2% w/v: 2 g FeCl$_3$ to 100 ml.

(h) APPARATUS AND OTHER MATERIALS

Urine samples.

Measuring cylinders, 50 ml, 100 ml, 250 ml: 10 of each.

Filter funnels: 10.

Beakers, 50 ml, 100 ml, 250 ml: 10 of each.

Plastic storage bottles, 100 ml: 100.

Paracetamol, 500 mg: 10 capsules.

Clocks: 10.

Test tubes, 120 mm × 15 mm: 400.

Marbles: 400.

UV–visible spectrophotometer (reading to 620 nm): 1.

Bench centrifuges: 10.

pH paper *or* pH meter: as available.

8.6 Problems

Propranolol, a β-adrenergic blocking drug, was administered both orally (80 mg) and intravenously (10 mg) on separate occasions to a patient (weight, 70 kg) and the following plasma levels of propranolol obtained.

Time after administration (h)	Plasma level (ng ml^{-1})	
	Oral	I.V.
0.5		52.5
1	80.7	46.0
2	95.2	33.5
3	100.0	25.0
4	83.6	18.3
5	69.5	13.6
6	57.7	10.2
7	48.0	7.5
8	40.0	5.6

(1) From the I.V. data determine the half-life ($t_{\frac{1}{2}}$), the rate constant of elimination (k_e) and the volume of distribution of propranolol. Comment on your results.
(2) From the oral data, determine the $t_{\frac{1}{2}}$ and k_e of propranolol.
(3) Determine the areas under the curve (AUCs) for propranolol following both oral and I.V. administration. (The AUC is a measure of the availability of the drug, i.e. how much of the drug reaches the systemic circulation. The AUC may be determined by various methods such as weighing the areas (on graph paper) or by the trapezoidal rule.) You must correct for the different amounts of drug given by the two routes. In this problem,

amount of orally administered drug reaching the systemic circulation

$$= \frac{\text{AUC (oral)}}{\text{AUC (I.V.)}} \times \frac{10}{80} \times 100\%$$

Suggest possible reasons for the different results obtained from both routes of administration.

8.7 Further reading and references

Aitio, A. (1974) *Int. J. Biochem.*, **5**, 325–30.
Åstrom, A. and de Pierre, J. W. (1982) 2-Acetylaminofluorene induces forms of cytochrome P-450 active in its own metabolism. *Carcinogenesis*, **3**, 711–13.
Bargar, E. M., Walle, U. K., Bai, S. A. and Walle, T. (1983) Quantitative metabolic fate of propranolol in the dog, rat and hamster using radiotracer, high pressure liquid

chromatography and gas chromatography/mass spectrometry techniques. *Drug Metab. Dispn.*, **11**, 266–72.

Bratton, A. C. and Marshall, E. K. (1939) A new coupling component for sulphanil-amide determination. *J. Biol. Chem.*, **128**, 537–50.

Burchell, B. (1974) Substrate specificity of UDP–glucuronyltransferase purified to apparent homogeneity from phenobarbital-treated rat liver. *Biochem. J.*, **173**, 749–57.

Burke, M. D. and Mayer, R. T. (1975) Inherent specificities of purified cytochromes *P*-450 and *P*-448 towards biphenyl hydroxylation and ethoxyresorufin de-ethylation. *Drug Metab. Dispn.*, **3**, 245–50.

Cummings, N., Martin, P. and Park, B. K. (1967) *Brit. J. Pharmacol. Chemother.*, **29**, 136.

Elshourbagy, N. A. and Guzelian, P. S. (1980) Separation, purification and charac-terization of a novel form of hepatic cytochrome *P*-450 from rats treated with pregnenolone-16α-carbonitrile. *J. Biol. Chem.*, **255**, 1279–85.

Falany, C. N. and Tephly, T. R. (1983) Separation, purification and characterisation of three isoenzymes of UDP–glucuronyltransferase from rat liver microsomes. *Arch. Biochem. Biophys.*, **227**, 248–58.

Gibson, G. G., Orton, T. C. and Tamburini, P. P. (1982) Cytochrome *P*-450 induction by clofibrate. Purification and properties of a hepatic cytochrome *P*-450 relatively specific for the 12- and 11-hydroxylation of dodecanoic acid (lauric acid). *Biochem. J.*, **203**, 161–8.

Guengerich, F. P. (1982) Microsomal enzymes involved in toxicology – analysis and separation. In *Principles and methods of toxicology* (ed. A. W. Hayes), Raven Press, New York, pp. 609–34.

Guengerich, F. P. and Martin, H. (1980) Purification of cytochrome *P*-450, NADPH–cytochrome *P*-450 reductase and epoxide hydrase from a single preparation of rat liver microsomes. *Arch. Biochem. Biophys.*, **205**, 365–79.

Guengerich, F. P. and Mason, P. S. (1980) Alcohol dehydrogenase-coupled spectro-photometric assay of epoxide hydratase activity. *Anal. Biochem.*, **104**, 445–51.

Habig, W. H., Pabst, M. J. and Jakoby, W. B. (1974) Glutathione-*S*-transferase, the first enzymatic step in mercapturic acid formation. *J. Biol. Chem.*, **249**, 7130–9.

Jacobson, M., Levin, W., Poppers, P. J., Wood, A. W. and Conney, A. H. (1974) Comparison of the *O*-dealkylation of 7-ethoxy-coumarin and hydroxylation of benzo[*a*]pyrene in human placenta. *Clin. Pharmacol. Ther.*, **16**, 701–10.

Kahn, G. C., Boobis, A. R., Murray, S., Brodie, M. J. and Davies, D. S. (1982) *Brit. J. Clin. Pharmacol.*, **13**, 637.

Kaminsky, L. S., Guengerich, F. P., Dannan, G. A. and Aust, S. D. (1983) Com-parisons of warfarin metabolism by liver microsomes of rats treated with a series of polybrominated biphenyl congeners and by the component purified cytochrome *P*-450 isoenzymes. *Arch. Biochem. Biophys.*, **225**, 398–404.

La Du, B., Mandel, H. and Way, E. (1972) *Fundamentals of drug metabolism and drug disposition*, Williams and Wilkins, Baltimore.

Lotlikar, P. D., Luha, L. and Zaleski, K. (1974) Reconstituted hamster liver microsomal enzyme system for *N*-hydroxylation of the carcinogen, 2-acetylaminofluorene. *Biochem. Biophys. Res. Commun.*, **59**, 1349–55.

Lowry, O. H.,, Rosebrough, N. J., Farr, A. L. and Randall, R. J. (1951) Protein measurement with the Folin phenol reagent. *J. Biol. Chem.*, **193**, 265–75.

Mallett, A. K., King. L. J. and Walker, R. (1982) A continuous spectrophotometric determination of hepatic microsomal azoreductase activity and its dependence on cytochrome P-450. *Biochem. J.*, **201**, 589–95.

Nash, T. (1953) The colorimetric estimation of formaldehyde by means of the Hantzsch reaction. *J. Biol. Chem.*, **55**, 416–22.

Nebert, D. W. and Gelboin, H. V. (1968) Substrate-inducible microsomal aryl hydroxylase in mammalian cell culture. I. Assay and properties of the induced enzyme. *J. Biol. Chem.*, **243**, 6242–9.

Oesch, F., Jerina, D. M. and Daly, J. (1971) A radiometric assay for hepatic epoxide hydrolase activity with (^{3}H)-styrene oxide. *Biochim. Biophys. Acta*, **227**, 685–91.

Ohnishi, K. and Lieber, C. S. (1977) Reconstitution of the microsomal ethanol-oxidising system. Qualitative and quantitative changes of cytochrome P-450 after chronic ethanol consumption. *J. Biol. Chem.*, **252**, 7124–31.

Parker, G. L. and Orton, T. C. (1980) Induction by oxyisobutyrates of hepatic and kidney microsomal cytochrome P-450 with specificity towards hydroxylation of fatty acids. In *Biochemistry, biophysics and regulation of cytochrome P-450* (eds J. Å. Gustafsson, J. Carlstedt-Duke, A. Mode and J. Rafter) Elsevier, Amsterdam, pp. 373–7.

Ryan, D. E., Thomas, P. E. and Levin, W. (1980) Hepatic microsomal cytochrome P-450 from rats treated with isosafrole. Purification and characterization of four enzymic forms. *J. Biol. Chem.*, **255**, 7941–55.

Sanchez, E. and Tephly, T. R. (1974) Morphine metabolism. Evidence for separate enzymes in the glucuronidation of morphine and *para*-nitrophenol by rat hepatic microsomes. *Drug Metab. Dispn.*, **2**, 247–53.

Schenkman, J. B., Remmer, H. and Estabrook, R. W. (1967) Spectral studies of drug interactions with hepatic microsomal cytochrome P-450. *Mol. Pharmacol.*, **3**, 113–23.

Schenkman, J. B., Sligar, S. G. and Cinti, D. L. (1981) Substrate interaction with cytochrome P-450. *Pharmacol. Ther.*, **12**, 43–71.

Schmassmann, H. U., Glatt, H. R. and Oesch, F. (1976) A rapid assay for epoxide hydratase activity with benzo[*a*]pyrene 4,5-oxide as substrate. *Anal. Biochem.*, **74**, 94–104.

Tredger, J. M., Smith, H. M. and Williams, R. (1984) Effects of ethanol and enzyme-inducing agents on the monooxygenation of testosterone and xenobiotics in rat liver microsomes. *J. Pharmacol. Exp. Ther.*, **229**, 292–8.

Tukey, R. H., Billings, R. E. and Tephly, T. R. (1978) Separation of oestrone UDP–glucuronyltransferase and *para*-nitrophenol UDP–glucuronyltransferase activities. *Biochem. J.*, **171**, 659–63.

Ullrich, V. and Weber, P. (1972) The *O*-dealkylation of 7-ethoxycoumarin by liver microsomes. *Hoppe-Seyler's Z. Physiol. Chem.*, **353**, 1171–7.

Wolff, T., Deml, E. and Wanders, H. (1979) Aldrin epoxidation, a highly sensitive indicator for cytochrome P-450-dependent monooxygenase activity. *Drug Metab. Dispn.*, **7**, 301–5.

Wood, A. W., Ryan, D. E., Thomas, P. E. and Levin, W. (1983) Regio- and stereo-selective metabolism of two C_{19} steroids by five highly purified and reconstituted rat hepatic cytochrome *P*-450 isoenzymes. *J. Biol. Chem.*, **258**, 8839–47.

Yang, C. S., Strickhart, F. S. and Kicha, L. P. (1978) Analysis of the aryl hydrocarbon hydroxylase assay. *Biochem. Pharmacol.*, **27**, 2321–6.

Ziegler, D. M. and Pettit, H. (1964) Formation of an intermediate *N*-oxide in the oxidative demethylation of *N*,*N*-dimethylaniline catalysed by liver microsomes. *Biochem. Biophys. Res. Commun.*, **15**, 188–93.

Index